Oxford Handbook of
Learning & Intellectual Disability Nursing

Edited by

Prof Bob Gates

Project Leader
Learning Disability Workforce Development
South Central Strategic Health Authority

and

Dr Owen Barr

Head of School
School of Nursing
University of Ulster

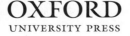

OXFORD
UNIVERSITY PRESS

OXFORD
UNIVERSITY PRESS

Great Clarendon Street, Oxford OX2 6DP

Oxford University Press is a department of the University of Oxford.
It furthers the University's objective of excellence in research, scholarship,
and education by publishing worldwide in

Oxford New York

Auckland Cape Town Dar es Salaam Hong Kong Karachi
Kuala Lumpur Madrid Melbourne Mexico City Nairobi
New Delhi Shanghai Taipei Toronto

With offices in

Argentina Austria Brazil Chile Czech Republic France Greece
Guatemala Hungary Italy Japan Poland Portugal Singapore
South Korea Switzerland Thailand Turkey Ukraine Vietnam

Oxford is a registered trade mark of Oxford University Press
in the UK and in certain other countries

Published in the United States
by Oxford University Press Inc., New York

© Oxford University Press, 2009

British Library Cataloguing in Publication Data
Data available

Library of Congress Cataloging in Publication Data
Data available

Typeset by Cepha Imaging Private Ltd., Bangalore, India
Printed in China
on acid-free paper by
Asia Pacific Offset

ISBN 978–0–19–953322–0

10 9 8 7 6 5 4 3 2 1

Preface

It is with considerable pride that the editors of this text, Bob Gates and Owen Barr, welcome you to the first edition of the Oxford Handbook of Learning and Intellectual Disability Nursing. This book represents the culmination of a two year project that has sought to involve leading practitioners and academics from the field of intellectual disabilities from the UK and the Republic of Ireland, in the production of an authoritative text able to offer essential facts and information on learning/intellectual disabilities. The editors set out on this task knowing that the landscape for the practice of learning/intellectual disability nursing has never been so complex. Learning disability/intellectual disability nurses can be found working and supporting people in a variety of different care contexts such as community learning disability teams, treatment and assessment services, outreach services, residential settings, day care services, respite services, health facilitation, mental health and challenging behaviour services, special schools, and specialist services for people who can be located on the spectrum of autistic disorders.

Additionally they can be found working for many different agencies such as health, social care, education and the independent sector (this comprises the private, voluntary and not for profit organizations), and also alongside numerous other professional disciplines including; clinical psychologists, social workers, occupational therapists, speech and language therapists, and consultant psychiatrists in intellectual disabilities, as well as a range of professionals within wider health, social services and education. Given this complexity of context and practice we believe that the Oxford Handbook of Learning and Intellectual Disability Nursing will offer students and newly qualified practitioners up to date, concise, practical, and theoretical information for use in the very many areas where learning/intellectual disability nurses are located. Notwithstanding that learning/intellectual disability nurses are the primary audience for this text, we firmly believe that a range of other health and social care professionals, who might need to seek an authoritative text that provides essential facts and information on learning/intellectual disability, might also find this book of considerable use.

In keeping with other handbooks in this series the underlying philosophy of this text is to be a guide adopting a 'person-centred' approach that has allowed space for the reader to record their own anecdotes, quotations, and notes. The reader will also find a small emergencies section at the back of the book that provides essential information for the management of, for example, status epilepticus, holding powers under the Mental Health legislation, and dealing with abuse. We believe that unique to this Oxford Handbook will be the attention that has been given to differences in legislation and social policy across the constituent countries of the UK and Ireland—subsequent editions will seek to further address this from a more international perspective.

It is important for us to make a brief note on terminology used in this text. Generally speaking within the UK the term 'learning disability' is used to describe that group of people who have significant developmental delay resulting in incomplete achievement of the 'normal' milestones of human development. The term is also used throughout the world but it holds a different meaning in many other countries, paradoxically so too in the UK as well. It is this difference in meaning that could cause confusion to an international audience of readers. This has prompted us to use a term for 'learning disability' that has greater international currency in meaning. Whereas we accept that 'naming is not a simple act' (Luckasson, 2003) the increasing internationalization of text books has led us to conclude that we needed to adopt a term to replace 'learning disability' that would enable this book to be seen as relevant to as wide a readership as possible. The term which we believe seems most appropriate to this text, the readership and to those who this book is principally about, and that which seems to have most universal consensus is 'intellectual disability'. Therefore, throughout the remainder of the text we will not repeat the rather clumsy term of learning/intellectual disability and from here on in this book will use the term intellectual disability; save where certain Acts or other technical works require the use of the term learning disability. The abbreviation ID is also used where appropriate in place of 'intellectual disabilities'.

We feel confident that the Oxford Handbook of Learning and Intellectual Disability Nursing will come to be a highly regarded textbook - not only in the field of intellectual disabilities but also more widely, and that it will be used by the many professionals and students from the broad range of different professional and academic backgrounds that have an interest in the lives of people with intellectual disabilities. Both editors also strongly believe that the excellent end product that you have before you is due entirely to the excellent contributions that have been made by our many friends and colleagues from across the UK and the Republic of Ireland, and we thank them for their trust in us by contributing to this textbook. We earnestly hope that all who read this book find it helpful, and that its use will assist us all in helping people with intellectual disabilities enjoy health and well being in their lives.

Bob Gates, Piccotts End, England
Owen Barr, Derry, Northern Ireland

Reference

Luckasson R. (2003) Terminology and Power. In: Her SS, Gostin LO, and Koh HH. *The Human Rights of Persons with Intellectual Disabilities*. Oxford University Press, Oxford.

Foreword

The phrase 'people with intellectual disabilities' encompasses a diverse range of people. It includes newly born infants and very elderly people who are nearing the end of their life. It includes men and women who possess a wide range of abilities and who fill a variety of roles including son, daughter, parent, friend, advocate, researcher, employee and carer. It includes people who are fit and well and also some who have complex and enduring health needs (although such health needs may not be adequately addressed). Indeed we are seeing demographic changes whereby young people with complex health needs are surviving into adulthood and generally people with intellectual disabilities are living longer and thus experiencing many of the diseases and conditions of ageing. Ensuring that such clients receive appropriate support may require the input of a number of professionals, and the family, as well as the individual, may be the focus of intervention.

It is in this context that we need to consider the role of the nurse working with people with an intellectual disability. This is not to argue that every person with an intellectual disability requires the support of an intellectual disability nurse, but rather to highlight that such nurses work with a diverse range of people in a diverse range of settings. If the care and support they deliver is to be 'person-centred' (Department of Health, 2007) then it follows that they need to call upon an extensive range of knowledge and skills in order to provide appropriate support.

Thinking back to my training as an intellectual disability nurse we had few relevant textbooks, and those we did have were very limited in scope. However, we live in an age where knowledge is constantly expanding and the amount of information we are confronted with can sometimes be overwhelming. There is thus a requirement to identify that knowledge which is central to our work and the need for a 'range of essential core competencies' has been highlighted (Department of Health, 2007). Thankfully we now have a better selection of textbooks but what this volume does extremely well, and what makes it different, is that it clearly identifies that core knowledge and presents it in a single, accessible volume. It is thus an important first point of reference and can assist in decision making in the clinical area (wherever this may be). However it goes beyond this and provides a basis for expanding knowledge by including not only references to support the text but also examples of further reading.

Intellectual disability nurses work in complex and dynamic settings. They have the ability to make positive changes in the lives of those they support. To do this they need to be able to call upon key knowledge and skills. This volume will, I am confident, assist them in this process and thus it will make a positive contribution to the lives of people with intellectual disabilities.

Ruth Northway
Professor of Learning Disability Nursing
University of Glamorgan

Reference

Department of Health (2007) *Good Practice in Learning Disability Nursing*. Department of Health: London.

Acknowledgements

Bob Gates would like thank his mother as well as Briege, Nicky, Lucy, David, Emily, Elise and Charlie.

Owen Barr would like to thank his parents, as well as Marie, Shannagh, Shane and Adam for all their support. He would also like to acknowledge the insights gained from the many people with intellectual disabilities and their families who have taught me many times about the importance of focusing on the individual.

We would also like to thank all the contributors and colleagues who offered help, advice and support throughout the completion of this book. We would also like to thank our colleagues at Oxford University Press for their continued help and hard work in bringing this book to fruition.

Acknowledgements

Contents

Detailed contents

Contributors

John Aldridge
Senior Lecturer,
The University of
Northampton

- Purpose and principles of assessment
- Framework for nursing assessment
- Assessment of independence and social functioning

Owen Barr
Head of School,
School of Nursing,
University of Ulster

- Principles and values of social policy and their effects on intellectual disability
- Defining families
- Family members of people with intellectual disabilities
- Explaining intellectual disabilities to family members
- The process of family adaptation
- Resilience in families
- Undertaking a nursing assessment
- Writing nursing care plans
- Interdisciplinary teamworking
- Interagency working
- Maternity services
- General hospital services
- Radiology departments
- Children's health services
- Dental services
- Planning for contact with health services
- Qualitative approaches
- Involving people with intellectual disabilities in the research process
- Mixed methods

Martina Bell
Nurse Manager,
Western Health and Social
Care Trust,
Londonderry

- Hearing
- Multisensory rooms
- Sensory integration
- Touch
- Art, drama, and music

Phil Boulter
Consultant Nurse (Learning
Disabilities), Surrey &
Borders Partnership NHS
Foundation Trust

- Risk assessment
- Quality of life
- Life experiences
- Risk assessment and management
- Risk management

Aoife N. Bradley
Lead Genetic Nurse/
Counsellor, Northern Ireland
Regional Genetics Centre,
Belfast City Hospital

- *Causes and manifestations of intellectual disability*
- *Common conditions among people with intellectual disability*
- *Antenatal screening and diagnosis*

Michael Brown
Nurse Consultant &
Lecturer, Napier University,
Edinburgh

- *Cardiorespiratory disorders*
- *Obesity*
- *Nutrition*
- *Mobility*
- *Exercise*
- *Diabetes*
- *Thyroid*
- *Cancer*
- *Stopping smoking*
- *Accidents*
- *Sexual health and personal relationships*
- *Gastrointestinal disorders*
- *Integration of sensory experiences*

Eddie Chaplin
Strategy Nurse, South
London and Maudsley
NHS Foundation Trust and
Section of Mental Health
Nursing, Health Services
and Population Research,
Institute of Psychiatry,
London

- *Promoting assertiveness*
- *Primary care*
- *Secondary care*
- *Tertiary care*
- *Mental health and emotional well being – introduction*
- *Self-harm*

Julie Clark
PhD Student, Research
Assistant,
Thames Valley University,
London

- *Profound and multiple learning disabilities*
- *Healthy skin*
- *Personal and intimate care*
- *Continence*

Janet Cobb
Associate Consultant, The
Foundation for People with
Learning Disabilities, London

- *UK-wide intellectual disability and health networks*

Christine Cole
Clinical Epilepsy Specialist
Nurse, Barnet Primary Care,
London

- *Independent nurse prescribers in intellectual disabiltiy*
- *Epilepsy specialist nurses*

Debbie Crickmore
Lecturer in Learning
Disability, University of Hull

- *Supporting people during transition*
- *Preschool children*
- *School-aged children*
- *Adulthood*

Caroline Dalton
Lecturer, University College
Cork, Ireland

- *Dysphagia*
- *PEG and PEJ feeding*
- *Nasogastric feeding*
- *Oral health*

Mary Dearing
Lecturer, The University of
Hull

- *Adolescents*
- *Puberty*
- *Adulthood*
- *Women and menopause*

Maurice Devine
Department of Health, Social
Services & Public Safety,
Nursing Officer - Mental
Health, Learning Disability
and Care of Older People,
Belfast

- *Medicines management*
- *Appropriate use of medication*

Matt Dodwell
Active Support and
Treatment/Assessment and
Treatment Matron, Surrey
& Borders Partnership NHS
Foundation Trust, Caterham

- *Risk assessment and management*
- *Risk management*

Bob Gates
Project Leader,
Learning Disability
Workforce Development,
South Central Strategic
Health Authority

- *The nature of intellectual disability – introduction*
- *Incidence and prevalence of intellectual disability*
- *Diagnosing intellectual disability*
- *Defining intellectual disability nursing*
- *The purist form of nursing*
- *Holism and working across the life span*
- *Physical health and well-being – introduction*
- *Residential alternatives*
- *Supported living and home ownership*
- *Village and intentional communities*
- *Quantitative approaches*
- *Ethical issues in research*
- *Involving people with intellectual disabilities in the research process*
- *QA statement of intellectual disability nursing*
- *Nursing and Midwifery Council (UK)*
- *Mencap and Enable*

Briege Gibbons
Clinical Nurse Specialist,
CAMHS, Western Health
& Social Care Trust, Derry,
Northern Ireland

- *Family therapy*

Alison Giraud-Saunders
Co-Director, Foundation for People with Learning Disabilities, UK

- *Foundation for People with Learning Disabilities*

Steve Hardy
Training and Consultancy Manager, Estia Centre, South London and Maudsley NHS Foundation Trust

- *Mental health and well being – introduction*
- *Promoting assertiveness*
- *Primary care*
- *Secondary care*
- *Tertiary care*
- *Self-harm*

Sue Hart
Mental Capacity/Deprivation of Liberty Safeguards Lead, Surrey Primary Care Trust, Leatherhead, Surrey

- *Health checks*
- *Screening of physical health*
- *Capacity and consent*
- *Health action plans and health facilitation*

Neil James
Senior Lecturer, Faculty of Health, Sport and Science, University of Glamorgan, Pontypridd

- *Allergies*
- *Adverse reactions to medications*
- *Medication error*
- *Needle stick/sharps injuries*

Robert Jenkins
Divisional Head of Learning Disability, Faculty of Health, Sport & Science, University of Glamorgan, Pontypridd

- *Unsafe standards of care*
- *Recording and reporting*
- *Complaints*
- *Self-harm*
- *Self-injury*

Paul Michael Keenan
Head of Intellectual Disability Discipline/Lecturer in Intellectual Disability Nursing, Trinity College Dublin, Ireland

- *An Bord Altranais–requirements*
- *Codes of practice*

Allyson Kent
Head of Profession; Learning Disability Nursing, Humber Mental Health Teaching NHS Trust, Hull

- *Personal relationships*
- *Marriage and family life*
- *Parents with intellectual disability*
- *Constipation*
- *Consent to treatment*
- *Making best interests decisions*
- *Vulnerability*
- *Child protection*
- *Adult protection*
- *Client held records*
- *Parenting groups*
- *Practice nurses*
- *Continence advisors*

Anne Kingdon
Consultant Nurse (Learning Disabilities), Cheshire & Wirral Partnership NHS Foundation Trust

- *People who have offended in law*
- *People in mainstream prison*
- *Rights of victims*
- *Rights of person offending*
- *Rights to a solicitor*
- *People with intellectual disabilities as witnesses*
- *Admission for treatment*
- *Admission for assessment*
- *Emergency holding powers*
- *Nurses holding power*
- *Mental Health Review Tribunal*
- *Mental Health Act Commission*
- *Use of restraint*
- *Keeping yourself safe*
- *Management in the community*
- *Working with criminal justice agencies*
- *Risk of suicide*
- *Missing person*

Elaine Kwiatek
Senior Lecturer and Teaching Fellow, Napier University, Edinburgh

- *Developing accessible information*
- *Communication passports*
- *Objects of reference*
- *Compiling life stories*
- *Care pathways*
- *Care programme approach*

Helen Laverty
Health Lecturer, University of Nottingham

- *Principles of working collaboratively with families*
- *Supporting siblings of people with intellectual disabilities*
- *People with intellectual disabilities as parents*
- *Family quality of life*
- *Respite services for people who have an intellectual disability*
- *Care management, case management, continuing care*

Stephanie Lawrence
Lecturer in Nursing, City University, Dublin

- *Retirement*

Jill Manthorpe
Professor of Social Work, Social Care Workforce Research Unit, King's College London

- *Families at risk*
- *Carers' assessment*
- *Older carers*
- *Service brokerage, direct payments, and self-directed support*
- *Commissioning*

Zuzana Matousova-Done
PhD student/Teaching Assistant at Thames Valley University and Deputy Manager at the Haven Children Respite Care Unit, London

- *Autistic spectrum disorders*
- *Intensive interaction*
- *Hydrotherapy*
- *Conductive education*
- *TEACCH*

Mary McCarron
Head of School of Nursing and Midwifery, Trinity College, Dublin

- *Older people with intellectual disability*
- *Older people with Down syndrome*
- *Dementia (in people with intellectual disability)*
- *Dementia nurse specialists*

Roy McConkey
Professor of Learning Disability, University of Ulster, N. Ireland

- *Productive work*
- *Supported employment*
- *Networks of support and friends*
- *Encouraging friendships*
- *Retirement options*

Steve McNally
Lecturer Practitioner, Ridgeway Partnership (Oxfordshire Learning Disability NHS Trust) and Oxford Brookes University, Oxford

- *Advocacy*
- *Therapeutic interventions – advocacy*
- *Citizenship*
- *Right to independent advocacy*

Stuart Mills
Information Officer, Down's Syndrome Association, Teddington

- *Down's Syndrome Association*

Duncan Mitchell
Professor of Health and Disability, Manchester Metropolitan University

- *Research – introduction*
- *Defining areas for research*
- *Undertaking a literature review*
- *Audit*
- *Evidence-based care*

James Mulkerrins
Clinical Nurse Tutor, Trinity College, Dublin

- *An Bord Altranais*
- *Codes of practice*

Aru Narayanasamy
Associate Professor and
Director of Diversity
Project, Ethnic, Diversity
and Spirituality (EDS) Hub,
University of Nottingham,
Faculty of Medicine & Health
Sciences, School of Nursing,
Midwifery & Physiotherapy,
Nottingham, UK

- *Cultural, religious and spiritual impact*
- *Spirituality*

Gavin Narayanasamy
MA Sociology Post Graduate
Student and Honorary
Research Assistant (Diversity
Project), School of Sociology
and Social Policy, University
of Nottingham, UK

- *Cultural, religious and spiritual impact*
- *Spirituality*

John Northfield
Project Lead, National
Library for Health, Learning
Disability Specialist Library,
Oxford

- *Learning Disability Specialist Library*

Edna O'Neill
Epilepsy Specialist Nurse
Learning Disability, South
Eastern Trust, Lisburn,
Northern Ireland

- *Epilepsy*
- *Supporting people with epilepsy*
- *Emergency management of a person in a seizure*

Peter Oakes
Clinical Psychologist,
Castlebeck/University of Hull

- *Identifying intellectual disability*
- *Degree of intellectual disability*
- *Definition of intellectual disability*

Sue Read
Senior Lecturer, Keele
University, Staffordshire

- *End of life*
- *End of life care, preferred place of care*
- *Responding to bereavement*
- *Support associated with loss and bereavement*
- *Tertiary care*
- *Palliative, end-of-life nurses*

Lesley Russ
Public Health Specialist
(Learning Difficulties), NHS
Bristol

- *Health inequalities*
- *Principles of health promotion*
- *Promoting public health*
- *Promoting physical well-being of individuals*
- *Physical health assessment of people with intellectual disability*
- *Blood pressure, temperature, pulse*
- *General practitioners*
- *Health visitors*
- *District nurses*
- *Community children's nurses*
- *School nurses*
- *Midwives*
- *Dentists*
- *Podiatrist*
- *Audiologist*
- *Dietitian*
- *Physiotherapy*
- *Occupational therapy*
- *Optical care*
- *Community nurses mental health*

Eamonn Slevin
Reader (Nursing), Institute of
Nursing Research & School
of Nursing, University of
Ulster, Northern Ireland

- *Behavioural interventions*

Natalie Smith
Senior Lecturer in Learning
Disability Nursing, Oxford
Brookes University, Oxford
and Practice Placement
Facilitator, Ridgeway
Partnership (Oxfordshire
Learning Disability NHS
Trust)

- *Person-centred planning*
- *Patient advice and liaison service*
- *Circles of support*
- *Life planning*

Margaret Sowney
Lecturer in Nursing,
University of Ulster,
Northern Ireland

- *Secondary care*
- *Outpatient clinics*
- *Accident and emergency departments*
- *Discharge planning*

Laurence Taggart
Lecturer, Institute of Nursing Research, University of Ulster, N. Ireland

- *Adaptive behaviour rating scales*
- *Screening of mental health problems*
- *Measurement of IQ*
- *Medicines management*
- *Promoting emotional well-being*
- *Prevalence rates*
- *Factors contributing to mental health*
- *Anxiety disorders*
- *Psychotic disorders*
- *Organic disorders*
- *Substance misuse*
- *Appropriate use of medication*

John Thompson
Information Manager, British Institute of Learning Disabilities, Kidderminster

- *British Institute of Learning Disabilties*

Jane Thompson-Hill
Macmillan Nurse Consultant in Palliative Care, University Hospital of North Staffordshire NHS Trust and Douglas Macmillan Hospice, Stoke-on-Trent

- *End of life*
- *End of life care, preferred place of care*
- *Palliative, end-of-life nurses*

Cath Valentine
Specialist Speech & Language Therapist, South Hams and West Devon Community Learning Disability Team, Devon

- *Promoting effective communication*
- *Verbal communication*
- *Non-verbal communication*
- *Providing information*
- *Active listening*
- *Principles in using augmentative and alternative communication*
- *Inclusive communucation*

Gaynor Ward
Nurse Consultant in Learning Disabilities & Mental Health, Derbyshire Mental Health Services NHS Trust, Derby

- *Psychopathology*

Michael Wolverson
Lecturer in Learning
Disabilities, University of
York

- *Anger management*
- *Cognitive behaviour therapies*
- *Counselling and psychotherapies*
- *Mental Health Act 1983*
- *Mental Health Act 2007*
- *Compulsory admission to hospital for assessment and treatment*
- *Emergency holding powers*
- *Mental Health Review Tribunals*
- *The Mental Health Act Commission*
- *Sexual Offences Act*
- *Disability Discrimination Act 2005*
- *Human Rights Act*
- *European Convention of Human Rights*
- *Race relations*
- *Diversion from custody schemes*
- *Appropriate adult*
- *The Representation of the People Act 2000*
- *Employment law*
- *Consent to examination, treatment, and care*
- *Mental Capacity Act 2005*
- *Healthcare Commission*
- *Common law and duty of care*
- *Safeguarding adults*
- *Medicines – the role of the nurse*
- *Dealing with abuse*
- *Physical assault*
- *De-escalation*
- *Use of restraint*

Jane Wray
Research Fellow, Faculty
of Health and Social Care,
University of Hull

- *Complementary and alternative therapies*
- *Gentle teaching*

Symbols and abbreviations

♂	male
♀	female
~	approximately
>	greater than
<	less than
📖	cross reference
🖥	website
A&E	accident and emergency department
A2A	Access to Acute
AAC	augmentative and alternative communication
ABA	applied behavioural analysis
ABA	An Bord Altranais
ABG	arterial blood gases
ABS	adaptive behaviour scales
ACE	adults facing chronic exclusion
ADD	attention deficit disorder
ADHD	attention deficit hyperactive disorder
ADR	adverse drug reaction
AED	anti-epileptic drug
AOT	Assertive Outreach Team
ASBO	antisocial behaviour order
ASD	autistic spectrum disorder
ASW	approved social worker
BILD	British Institute of Learning Disabilities
BNF	British National Formulary
BSID	Bayley Scales of Infant Development
CAB	Citizens' Advice Bureau
CAMHS	Child and Adolescent Mental Health Services
CAT	cognitive analytical therapy
CCN	community children's nurse
CE	conductive education
ChA-PAS	Child and Adolescent Psychiatric Assessment Schedule
CIOS	Caregiver Interactional Observation System
CMHT	community mental health team
CLDT	community learning disability team
CMP	clinical management plan

CNMH	community nurses mental health
CNS	central nervous system
COAD	chronic obstructive airways disease
COP	code of practice
CPA	Care Programme Approach
CPS	Crown Prosecution Service
CRB	Criminal Records Bureau
CSCI	Commission for Social Care Inspection
CVS	chorionic villus sampling
DAI-10	Drug Attitude Inventory
DAMP	deficit in motor coordination, attention, and perception syndrome
DASH	The Diagnostic Assessment for the Severely Handicapped
Db	decibel
DDA	Disability Discrimination Act
DISCUS	Dyskinesia Identification System: Condensed User Scale
DisDaT	Disability Distress Assessment Tool
DLA	disability living allowance
DPII	Developmental Profile II
DSA	Down's Syndrome Association
DTP	deep touch pressure
ECHR	European Convention of Human Rights
ECI	Early Coping Inventory
ECG	electrocardiogram
ECT	electroconvulsive therapy
EEG	electroencephalogram
ELP	essential lifestyle planning
ELTS	English Language Testing System
EMP	epilepsy management plan
FAAR	family adjustment and adaptation response
FACE	Functional Analysis in the Care Environment
FE	further education
FPLD	Foundation for People with Learning Disabilities
GORD	gastro-oesophageal reflux disorder
GP	general practitioner
GT	gentle teaching
HALO	Hampshire Assessment for Living with Others
HAP	Health Action Plan
HASI	Hayes Ability Screening Index
HC	Healthcare Commission

HF	health facilitator
HFA	high-functioning autism
HPC	Health Professions Council
HPT	heat–pain threshold
hr(s)	hour(s)
HRT	hormone replacement therapy
IB	incapacity benefit
ID	intellectual disability
IMCA	independent mental capacity advocate
IQ	intelligence quotient
IS	income support
JCHR	Joint Committee on Human Rights
JSNA	joint strategic needs assessment
Kg	kilogram
KSF	knowledge and skills framework
L	litre
LAA	local area agreement
LDSL	Learning Disability Specialist Library
LREC	Local Research Ethics Committee
LSP	Local Strategic Partnerships
LTP	light touch pressure
LUNSERS	Liverpool University Neuroleptic Side Effect Rating Scale
M	metre
MAPPA	multiagency public protections arrangements
MAPS	McGill Action Planning System
MCA	Mental Capacity Act
MELAS	mitochondrial encephalopathy-lactic-acidosis Storkes
MERRF	myoclonic epilepsy with ragged red fibres
MHA	Mental Health Act
MHC	Mental Health Commission
MHRA	Medicines and Healthcare Products Regulatory Agency
MHRT	Mental Health Review Tribunal
min(s)	minute(s)
Ml	millilitre
MMSE	Mini-Mental State Examination
MREC	Multicentre Research Ethics Committee
MRI	magnetic resonance imaging
mth(s)	month(s)
NG	nasogastric
NHS	National Health Service

NICE	National Institute for Health and Clinical Excellence
NMC	Nursing and Midwifery Council
NLH	National Library for Health
NNLDN	National Learning Disability Nurses Network
NOMS	National Offender Management Service
NPSA	National Patient Safety Agency
NSF	National Service Frameworks
OCD	obsessive–compulsive disorder
OT	occupational therapist
PADS	Pain and Discomfort Scale
PALS	Patient Advice and Liaison Service
PAS-ADD	psychiatric assessment schedules for adults with developmental disabilities
PATH	Planning Alternative Tomorrows With Hope
PBS	positive behavioural support
PCT	Primary Care Trust
PECS	pictures exchange communication system
PEG	percutaneous endoscopic gastrostomy
PET	positron emission tomography
PFP	personal futures planning
PHCT	primary healthcare team
PIMRA	Psychopathology Instrument for Mentally Retarded Adults
PIOS	Person Interactional Observation System
PKU	phenylketonuria
PMLD	profound and multiple learning disabilities
POCVA	protection of children and vulnerable adults
POVA	protection of vulnerable adults
PPC	Preferred Place of Care
PPC	Preferred Priorities of Care
QOF	quality outcomes framework
RCT	randomized controlled trial
RET	rational emotive therapy
RMO	responsible medical officer
RNLD	Registered Nurse Learning Disability
RPA	Representation of the People Act
RSCN	Registered Sick Children's Nurse
SD	standard deviation
s	seconds
SDA	severe disability allowance
SEN	special educational needs
SIB-R	Scales of Independent Behaviour: Revised

SSRI	serotonin specific re-uptake inhibitors
SOPO	sex offender prevention order
STI	sexually transmitted infection
TEACCH	The Treatment and Education of Autistic and Related Communication-handicapped Children
TOEFL	Test of English as a Foreign Language
TSE	Test of Spoken English
TSH	thyroid stimulating hormone
TWE	Test of Written English
UTI	urinary tract infections
VABS	Vineland Adaptive Behaviour Scale
VABS-II	Vineland Adaptive Behaviour Scale-II
wk(s)	week(s)
YOI	young offender institutions
yr(s)	year(s)

The nature of intellectual disability

Introduction

In this chapter the term intellectual disability (ID) will be defined. It will be shown that ID is identified by the presence of a significantly reduced ability to understand new or complex information (impaired intelligence) with the reduced ability to cope independently (impaired social functioning), which started before 18yrs of age.[1]

The chapter outlines that there is general agreement that 3–4/1000 of the general population will have a severe ID, and that 25–30/1000 of the general population will have a mild ID.

Also outlined are the various ways in which a diagnosis, or assessment, of ID is made. A range of known causes and manifestations of ID will be provided.

Above all else it will be emphasized that people with ID, regardless of the impact of their disabilities, share a common humanity with that of their fellow citizens in their communities, and in the wider society in which they live. Most people desire love and a sense of connection with others; they wish to be safe, to learn, to lead a meaningful life, to be free from ridicule and harm, to be healthy, and free from poverty, and in this respect people with ID are no different to any of us.

All health and social care workers, especially ID nurses, have a professional responsibility to bring about their inclusion, into their communities, by adhering at all times to a value base that respects them as fellow citizens.

This value base leads this chapter to conclude by articulating the nature of ID nursing, and how this group of professionals work to support the whole person throughout their lives when they are in need of such support.

1 DHSSPS (2005). *Equal Lives*. DHSSPS: Belfast.

Identifying intellectual disability

It is essential to stress at the outset of this section that each person with an ID is a unique human being. Like everyone else, each person has their own personality along with a profile of abilities and disabilities that can only be understood in the context of their culture, history, and relationships.

ID manifests in a number of different ways for each individual.

Intellectual profile

Fundamental to ID is a difficulty in learning and processing information. The following intellectual abilities may be impaired:

Verbal abilities

- Memory—including immediate recall of people, objects or events, and the ability to store and process information
- Comprehension—this means understanding situations, knowing socially accepted norms and being able to weigh up possible options
- Language—vocabulary may be limited and some people may not understand words at all. Others may recognize words but struggle to understand more subtle meanings
- Abstract thinking—people may find it hard to separate themselves from the thing they are thinking about. Hypothetical situations are particularly difficult.

Non-verbal abilities

- Speed of processing—an individual may take a long time to work out what is going on in a situation
- Reasoning—shapes, patterns and numbers may be confusing and people can find it hard to put things in order
- Coordination – there may be difficulty in coordinating movement or using fine motor skills.

Coping with everyday life

These difficulties in intellectual function can have an impact on a person's ability to cope with everyday life. This means that a person may have a range of difficulties that require support:

- Self care—including everything from getting up, washing, and dressing, through to going to bed
- Domestic skills—looking after clothes, cooking, and cleaning are all included here
- Community living skills—getting out and about, managing simple social interactions, and using shops and public services
- Communication—getting on with people and being able to communicate needs and wishes
- Work and leisure—using time purposefully, having fun, and pursuing personal goals.

Behavioural phenotypes

As will be seen later, most people with ID have a general ID that manifests in the ways shown above. There are a number of people with specific syndromes, and these syndromes may be associated with a particular profile of verbal and non-verbal abilities. For example people who are on the autistic spectrum of disorders are characterized by specific difficulties with social communication and information processing. Information about specific syndromes is important, therefore, in understanding and predicting possible manifestations of ID.

Additional needs

People with ID are more likely to have a range of additional needs. Of particular note are:
- Sensory impairments
- Gastro-oesophageal reflux disorder (GORD)
- Epilepsy.

Context

As mentioned above, each person with ID presents with a history and background, and it is essential to understand these alongside the immediate disabilities. People with ID are likely to be receiving support from their family or from other carers, and these people will have a key role to play in any assessment or intervention.

Further reading

American Association for Mental Retardation (2002). *Mental Retardation, Definition, Classification and Systems of Support.* 10th edn. AAMR: Washington.

Hogg J, Langa A (2005). *Assessing Adults with Intellectual Disabilities: A Service Providers Guide.* Blackwell Publishing: Oxford.

Prasher V, Janicki M (2002). *Physical Health of Adults with Intellectual Disabilities.* Blackwell Publishing: Oxford.

Degree of intellectual disability

For many years, ID has been divided into a number of categories to reflect its nature and extent. These tended to range from 'borderline' through 'mild', 'moderate' and 'severe', to 'profound'. This represents one understanding of ID but there are others. This understanding uses the World Health Organization classification system that defines the degree of disability according to how far an individual is from the normal distribution of IQ for the general population. Using this system, an individual who consistently scores more than 2 Standard Deviations (SD) on an IQ test, that is, a measured IQ of <70, is said to have ID. Individuals whose IQ is 50–69 are generally identified as having mild ID (F70); those with an IQ of 71–84 are said to be on the borderline of intellectual functioning; moderate ID (F71) is identified when the IQ is 35–49; the term 'severe intellectual disability' (F72) is reserved for people whose IQ is 20–34; finally, the term 'profound intellectual disability' (F73) refers to those with an IQ of <20. There are also other classifications. These are not identified here but most rely on the use of standardized tests offering high validity and reliability. An alternative approach is based on a model of ID that sees it as an interaction between a person, the support they receive, and the environment they are in (Fig.1.1). For example:

Andrew has very significant ID. He has to use a wheelchair, he cannot speak or understand words, and he has not been able to look after even his most basic needs. He needs a great deal of support to provide his basic care, and to understand what he is trying to communicate. He also needs an environment with special equipment, and opportunities to get out and meet new people, which he loves to do.

Elizabeth has Down syndrome and can communicate very well with words. She looks after herself and can cope well in the community. She has to do things one at a time and can get overwhelmed if she feels there is too much to do. Elizabeth needs someone to visit her once a day to make sure she has remembered everything, including her epilepsy medication, and to make sure she is not getting overwhelmed. She needs an environment where she has just one task at a time to get through the day, and the opportunity to meet her family at least once a week.

These examples show that each individual has a unique profile of ID that impacts on everyday life in different ways. Assessment of the degree of ID will identify the level of support a person needs, as well as the kind of environment and opportunities that they need.[1] There is a system for categorizing the amount of support people need on 4 levels:
- Intermittent—this is time limited support at key times in life such as loss of key relationships or transition
- Limited—consistent need of support for specific tasks, such as employment training; still time limited

- Extensive—regular long-term direct support in at least one setting
- Pervasive—constant high-intensity support across all settings.

To this is added an assessment of the kind of environment a person needs, and the opportunities that are important for them to be healthy and to achieve their personal goals. It is always important to remember that quality of life and relationships are very important to everyone whatever the degree of ID.

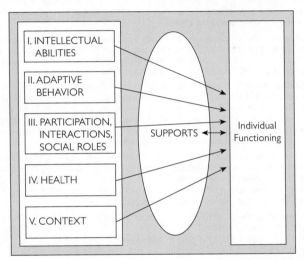

Fig. 1.1 American Association for Mental Retardation (2002). *Mental Retardation, Definition, Classification and Systems of Support.* 10th Edn. AAMR: Washington.

Reference and further reading

1 American Association for Mental Retardation (2002). *Mental Retardation, Definition, Classification and Systems of Support.* 10th edn. AAMR: Washington.

Hogg J, Langa A (2005). *Assessing Adults with Intellectual Disabilities: A Service Providers Guide.* Blackwell Publishing: Oxford.

Definition of intellectual disability

ID has been understood from a number of different theoretical perspectives. Three key perspectives have led to modern definitions of ID:

Sociological—people who fall outside accepted norms and expectations in society. From this perspective intellectual disability can be seen as deviance, where the task of services is to enable people to be included in community life. The alternative is to see ID as a subculture that is distinct and different from other groups in society. Here services are intended to empower and support the group.

Medical—this focuses on the possibility that there is an underlying disease or pathology that might at some point be identified, understood, and treated as a medical condition. There is also a controversial notion that prevention of ID might be an important and valid aim.

Statistical—here it is assumed that any aspect of human behaviour can be measured and will have a mean and standard deviation. In the case of ID there are two aspects of measurement—intelligence as measured by intelligence tests to arrive at an IQ, and adaptive behaviour: the ability to cope with the challenges of everyday life. People with ID are defined as those who fall below one SD below the mean on these measures.

These perspectives have produced a common understanding that ID is defined as an interaction between the person and the community. A person may have significant deficits but cope well in the right environment and with the right support. Minor difficulties can be massively handicapping in a world where the person is isolated and unsupported.

These ideas have led to an accepted definition of ID in the UK. There are 3 main components:
- A significant lifelong difficulty in learning and understanding
- A significant difficulty in learning and practising the skills needed to cope with everyday life
- That there is evidence that these difficulties started before adulthood.[1,2]

These definitions have been worded very carefully from a political perspective but they are not sufficiently precise for professional practice. It is important, therefore, to add the internationally accepted definition of ID, the latest revision of which was drawn up in the USA in 2002. The same social model is used and ID refers to:

"Substantial limitations in present functioning. It is characterized by significantly sub average intellectual functioning, existing concurrently with related limitations in two or more of the following applicable adaptive skill areas: communication, self care, home living, social skills, community use, self direction, health and safety, functional academics, leisure and work. Mental retardation manifests itself before age 18."

Intellectual function is generally measured by intelligence tests, but although this may be necessary it is not sufficient to define ID. Coping with everyday life is broken down into 10 key areas, of which 2 must be significantly impaired.

The rigid application of assessments based on this definition is not helpful. Rather it is important that practitioners consider the individual circumstances of each person, including culture, personal history, socio-economic, and psychological factors. There is increasing attention now being paid to the role of economic factors in determining ID in general and health inequalities in particular.

Further reading

American Association for Mental Retardation (2002). *Mental Retardation, Definition, Classification and Systems of Support*. 10th edn. AAMR: Washington.

1 Department of Health (2001). *Valuing People: a New Strategy for Learning Disability in the 21st Century*. Cmnd 5086. HMSO: London.

2 Scottish Executive (2000). *The Same as You: a Review of Services for People with Learning Disabilities*. Scottish Executive: Edinburgh.

3 American Association for Mental Retardation (2002). *Mental Retardation, Definition, Classification and Systems of Support*. 10th edn. AAMR: Washington.

Incidence and prevalence of intellectual disability

Calculating the incidence of ID is difficult because there is no way of detecting the vast majority of those infants who have ID at birth. Therefore to arrive at any estimate one has to use cumulative incidence, and this has been calculated at 8yrs of age as 4.9/1000 for severe ID and 4.3/1000 for mild ID.[1]

It is only the obvious manifestations of ID that can be detected at birth—e.g. Down syndrome (see 📖 Carers' assessment, p.38), and for these conditions it is possible to calculate incidence.

It is more usual, therefore, to refer to the prevalence of ID, and where there is no obvious physical manifestation at birth, diagnosis must be delayed in order to await significant developmental delay along with other manifestations to diagnose ID; therefore, it is more common to talk about prevalence.

Prevalence is concerned with an estimation of the number of people with a condition, disorder or disease as a proportion of the general population.

If IQ is used as an indicator of intellectual disability, then it can be calculated that 2–3% of the population is likely to have an IQ <70. Given that a large proportion of the people with such an estimated IQ never come into contact with a caring agency, it is more common to refer to 'administrative prevalence', which refers to the number of people provided with some form of service from caring agencies.

Historically, there has been a general consensus that the overall prevalence of severe learning disabilities is approximately 3–4/1000 of the general population.[2]

The Department of Health has suggested that mild learning disability is quite common; prevalence has been estimated to be in the region of 20/1000 of the general population. In the UK it has been further calculated that, of the 3–4/1000 population with an intellectual disability, ~30% will present with severe or profound learning disabilities. Within this group it is not uncommon to find multiple disabilities, including physical and/or sensory impairments, or disability as well as behavioural difficulties.

Emerson et al., drawing on extensive epidemiological data, have confirmed the estimation of prevalence for severe learning disabilities.[1] They state it to be somewhere in the region of 3–4/1000 of the general population. The prevalence rate Emerson et al. give for the intellectually disabled population referred to as having mild ID is much more imprecise. It is estimated that it might be 25–30 people/1000 of the general population. Based on these estimates it can be assumed that there are some 230,000–350,000 persons with severe ID, and possibly 580,000–1,750,000 persons with mild ID in the UK.

There is a slight imbalance in the ratio of males to females in people with both mild and severe learning disabilities, with males having slightly higher prevalence rates. Also there is some evidence of slightly higher prevalence rates among some ethnic groups, and this includes Black Groups in the USA, and South Asian Groups in the UK.[1]

Further reading

Grant G, Goward P, Richardson M, Ramcharan P (2005). *Learning Disability: a Life Cycle Approach to Valuing People*. Open University Press: Milton Keynes.

Learning About Intellectual Disabilities and Health ▣ http://www.intellectualdisability.info/home.htm [accessed March 2009]

1 Emerson E, Hatton C, Felce D, Murphy G (2001). *Learning Disabilities: The Fundamental Facts*. The Foundation for People with Learning Disabilities: London.

2 Department of Health (2001). *Valuing People: a New Strategy for Learning Disability for the 21st Century*. CM 5086. HMSO: London.

Diagnosing intellectual disability

That this section concerns the diagnosis of ID would seem to imply that people with ID are the preserve of the medical model: this is not so. In the context of this section it will be shown that sometimes identifying an ID is arrived at in a number of ways and by different professionals, and this may or may not include a medical diagnosis.

Diagnosing or identifying intellectual disabilities

The vast majority of parents will have no evidence that their child will have ID before the birth. Only a minority of parents have advance warning, possibly from screening investigations such as blood tests and ultrasound scans, or diagnostic investigations such as amniocentesis, chorionic villous sampling or other tests undertaken because the parents are perceived as being at a high risk.[1]

Unless a definite physical abnormality or characteristic signs (as in children with Down syndrome) are present at birth, or a traumatic delivery has taken place, ID is seldom suspected or diagnosed at birth. A diagnosis can vary from the confirmation of the presence of a specific condition (e.g. Down syndrome) to a much broader diagnosis of developmental delay with no specific condition identified.

ID is usually identified during childhood or sometimes later during adolescence, but in order to meet most criteria for being classified as intellectually disabled this should be before 18yrs of age, or if identified later in life there should be sufficient evidence available that this started before 18yrs. Those children with severe or profound ID are likely to be more noticed as having learning disabilities at a younger age than those with mild to moderate ID. Therefore ID is most often diagnosed in early childhood when a child fails to reach 'normal' developmental milestones.

During this period, parents may have expressed concerns over the nature of their child's progress and suspect that a problem exists. It is unprofessional and potentially dangerous if those in contact with the parents at this time (e.g. GP, health visitor, paediatrician or other nurses) dismiss parental concern and label them as 'overanxious' or 'overprotective'. Such judgements are prejudicial and negate parents' concerns subsequently; they have no place in family centred services.[1] Rather a regular check should be kept on the child's progress, more frequently than the usual screening checks, and records kept. It is a relief to both parents and professionals, after a period of observation, to be able to show that the child is reaching normal milestones. The prospects of active family involvement will be damaged in the short term, and possibly for several years, when a diagnosis of ID is confirmed despite repeated concerns having been previously raised only to be dismissed or largely ignored.

Finally it is important to identify the nature and extent of ID and either exclude or include other more specific developmental disorders that are sometimes present, for example ASD, ADHD, or dyspraxia (developmental coordination disorder).

Conclusion

Identification of the cause of ID and the provision of an early diagnosis are crucial to:

- limit the feelings of self blame that may be experienced by some parents of children with ID
- reduce the possibility of inadequate adaptation by the parents to their child and thereby hopefully avoid rejection.

Other reasons for identifying the presence of ID and diagnosis include a need to:

- understand the possible manifestation of the identified condition over a defined period of time
- identify the range of therapeutic approaches that may be used to ameliorate the effects of the condition, including the mobilization of specific resources
- establish, in some cases, the degree of risk to other family members of the condition reoccurring in their siblings and offspring.

Further reading

Grant G, Goward P, Richardson M, Ramcharan P (2005). *Learning Disability: a Life Cycle Approach to Valuing People*. Open University Press: Milton Keynes.

Overview of Learning (Intellectual) Disability in Children ⌨ http://www.intellectualdisability.info/families/ldchildren_ml.htm [accessed March 2009]

1 Barr O (2007). Working effectively with families of people with learning disabilities. In: Gates B (Ed). *Learning Disabilities: Toward Inclusion*. 5th edn. Churchill Livingstone: Edinburgh, 567–598.

Causes and manifestations of intellectual disability

ID is a major health condition thought to affect an estimated 150,000 infants/year either born with, or later diagnosed as having ID.[1] The reported frequency of ID varies across studies, but overall rates of 1–3% of the general population have been found, with a male:female ratio of 1.3:1, mainly attributed to X-linked ID.[2]

In 40–80% of individuals with ID the cause cannot be determined.[1] The aim should be to try to establish any cause of ID so that accurate information about any diagnosis reached can be given, as well as precise rather than empiric recurrence risks.[2]

ID can result from experiences in the prenatal environment that interfere with brain and CNS development and functioning. ID is a feature of hundreds of congenital conditions, but 5–15% are thought to result from genetic disorders. Abnormalities associated with chromosomes and/or genes can often disrupt physical and/or intellectual development.

ID can result from a combination of the following factors:

Genetic abnormalities

Genetic abnormalities may be subdivided into chromosomal, single gene, multifactorial, mitochondrial, and/or somatic cell disorders. Recognized Mendelian patterns of inherited disorders include autosomal dominant, autosomal recessive and X-linked (see 📖 Common conditions among people with intellectual disability, p.16).

Exposure to environmental agents/teratogens

Environmental agents that cause disruption in normal prenatal development are known as teratogens. Fetal development can be disrupted by teratogenic exposure to chemicals, drugs or diseases.

Chemicals: Examples of chemicals with known teratogenic effect include excessive radiation, smoking, and alcohol.

Drugs: Examples of drugs include so-called 'recreational' illegal substances, and also prescribed drugs, which may have teratogenic effects (e.g. thalidomide or phenytoin).

Diseases: Examples of diseases with known teratogenic effect include rubella.

It is now recognized that an embryo may be susceptible to virtually any substance if exposure to the substance is sufficiently concentrated. A number of broad generalizations have emerged from research into teratogens, for example, some individual embryos and pregnancies are more *susceptible* to exposure, and/or there may be developmental periods which are *critical or sensitive* with regard to specific teratogen exposure.

Intrauterine or birth trauma

Where there is a clear biological cause of ID, for example, oxygen deprivation at birth or placental insufficiency.

Prematurity

ID caused by premature birth due to interruption of the normal course and duration of maturation in the uterine environment or due to trauma(s) experienced in the perinatal period following premature birth.

Postnatal developmental period

ID may be caused in the immediate postnatal period, if there is interruption, disruption or damage of a sufficient, significant level to the normal course of development. Examples would include infections such as meningitis, or trauma such as severe or intractable epilepsy or head injury.

1 Wynbrandt J, Ludman MD (2000). *Genetic Disorders and Birth Defects*. Facts on File Inc.: New York.

2 Firth HV, Hurst JA (2005). *Oxford Desk Reference. Clinical Genetics*. Oxford University Press: Oxford.

Common conditions among people with intellectual disability

Genetic diseases and disorders with associated ID may be subdivided into chromosomal, single gene, multifactorial, and mitochondrial disorders. Recognized Mendelian patterns of inherited single gene disorders include autosomal dominant, autosomal recessive and X-linked inheritance.

Chromosomal disorders

The normal chromosome complement is 46 chromosomes occurring in pairs. Pairs 1 to 22 are called autosomes and are common to both genders. The 23rd pair are the sex chromosomes because they relate to gender. Thus normal male chromosome complement is 46 XY whereas female chromosome complement is 46 XX. An abnormal chromosome complement can be the result of loss, duplication, or rearrangement of genetic material.

Aneuploidy is the condition in which the chromosome number in the cells of an individual is not an exact number of the typical chromosome complement of 46 XX or 46 XY. There may be a full extra chromosome, called trisomy, or there may be a complete loss or absence of a chromosome, called monosomy.[1] Examples of trisomy include trisomy 21 (Down syndrome), trisomy 18 (Edwards syndrome), or trisomy 13 (Patau syndrome). An example of monosomy that may be but is not always associated with ID is monosomy X (Turner syndrome).

Single gene disorders

Genes located on the X chromosome are referred to as X-linked genes and those on the autosomes as autosomal genes. Of each of the pairs in a chromosome set, one is derived from each parent, so each pair of chromosomes will have a comparable gene located at the same position on each chromosome pair, which may be referred to as alleles. Therefore, with the exception of the X and Y chromosomes in males, each gene is present in two copies, one from each parent. A gene mutation indicates a changed or altered gene.[2] These principles of dominant, recessive and X-linked inheritance patterns reflect Mendelian laws of inheritance.[2]

Autosomal dominant—a gene mutation in one of a pair of genes, which produces an abnormal characteristic despite the presence of the other normal or unaltered copy, is referred to as dominant. Examples of autosomal dominant disorders often associated with differing degrees of ID include Apert syndrome, myotonic dystrophy (early onset and congenital cases frequently associated with ID, though adult onset infrequently associated with ID), tuberous sclerosis.

Autosomal recessive—a gene mutation that causes an abnormal characteristic only when present in both copies of a gene is referred to as recessive. Examples of autosomal recessive disorders causing, or often associated with, differing degrees of ID include galactosaemia, Sanfilippo syndrome, Tay–Sachs disease, phenylketonuria.

X-linked—The sex chromosomes consist of two X chromosomes in a normal female, and one X and one Y chromosome in a male. Therefore females have two copies of each X chromosome gene, one from each parent, but males have only one copy of each gene on the X chromosome. Mutations on the X chromosome may be described as dominant or recessive. X-linked dominant mutations may manifest obvious clinical effects in both males and females, whereas X-linked recessive mutations usually manifest in males but have minimal, or no, effect on (carrier) females. Examples of X-linked disorders causing, or often associated with, differing degrees of ID include fragile X syndrome, Coffin–Lowry syndrome, adrenoleucodystrophy.

Multifactorial/polygenic disorders

In multifactorial/polygenic disorders, both genetic and environmental factors combine to influence the manifestation of the disorder. Such disorders, although frequently exhibiting familial clustering and raised recurrence risks in relatives, do not conform to Mendelian laws of gene transmission. Examples of multifactorial disorders include neural tube defects, orofacial clefting, and pyloric stenosis.

Mitochondrial disorders

Mitochondria of cells contain DNA, which has unique features that distinguish it from nuclear DNA. Mitochondrial DNA is exclusively maternally inherited, with few, very rare, exceptions. Paternal mitochondria enter the egg on fertilization only in miniscule proportions and are usually rapidly eliminated early in embryogenesis.[3] Examples of mitochondrial inherited disorders include MERRF and MELAS.

Further reading

Harper P (2004). *Practical Genetic Counselling*. 6th edn. Arnold: London.

1 Field RC, Stansfield WD (1997). *A Dictionary of Genetics*. 5th edn. Oxford University Press: Oxford.

2 Jones KL (2006). *Smith's Recognizable Patterns of Human Malformation*. 6th edn. Elsevier Saunders: Philadelphia.

3 Firth HV, Hurst JA (2005). *Oxford Desk Reference. Clinical Genetics*. Oxford University Press: Oxford.

Defining intellectual disability nursing

Twelve years ago Gates provided the first comprehensive definition of ID nursing that stated its purpose to be:

'To skillfully assess the social and health care needs of people with intellectual disabilities and/or their families, in order to assist them to live as independently as possible. The nurse will achieve this by marshalling skills as manager, enabler and co-coordinator of services, and will demonstrate that her evidence based interventions lead to health maintenance and/or gain. The nurse will practice her craft autonomously yet interdependently with other colleagues from a variety of other academic disciplines and service agencies in a variety of settings, in partnership with people with intellectual disabilities to assist them to lead valued life styles. This role will require her to develop and refine her knowledge and competence in a range of skills in order to meet the changing needs of people with intellectual disabilities.' [1]

What is intellectual disability nursing?

'Learning disability nursing is a person-centred profession with the primary aim of supporting the well-being and social inclusion of people with learning disabilities through improving or maintaining physical and mental health'. [2]

What do intellectual disability nurses do?

Nowadays much of the care planning and delivery of ID nursing no longer takes place in the old long-term ID hospitals, rather it occurs in a landscape of complex service provision that includes: residential care homes, independent living homes, supported living, and people with ID living in their own home as well as family homes.

Also to be found are larger service configurations and/or very specialist settings such as treatment and assessment services and challenging behaviour units. They may also reside in other specialist health or social care settings such as hospices or homes for older people.

Wherever people with ID live, if they are in receipt of nursing care, whether this comprises short intensive nursing interventions or long periods of care and support, then this care should be guided by a care plan. ID nurses must be competent in preparing robust, professionally prepared care plans based on a systematic nursing assessment. Much evidence exists of the positive contribution of ID nurses to the lives of some people with ID. [3] The authenticity and validity of such a claim continue to be validated by the many examples of excellent practice highlighted in the recently published *Good Practice in Learning Disability Nursing.* [2]

Intellectual disability nursing today

ID nurses currently work in a wide range of organizational settings that include: NHS, local authority, private, statutory, and third sector. Typically they are likely to work in inter-professional teams and for a variety of agencies. Recent changes are beginning to dictate a range of new roles that are undertaken by ID nurses, for example nurses working in health-care teams such as in acute hospitals, mental health services, and primary care. In England the *Good Practice in Learning Disability Nursing* publication[2] has asserted that most ID nurses still employed by the NHS can be described as working in one of three practice areas:

- Health facilitation—supporting mainstream access
- Inpatient services—for example, assessment and treatment, and secure services
- Specialist roles—in community teams.

Other, broader developments in healthcare roles, such as the modern matron and nurse prescribing openings, have provided new opportunities in ID services. Also to be found are ID nurse consultant roles who are able to offer valuable clinical, supervisory expertise along with regional and national professional leadership.

Further reading

Turnbull J (2004). *Learning Disability Nursing*. Blackwell Publishing: Oxford.

Department of Health (2007). *Good practice in learning disability nursing*. Department of Health: London. ▣ http://www.dh.gov.uk/en/Publicationsandstatistics/Publications/PublicationsPolicyAnd Guidance/DH_081328

Northway R, Hutchinson C, Kingdon A (2006). *Shaping the Future: A Vision for Learning Disability Nursing*. UK Learning Disability Consultant Nurse Network: UK. ▣ http://www.ntw.nhs.uk/ uploads/documents/doc203.pdf

1 Gates B (Ed) (1997). Understanding learning disability. In: *Learning Disabilities* 3rd edn. Churchill Livingstone: Edinburgh, 16–17.

2 Department of Health (2007). *Good Practice in Learning Disability Nursing*. Department of Health: London.

3 Alaszewski A, Gates B, Ayer S, Manthorpe G, Motherby E (2000). *Education for Diversity and Change: Final report of the ENB-funded project on educational preparation for learning disability nursing*. Schools of Community and Health Studies and Nursing. The University of Hull: Hull.

The purist form of nursing

The context of intellectual disability nursing

The practice setting for ID nursing is located in a complex landscape of service provision. This includes, for example, residential care homes, independent living homes, supported living arrangements, and people with ID living in their own homes as well as family homes. There are also larger service configurations and very specialist settings such as treatment and assessment services, challenging behaviour units, as well as specialist health or social care settings, such as hospices for children with life-limiting conditions, or homes for older people. ID nurses work with people from birth through to death, who require a range of supports throughout their lives that will range from none, or minimal, support through to intensive holistic nursing aimed at meeting the multidimensional needs of people with ID. This is why ID nursing is often referred to as the purist form of nursing; unlike our colleagues in other branches of nursing, we do not concentrate on specific manifestations of physical ill health or trauma, nor do we just focus on mental health and well-being, or children, or childbirth for that matter; rather we offer support to people with ID and their families that is all embracing and quite literally from the cradle through to the grave.

The purist approach

In order to offer comprehensive nursing interventions that meet the multidimensional needs of people with ID, it is necessary to adopt a structured approach. A comprehensive needs assessment (physical, psychological, social, spiritual, and emotional) has to be completed. If a nurse is required to work with someone with ID and their families, it is necessary that their needs are assessed and incorporated into an individual care plan, taking their desires, wishes, and aspirations into account. The nurse must work closely with the client's family, care providers, and other professionals, as this broad approach may bring very important and essential information to light for assessment, as well as care plan development, its approach, delivery, and management. This is followed by construction of a written care plan that is then implemented and followed, with ongoing review and evaluation. It is this very structured approach, with partnership working and a consideration of the multidimensionality of people coupled with person-centred planning, that allows us to make claim, as well as others, to validate, that what we do is the purist form of nursing.

A modelled approach

In response to social and political influences, the arena of ID care models, and that of care planning, have changed considerably; so, therefore, has the practice of ID nurses.[1] For example, during the last century, ID services were dominated by a medical model of care that emphasized the biological needs of people and the need to 'cure' physical problems in order to allow a person to function in society. Most people with ID have now moved out of long-stay hospitals, but there remains a concern that the powerful effects of the medical model continue to influence care provided in smaller community based residences. Klotz has argued that the use of the medical model has pathologized and objectified people with

ID, leading to them being seen as 'less human'.[2] Therefore, nurses need to consider adopting a nursing model to guide their care in practice, to ensure that what they offer is holistic and is the purist form of nursing. It must be remembered, therefore, that the use of such a model must hold the person with ID as central to the care-planning process, and that the nurse must be mindful they use such a model to promote what is best for that person. There are numerous nursing models that can be adapted and used in a variety of health and social care settings. Some nursing models, such as Orem's self-care[3], Roper's (2002) activities of daily living,[4] and Aldridge[5] are all well known and seemingly most used in ID nursing. It should be remembered that they may not be seen as relevant or ideal for all people with ID, but they can generally be adapted relatively easily and then become ideal frameworks for the assessment of health as well as more general needs.

Further reading

Gates B (2006). *Care Planning and Care Delivery in Intellectual Disability Nursing*. Blackwell Science: London.

1 Alaszewski A, Motherby E, Gates B, Ayer S, Manthorpe J (2001). *Diversity and Change: The Changing Roles and Education of Learning Disability Nurses*. London: English National Board.

2 Klotz J (2004). Sociocultural study of intellectual disability: moving beyond labelling and social constructionist perspectives. *British Journal of Learning Disabilities* **32**, 93–4.

3 Orem DE (1991). *Nursing: Concepts of Practice*. St Louis: Mosby.

4 Roper N, Logan W, Tierney A (2002). *The Elements of Nursing*, 4th edn. Churchill Livingstone: Edinburgh.

5 Aldridge J (2004). Intellectual disability nursing: a model for practice. In: Turnbull J (Ed). *Learning Disability Nursing*. Blackwell Publishing: Oxford.

Principles and values of social policy and their effects on intellectual disability

Since 2000, each of the countries of the UK have published substantial reviews of their policy guiding the development and delivery of ID services.[1,2,3,4] These highlight the importance of supporting people as individuals, and giving due regard to their human, civil and legal rights.

Scotland: *Same as You?*[1]

- People should be valued. People are individuals and they should be asked about the services they need and be involved in making choices about what they want
- People should be helped and supported to do everything they are able
- People should be able to use the same local services as everyone else, wherever possible
- People should benefit from specialist social, health, and educational services
- People should have services that take account of their age, abilities, and other needs.

England: *Valuing People*[2]

Legal and civil rights—all services should treat people with ID as individuals with respect for their dignity, and challenge discrimination on all grounds including disability. People with ID will also receive the full protection of the law when necessary.

Independence—the starting presumption should be one of independence, rather than dependence, with public services providing the support needed to maximize this. Independence in this context does not mean doing everything unaided.

Choice—this includes people with severe and profound disabilities who, with the right help and support, can make important choices and express preferences about their day-to-day lives.

Inclusion—enabling people with ID to do ordinary things, make use of mainstream services, and be included fully in the local community.

These original principles were revised in 2009, placing a greater emphasis on the outcomes that need to be achieved:[5]

Personalization—people have real choice and control over their lives and services.

What people do during the day (and evenings and weekends)—helping people to be properly included in their communities, with a particular focus on paid work.

Better health—ensuring that the NHS provides full and equal access to good quality healthcare.

Access to housing that people want and need, with a particular emphasis on home ownership and tenancies.

Making sure that change happens and the policy is delivered, including making partnership boards more effective.

Wales: *Fulfilling the Promises*[3]

- Provide comprehensive and integrated services to achieve social inclusion, be person-centred, and improve empowerment and independence
- Ensure effortless and effective movement between services and organizations at different times of life
- Be holistic in approach and delivery, taking into account an individual's preferences, hopes and lifestyle, and ensure a range of appropriate advocacy services is available for people who wish to use them
- Be accessible in terms of service users and their carers and families having full information, and have fully developed collaborative partnerships to deliver flexible services that have been developed on evidence of their effectiveness, and have transparency for costs
- Be delivered by a competent, well informed, well trained, and effectively supported and supervised workforce
- The early completion of the National Assembly's resettlement programmes to enable all people to live in the community.

Northern Ireland: *Equal Lives*[4]

Citizenship—people with ID are individuals first and foremost, and each has a right to be treated as an equal citizen.

Person-centred—people with ID should be supported in ways that take account of their individual needs.

Participation—people with ID should be consulted about the services they want. They should be actively involved in making choices and decisions affecting their lives.

Interdependence—people with ID should be valued and encouraged to contribute to the life of the community.

Equality—people with ID should be able to use the same services and have the same entitlements as everyone else.

1 Scottish Executive (2000). *The Same as You? A Review of the Services for People with Learning Disabilities*. Scottish Executive: Edinburgh.

2 Department of Health (2001). *Valuing People. A New Strategy for Learning Disability for 21st Century*. Department of Health: London.

3 Welsh Office (2001) *Fulfilling the Promises*. Welsh Assembly: Cardiff.

4 Department of Health, Social Services and Public Safety (2005). *Equal Lives*. Department of Health, Social Services and Public Safety: Belfast.

5 Department of Health (2009). *Valuing People Now. A New Strategy for People with Learning Disabilities* Department of Health: London.

Holism and working across the life span

Holistic nursing for health

Holistic approaches to nursing seek to promote nursing interventions that adopt a whole-person approach. This means providing nursing that responds to the various dimensions of being, and these typically include attention to the physical, emotional, social, economic, and spiritual needs of people.

Working holistically across the life span

Being healthy is a positive state of being that we all seek. We are constantly exposed to factors throughout our lives that have the potential to compromise our health. Thus the health of all individuals, but in particular those with ID, are susceptible to health loss. To seek health gain and health maintenance for this group will sometimes require the support of an ID nurse.[1] Throughout the life span from childhood to old age, and even in end of life care, ID nurses can be found supporting people with ID, and wherever they practice they must remember that holistic care planning and delivery form an essential part of their everyday practice. ID nurses can enable people with ID to obtain good quality care. But in order to do this they must reflect on their practice and use the best possible evidence to meet the multidimensional needs of people—thus providing person-centred holistic care. ID nurses have many dimensions and responsibilities within their role; however, supporting people with ID to reach their goals in the form of living their lives as fully and independently as possible is by far the most vital. As registered professionals they have a duty of care, and they have to act within the best interests of their clients at all times. This necessarily includes the planning and delivery of care that attends to the holistic nature of the people they are supporting.

Further reading

Allan E (1999). Learning disability: promoting health equality in the community. *Nursing Standard* 13(44), 32–37.

Journal of Holistic Nursing. Available at ▣ http://www.sagepub.co.uk/journalsProdDesc. nav?prodId=Journal200847

1 Gates B, Beacock C (Eds) (1996). *Dimensions of Learning Disability*. Baillière Tindall: London.

Working with families

Defining families

Families of people with ID can be major influences in their lives and in many situations they provide most of the care and support to people with ID. The need for nurses to work collaboratively with family members is intregral to current government policy within ID services, and a key professional requirement by the Nursing and Midwifery Council.

In using the word 'family' there is often a perceived common understanding of what we mean by the term. There is often common language used when talking about family members and relatives within the wider family. The nature of these relationships, however, and the importance attached to them can differ considerably between different individuals within the same family, and people across different families. Although considerable variation may occur between family structures, overall the family unit is still recognized as a core unit within society that has a major influence on the development and overall functioning of its individual members, as well as on local communities.[1]

The meaning of what a family is has altered considerably over the past 30yrs. Although most children, including those with ID, grow up within a family environment, the stereotypical definition of a family of 2 married parents and 2 children growing up together no longer reflects the range of possible family structures within current society in the UK or the Republic of Ireland.

As a consequence, defining the nature of families is not as straightforward as it may first appear. There are a growing number of possible differences to be considered, for instance: number of parents present, marital or legal relationships between parents, biological and legal relationships between children and adults within the family, gender of parents, number of children, and number of generations present within the one family unit as defined by family members. Given the considerable evolution of the nature of families over the past 30yrs, it is reasonable to expect that there will be further developments in the structure and function of families over the years to come. However, despite variations in family structures and roles of members it is generally accepted that a family involves the following key components:
• A defined membership
• Agreed group values
• Relationships between members
• Roles
• Structure
• Functions
• Stability over time[2]

Nurses need to learn the legal definitions of families and family relationships, such as next of kin, partners, parental responsibility, and civil partnerships used within the jurisdiction in which they are working, and consider the practical implications of these and how they should be applied within their role. Such definitions can be found in mental health legislation, children-based legislation such as the relevant Children's Act or Order, as well as in guidance on consent and child protection. Nurses should make time to review and remain up to date with these definitions, because often, when they need to make decisions, for instance about the role of parents or other family members in relation to consent or admission to care, or child protection issues, there may be limited opportunity to consult legal documents or seek a legal opinion at that time.

Nurses working with people with ID need to be aware of the changing nature of the demography of people with ID, and the structure and membership of families. There is growing diversity of family arrangements, spanning small nuclear family groups to more extended networks, and the social, cultural, and religious factors that may influence these arrangements. It is also important to be alert to the potential differing rules and roles within families, yet treat all families with respect and do not discriminate against families or the members within them due to their family structures and functioning.

1 Haralambos M, Holburn M (2004). Sociology. *Themes and Perspectives* 6th Edn. Collins Educational: London.

2 Barr O (2007). Working effectively with families of people with learning disabilities. In: Gates B (Ed). *Learning Disabilities: Towards Inclusion,* 5th edn. Churchill Livingstone: London.

Family members of people with intellectual disabilities

Family membership—a lifetime bond?

All people with ID are born into families of some description. It is accepted that the composition and structure of the families may vary considerably, depending on the number of parents living together, other siblings, extended family networks, together with other social and cultural influences. However, most people recognize themselves as family members, with the roles and responsibilities that brings during their life. It is important to acknowledge that a person with ID may also be a brother, sister, cousin, grandchild, aunt, uncle, and increasingly parents. In situations when a person with ID is adopted or fostered, they will usually still see themselves as 'belonging' to a family.

Furthermore, just like most people who do not have ID, individuals with ID will normally view themselves as family members, even after they have left home and possibility move some miles away. Likewise, other family members will continue to see the person with ID as a family member, and will often wish to continue to maintain contact and may wish to be involved in providing some ongoing support.

Nurses need to recognize that family members will provide most of the support for people with ID during their lifetime, and that successful collaborative working arrangements with family members is key to being able to provide effective professional support. Furthermore, while it is accepted that working with family members can at times be difficult, the need to seek ways to work effectively with families is a professional requirement for all nurses and is never an optional extra.[1]

Impact of having family member(s) with intellectual disabilities

Much has been written about the impact of having a family member with ID, and the picture that emerges from the research is very mixed. Depending on the literature you are reading and the focus of the research undertaken, nurses could at times almost be forgiven for believing that the impact on other family members is almost universally negative.

However, this is not an accurate picture, and is in many ways more reflective of the research focus taken and the pathological view of families held by some professionals. This is not to deny that at times families may have difficulties, but consider how many families of people with ID manage very well most of the time, and with limited need for ongoing professional support.

For many families the impact is mixed, a combination of positive and negative experiences. At times extra challenges may arise as a consequence of having a person with ID in the family, for instance, additional physical care needs, concerns over further education and development, and reduced opportunities for flexibility in family activities. In contrast, parents have reported positive impacts, including increased knowledge and skills, increased confidence, and stronger family cohesion.[2]

The impact on the family is evolving and will change as the abilities and needs of other family members and the person with ID changes. For example, as parents get older they may require more support; on some occasions the person with ID may play an important role in supporting other family members. In seeking to develop effective collaboration with family members, nurses need to take time to understand the strengths and challenges for each family and avoid making stereotypical judgements about the support that all families may need. While nurses cannot always 'make things better' for families and most family members understand that, we should always seek not to make things worse by our actions or omissions.

Acknowledging family membership

In acknowledging the person with ID as a family member, nurses should seek to support the person with ID to maintain contact with other family members. Practical examples may include knowing the birthdays of other family members and supporting the person with ID to send a card if they wish, supporting people with ID to be included in important family events such as birthday parties, wedding ceremonies, and other family celebrations of a religious or cultural significance.

It is also important to recognize the other roles people with ID may have in the family, such as aunt, uncle, or cousin. Many people with ID wish to have the opportunity to 'maintain contact' with dead family members, and for this reason it is also important they have the opportunity if they wish to remember anniversaries and visit burial sites, as is culturally appropriate.

Further reading

Grant G, Ramcharan P, McGrath M *et al.* (1998) Rewards and gratifications among family caregivers: towards a refined model of caring and coping. *Journal of Intellectual Disability Research* **42**(1), 58–71.

1 Nursing & Midwifery Council (2008). *The Code: Standards of conduct, performance and ethics for nurses and midwives.* NMC: London.

2 Maxwell V, Barr O (2003). With the benefit of hindsight: a mother's reflection on raising a child with Down Syndrome. *Journal of Learning Disabilities* **7**(1), 51–64.

Explaining intellectual disabilities to family members

Changing understandings and terminology

To some degree the changing names used to describe people with ID reflect a developing understanding of the nature of ID, as it becomes more understood as a condition that could be ameliorated by education, support, and effective healthcare, in contrast to a previous view that a child or adult would learn little and have little chance of becoming independent, with many people going to live in large hospitals or other congregated living settings. Indeed in planning this book much discussion took place on the title and terminology to be used as noted in the introductory section of the book. However, for people not familiar with the history of these debates and discussions of the fine differences between terms, their understanding of ID may be quite varied, with a mixture of previous understandings and terms being used.

It is likely that new terms will become used in the years to come as further debate and discussion occurs. Indeed conditions that have previously been linked to ID may be viewed as separate, for instance, autism, Asperger's syndrome, and cerebral palsy, as ID is not always a key feature of these conditions.

Need for a common understanding

Given the potential for debate about the meaning of terms, a useful starting point in explaining the nature of ID is the definition used within current policy documents. Within the UK, Republic of Ireland and internationally, the term intellectual disabilities has three key components:
- A significantly reduced ability to understand new or complex information (impairment intelligence)
- A reduced ability to cope independently (impaired social functioning)
- Started before adulthood with a lasting effect on development.

The need for an explanation

Despite having a largely agreed policy based definition this will not be familiar to many parents or other family members of children with ID. In fact, even the term intellectual or learning disability may have limited agreed understanding across family networks, even after a diagnosis has been provided. It is important, therefore, to provide opportunities for further discussion about what such terminology means, so that parents, siblings, other family members, and professionals are all using the term to mean the same thing.

It is necessary to tailor any explanation to the audience, be that mothers, fathers, parents together, siblings, or members of the extended family. Although, nurses will largely be involved in discussions with members of the immediate family, the words and explanations that parents and siblings may use with other people can be a useful investment of time. Although parents may be aware of the terminology and have received a diagnosis, how effectively a diagnosis and an explanation is provided can have lasting effects on the future relationships parents and other family members may have with professionals.

Key points to remember

- Not being told should not be mistaken for not knowing; just because a confirmed diagnosis has never been provided does not mean parents are not aware that some difficulties may exist, even if they have never mentioned them.
- Family members' concerns should be fully discussed and investigated— they know their child best. Their concerns must not be dismissed as being 'over anxious' or fobbed off as 'each child developing at different rates', or 'sometimes people with intellectual disabilities do things like that'.
- At times more detailed explanations of complex conditions are necessary in relationship to origins and care needs. An assessment of family members' training needs should be undertaken in relation to caring for the person with ID, and this used as a basis for further skills teaching.
- The potential of any individual to learn is largely influenced by the opportunities they have to learn, therefore any explanation should include hope that individuals will continue to learn and avoid categorical statements about final outcomes, such as 'he/she will never…'.
- Siblings need explanations in a language they can understand; it is often helpful to explain this as people learning slower, and may be having different abilities from each other. Balance against confidentiality of personal information.
- Adult siblings may need further explanations as the care of the person may change, and parents may have provided limited detailed explanation of their sibling's condition or future care needs as an adult.
- Provide opportunities for grandparents to ask questions; they may not have had a reason or opportunity to update their previous views towards ID and understanding of interventions.
- Never lose sight of the fact that the person with ID is still first and foremost a family member—a son, daughter, brother, sister, or grandchild—build on strengths.

Further reading

Foundation for People with Learning Disabilities ◲ www.learningdisabilities.org.uk

Mencap ◲ www.mencap.org.uk

Down's Syndrome Association ◲ www.dsa.org.uk

1 Scottish Executive (2000). *The Same as You? A Review of the Services for People with Learning Disabilities.* Scottish Executive: Edinburgh.

2 Department of Health (2001). *Valuing People. A New Strategy for Learning Disability for 21st Century.* Department of Health: London.

3 Department of Health (2007). *Valuing People Now. From Progress to Transformation.* Department of Health: London.

The process of family adaptation

Parents and other family members (on the news of a pregnancy within the family) often start planning the birth of a child well in advance of the day it is born. Even with the developments in antenatal screening very few families expect the birth of a child with, or the subsequent diagnosis of ID.

The diagnosis of a condition linked to ID can be made within a few weeks of birth only in a small number of conditions with clearly recognized syndromes and diagnostic tests available. For most parents, the presence of ID becomes visible over a period of months, often years, before a diagnosis is confirmed.

Bereavement reaction—a note of caution

Previously a comparison has been made between the bereavement process and the birth of a child with ID, the rationale being that parents and other family members 'grieve' the loss of the expected child without ID. Although parents have reported shock and a sense of loss at the diagnosis of a child with ID, caution is needed when using a bereavement model to explain the process of family adaptation.

A fundamental difference exists in that when a child with ID is born, no child actually dies and the parents and other family members have the task of caring for and supporting the child who was born. Following on from this, parents do not reach an end stage of 'acceptance' as outlined in earlier bereavement models, rather they continue to work through a process of adaptation as the abilities and needs of the child and other family members change. Therefore, nurses and other professionals need to be very careful about what they mean if they choose to use the word 'acceptance' of the birth or diagnosis of ID in a child.

Adaptation as a process

The birth or diagnosis of ID does come as a shock to parents and other family members, whether this information was suspected during pregnancy, confirmed during pregnancy, or when the child was a few weeks, months or years old.

A number of models have been presented to explain the stages parents may go through in seeking to adapt to this news. While some differences exist in the terminology used and the numbers of stages within individual frameworks the overall process outlined is largely the same.

One four-stage model developed by Miller and mothers of children with a range of disabilities, although written some years ago, still provides important understandings.[1]

- The first stage is that of 'surviving', and is characterized by mixed emotions of shock, fatigue, feelings of weakness, fragility, vulnerability, grief, helplessness, confusion, self-doubt, shame and embarrassment, resentment, and feelings of betrayal. Parents may find themselves preoccupied with their child, worrying about the uncertainty of the future, asking questions that appear to have no answers
- The second stage has been called 'searching', and often involves a focused search of a more confirmed diagnosis and a 'label' for the condition beyond ID. While at the same time parents are gaining increased knowledge and skills in caring for their child. Parents may also find that

they reconsider their priorities in life and start to ask more realistic questions about their child's abilities, without giving up hope
- With the realization that there are no quick answers or cures, parents enter a stage of 'settling in', during which they recognize the progress their child has made and you become aware of regular progress and realize that some questions they have been asking do not have answers. Parents may also make further adjustments to their own life goals, continue to develop knowledge, skills, and flexibility, and start to know what works for them in supporting and caring for their child
- Finally, as parents move to the next stage they start to give over some control to the child and others, admitting that they cannot make the disability go away, and yet take pride in seeing their child achieve goals. This stage is called 'separating'.

Supporting the process of adaptation

In seeking to support the effective adaption process for families, nurses need to remember:
- No two families will follow exactly the same journey; factors inside and outside each family will influence it
- The model presented is a broad framework and not a rigid structure; parents do not experience all emotions
- Progression through the stages is not linear—it may be two steps forward and one back at times
- Both parents and each family member is an individual, and they will often go through the process at different speeds
- There is a need to recognize where each parent is in the process and provide relevant tailored support; there is no point is assuming 'settling in', if parents are clearly still 'surviving'.

1 Miller NB, Burmester S, Callahan DG, Dieterle J, Niedermeyer S (1994). *Nobody's Perfect*. Paul H Brookes: Baltimore.

Resilience in families

Resilience

Resilience is the ability to adapt successfully to challenges in the face of ongoing adversity. Initially the study of this area focused on the ability of individuals, but since the mid 1990s there has been a growing recognition of the ability of families to adapt successfully, and an acknowledgement of the internal and external factors that may assist in that process.[1]

The changing view of families of people with intellectual disabilities

Until the 1990s, much of the literature about the families of people with ID portrayed the family and its members within a largely pathological frame of reference. Much of the research investigated the 'burden' on families and the negative emotional impact such as 'chronic grief', stress in families, and difficulties for siblings. While some of this type of research continues, it is now somewhat balanced by studies and personal accounts of relatives about the way they have successfully managed to adapt and cope with challenges.

Such a view is often evident in my experience when you ask professionals an open question 'What do you think the impact of having a family member with intellectual disabilities is?' In my experience over the past 15 years almost every time I ask this question of a group of professionals working in ID services, 10 or more negative attributes are called out before any potentially positive aspects are noted. On the rare occasions that a positive aspect is noted within the first 10 comments, a family member of a close relative with ID has been in the group. Nurses and other professionals need to be careful that they recognize the full range of abilities and needs of families of people with ID, and do not become restricted to seeing families as always 'in need'. They need to recognize that although this may be reflective of the families that they as professionals may come in contact with, that many families with whom they do not have regular contact manage well within their family and social support networks.

A revised view of families now recognizes that many families of people with ID manage successfully most of the time and largely require support at times of particular difficulty, for instance in the early stages of adapting, during key transition points to and from school, and when the ability of the family to continue providing care is challenged due to changes within the family. Effective service planning seeks to recognize the potential difficulties for families at these times and to work with them to plan ahead.

It is not the presence of a person with ID in the family that causes difficulties for families, but rather the reaction of family members, friends and members of the local community that may present the largest challenges. The stress of family members can be added to considerably by having contact with professionals, particularly if they feel they have to 'fight for services'.

Supporting families develop and maintain resilience

The emerging view of families highlights their ability to cope successfully given the necessary opportunities. Patterson has developed a model known as the Family Adjustment and Adaptation Response (FAAR) model to explain how services can effectively support families.[2]

Within the first phase of this model, families work through the process of adjustment, during which time demands on the family outweigh their coping resource. The emphasis of intervention is to increase individual, family, and community resources in order to facilitate families to develop, establish, and maintain successful coping behaviours. The focus is on developing strength and resilience within families and their communities, rather than dealing only with crises that may arise for families.

As families increase their range of coping behaviours, the demands on the family are dealt with successfully, and equilibrium between demands and resources is achieved. The aim of intervention is empowerment of family members and professionals involved; this has been defined as the 'increased ability to meet the needs and goals while maintaining autonomy and integrity'.[2] Such a model is consistent with the requirements of working in partnership with families and to facilitate their development.

The last words...

The importance of supporting families developing and maintaining their abilities to respond successfully are captured in the words of a parent, who on reflecting on her experience of what helped in a real way noted that: 'the journey has been made easier for us by friends and professionals who took time to listen to what I was saying, knowing I only wanted the best for Peter, and attempting to find it for me. By friends who allowed me to cry when I needed, and to rejoice when he achieved some particular goal no matter how small. By the school and its teachers who have kept on working with Peter over the years and watch with satisfaction his achievements...'[3]

1 McCubbin H, Thompson E, Thompson A, and Futrell J (eds) (1999). *The dynamics of resilient families*. Sage: Thousand Oaks, California.

2 Patterson J (1995). Promoting resilience in families experiencing stress. *Pediatric Clinics of North America* 42(1), 47–63.

3 Maxwell V, Barr O (2003). With the benefit of hindsight: a mother's reflection on raising a child with Down's Syndrome. *Journal of Learning Disabilities*. 7(1), 51–64.

Families at risk

This term is increasingly applied to families with multiple disadvantages in the UK. Among these families are children and parents with ID who, like others placed in this group, are said to experience multiple disadvantages. According to one government overview, about 2% of families with children experience five or more disadvantages;[1] these include low income, parents with long-standing limiting illnesses or disabilities, poor housing, and unemployment. The children of such families are said to be at great risk of social exclusion and at risk of this being perpetuated into adulthood.

The Social Exclusion Action Plan argued that specific approaches are needed to tackle social exclusion among people facing multiple and complex issues that require specialized interventions and support.[2] Though a minority of this group have ID, like others they may place themselves at risk and in some cases heighten risks to those around them. Services provision is expensive when people bounce between services or drop through safety nets, often not receiving the help they need until a crisis is reached.

What is distinctive about this group of people is that they often face multiple problems that cross several agencies and professional groups, with long-term issues such as childhood abuse, addictions, mental health problems, and homelessness, combined perhaps with relationship breakdowns or loss of social supports. This necessitates a birth-to-adult approach to social exclusion, but also underscores the importance of early intervention programmes aimed at the early months and years of children's lives such as Family Nurse Partnerships supporting vulnerable pregnant women and their babies.

Adults facing chronic exclusion often experience:
- Poor health prospects—mental and/or physical health issues
- A history of exclusion, institutionalization or abuse
- Behaviour and control difficulties
- Skills deficit—unemployment and poor educational achievement
- Addictions.

Adults Facing Chronic Exclusion (ACE) pilots launched in 2007 include one project that focuses on adults with learning disabilities, autism, or mental health problems. It is helping them to access, for example, housing, social and health care, learning, employment, leisure, and financial services, focusing on those who experience chronic exclusion, as well as those with histories of 'bouncing' in and out of services. Among these people are those with autism and Asperger's syndrome, which is often undiagnosed. Their needs may have been neglected for many years, and they may have been considered as ineligible for services or referred to general services covering intellectual disability or mental health. The aims of such new approaches are to provide individualized support, through person-centred plans, mentoring, and advocacy. System change is part of the conceptual base of this approach, and this involves:
- Simplifying the complexities associated with several statutory services working collaboratively (e.g. housing, social care, benefits, health and criminal justice system) to offer coordinated support to someone with multiple needs

- Helping people to negotiate difficult times or transition points in their lives such as leaving prison, leaving the care of local authorities, or fleeing domestic violence
- Offering practical help to people to access several services or manage their own support at one time, through providing a named worker or navigator through services.

Adults with moderate to severe ID are a government priority as outlined in the Public Sector Agreements for England.[3] Specific commitments have been made to increase the proportion of adults with intellectual disabilities in settled accommodation and the proportion of adults with intellectual disabilities in employment. Much of this confirms the *Valuing People* White Paper: the government wants access to paid work for adults with intellectual disabilities to be a greater priority for local areas, as well as recognition that people with intellectual disabilities can live in all types of housing.

As long-stay hospitals and large residential care homes close, it is important that mainstream housing, with appropriate support, is available for people with ID. Adaptations for disabilities will be necessary, and widening opportunities will be important. Many adult education and training initiatives for people with ID do not lead to employment and this can be frustrating. More initiatives around moving on and transition into employment are likely to be provided.

Nurses working with families and individuals who are at risk of social inclusion should:

- Familiarize themselves with current policy—often outside traditional health knowledge and practice zones
- Contribute to the monitoring of targets to ensure that people with ID are not excluded or neglected because they have a lower profile than many other excluded groups
- Work with other agencies to improve processes of collaboration but with a strong and well-developed sense that it is the outcome of this collaboration that is important and not just the process
- Be aware of the multiple meanings of risk.

1 Social Exclusion Task Force (2007).
http://www.cabinetoffice.gov.uk/social_exclusion_task_force/ [accessed April 2009]

2 Cabinet Office (2006). *Social Exclusion Action Plan.* HMSO: London.

3 HM Government (2000). *PSA Delivery Agreement 16: Increase the proportion of socially excluded adults in settled accommodation and employment, education or training.* HM Government: London.

Carers' assessment

Rights to a carers' assessment were established in England and Wales in 1995. Three pieces of legislation underpin carers' rights to be assessed.

- Carers (Recognition and Services) Act 1995
- Carers and Disabled Children Act 2000
- Carers (Equal Opportunities) Act 2004

The Acts cover carers of all ages and parents of disabled children.

Under the Carers Act 1995 and enhanced by the Carers and Disabled Children Act 2000, carers have rights to an assessment by the local authority if they provide substantial and regular care. None of the Acts define what is meant by this term so there is a certain amount of discretion in the way in which this term is interpreted. This assessment should cover the carer's perceptions of the situation, the carer's relationship with the person they support, the caring tasks, the carer's willingness and ability to continue to provide care, their other commitments, and their coping strategies. If appropriate this will lead to a care plan that is monitored and reviewed, with agreed and identified outcomes. Local Authorities can delegate their powers of carers' assessment to health service staff (in Northern Ireland these may be undertaken by health service staff as joint Health and Social services structures exist). The passage of the Carers (Equal Opportunities) Act 2004 placed new duties on local authorities to inform carers of their rights to an assessment, to consider carer's other preferences for employment and leisure, and to involve other sectors in providing support for carers.

In Scotland, carers also have a right to request an independent assessment under the Community Care and Health Act 2002. Local NHS Boards in Scotland have a duty to produce a Carer Information Strategy that will cover a wide range of relevant material.

Nurses working with carers throughout the UK should ensure that they:

- provide information leaflets about carers' assessment and are familiar with the process
- are confident in explaining the purpose of carers' assessments
- are encouraging of carers' rights to an assessment (even if the person they are supporting refuses to be assessed)
- are sensitive to the needs and wishes of a carer to being assessed separately and in private, away from the person they are supporting
- understand local definitions of *regular* and *substantial*, and can challenge misinformation
- are able to discuss with carers desired outcomes
- record the existence of a carers' assessment in their documentation and use it to influence their work
- are sensitive to the possible anxieties surrounding the term 'assessment' as making judgements upon someone
- are mindful of carer's possible worries about involvement with social services (e.g. for fear of stigma)
- encourage carers to make sure that they receive written copies of their assessments and care plans, possibly asking for permission to have a copy for health service records if this does not appear to have been shared

- recommend carers ask for a review if needs/circumstances alter
- offer assistance or explanation, if required, with elements of the assessment that involve self-completion by the carer
- are aware of the circumstances in which carers may be at risk of additional stress, for example at times of illness, when the person for whom they care is first diagnosed, if his or her condition deteriorates suddenly, or he or she becomes terminally ill
- are aware of the nature and extent of the support systems that the carer has and their care plans reflect these.

At system level, processes for starting a carer's assessment should be incorporated into strategic documents such as local Carers' Strategies. Joint information may be a useful product of collaboration between agencies. Joint (multi-agency and multidisciplinary) training around carers' assessment may foster closer collaboration. Carers with experience of assessment may be important contributors to training, information provision and auditing.

Research on carers' assessments has found that many social workers feel that carers' assessments will raise expectations that cannot be met and lead to disappointment.[1,2] This might explain the limited number of carers' assessments. Carers themselves may limit the amount of help for which they ask because they recognize that resources are often limited.[3,4] Nonetheless such assessments are important ways of focusing attention on carers and may allow carers greater control than traditional social care services, for example, by suggesting that direct payments may be suitable for their needs. Nurses therefore have a key role in working with carers to promote their rights in acknowledging their expertise, and in using aggregated information to inform local commissioning of services.

Further reading

Carers UK ▣ http://www.carersuk.org/Home

Princess Royal Trust for Carers - Learning Disabilities Links
▣ http://www.carers.org/articles/learning-disabilities-links,73,CA.html

Directgov - Information for Carers
▣ http://www.direct.gov.uk/en/CaringForSomeone/DG_071391

CarersScotland - Research
▣ http://www.carerscotland.org/Policyandpractice/Research

1 Seddon D, Robinson C (2001). Carers of older peoples dementia: assessment and the Carers Act. *Health and Social Care in the Community,* **9**(3), 151–8.

2 Nicholas E (2003). An outcomes focus on carers assessments and review: value and challenge, *British Journal of Social Work* **33**, 31–47.

3 Arkse H (2002). Rationed care: assessing the support needs of informal carers in English social services authorities. *Journal of Social Policy*, **31**(1), 81–101.

4 Robinson C, Williams V (2002). Carers and people with learning disabilities and their experiences of the 1995 Carers Act. *British Journal of Social Work* **32**,169–83.

Principles of working collaboratively with families

Key phrases and considerations:
- Partnership as an outcome
- Partnership as a means of achieving goals
- Collaboration
- Decision making processes
- Seamless webs of care

What defines a family?

The family is a basic unit of society that represents racial, ethnic, cultural, and socioeconomic diversity. It is also important to reinforce that people grow both individually and as part of a family.[1] Therefore families will use a whole raft of coping strategies, and expect (or not) partnership/collaboration at different levels. Collaboration = team work; partnership; group effort; alliance; relationship; cooperation.

Working in partnership

Valuing People[2] define partnership as 'people and organizations working together' but hinge most of their discussion around Partnership Boards, and while these have brought about some real empowerment in the lives of individuals who have an ID the principles of working collaboratively with families needs exploring further.

Such partnerships need to recognize that parents and other family members can often be important informal and formal educators of professionals in their training and in practice.[3] Professionals need to learn to listen to the views of parents and learn from their experience, avoiding the belief that they have the all the answers as professionals.

The essential principles of collaborative working have their roots and origins firmly linked to the principles of beneficence and non-maleficence (i.e. the duty to produce good and avoid harm) of Ashworth, in identifying the aims of nursing identifies 5 principles that bring about effective partnerships in 'patient' care.[4] The essence of these principles is integrated into the following discussion on the principles of working collaboratively with families.

- Relationship building—a positive goal or outcome will only be achieved if the professional establishes a firm base for the relationship. This could involve setting a timeframe; being clear about what it is possible to achieve; by not making unrealistic promises; being willing and proactive to try non-traditional ways of working; listening, accepting and responding to the other party's points of view; valuing the other members of the partnership as equals, who have worth and a valid opinion
- Needs based services/approaches—demonstration of a willingness to listen to the needs of the individual and their family. Responding appropriately to expressed needs by family carers, while making accessible the focus of the professional's intervention (for example it is important to remember that assessment or evaluation data is not about secrets!)

- Care decisions have to be based in the real world, not just in services. Families need to be clear about the role a professional will take in the seamless web of care provided to a relative. Individuals need a benchmark by which they can assess the success of the partnership
- Independence—the ultimate aim of any professional intervention should be to promote an individual level of independence with the person in receipt of care. To do this collaboratively families and people with ID should be given the opportunity to develop their own sustainable solutions through appropriate packages of education
- Conflict resolution.

Use Table 2.1 to explore issues that you have come across that are barriers to collaborative working in your practice experience.

Table 2.1 Conflict resolution

Issue	Sticking point	Partnership resolution
	Interests—the difference between what you want and I want	
	Understanding—the difference between what I understand and what you understand	
	Values—the difference between what is important to me and what is important to you	
	Style—the difference between the way I do things and the way you do things	
	Opinion—the difference between what I think and what you think	

Further reading

Bigby C (2007). *Planning and Support for Individuals with Intellectual Disabilities*. Jessica Kingsley Publishers: London.

Lacey P, Ouvry C (2006). *People with Profound and Multiple Learning Disabilities: A Collaborative Approach to Meeting Complex Needs*. David Fulton Publishers Ltd: Oxford.

References

1 Pillitteri A (1999). *Child Health Nursing*. Lippincott: London.

2 Department of Health (2001). *Valuing People: a New Strategy for Learning Disability in the 21st Century*. Cmnd 5086. HMSO: London.

3 Maxwell V, Barr O (2003). With the benefit of hindsight: a mother's reflection on raising a child with Down Syndrome. *Journal of Learning Disabilities*. **7**(1), 51–64.

4 Ashworth P (1980). *Care to Communicate*. RCN: London.

Supporting siblings of people with intellectual disabilities

Is there a need for specialist sib groups?

Over the past 10yrs there has been a growing awareness that there is a need to effectively support the siblings of individuals who have ID. The growing interest in the stories of people who have a 'looked after' life[1] has heightened a recognition of the needs of these brothers and sisters. Unfortunately there is not yet a great body of knowledge to inform and underpin the professional support we offer, although more regions are seeing the development of 'sibs clubs'. The question that needs debating is whether these actually serve a positive purpose or reinforce a feeling of being different and isolated in a crowd.

Wilson[2] tells the story of Lily and her sister Daisy, with a profound ID, and while the story is written for children as informative entertainment there are lessons we as professionals need to learn from the text in relation to the way we support siblings.

The experience of being a sibling of a person with ID can be mixed, and no two siblings should be viewed as the same. While the experience of siblings can be difficult at times, depending on how the wider family reacts to and manages the presence of a person with ID, there can be positive impacts also. Professionals should remember this when seeking to provide holistic support to siblings. Siblings may have a range of feelings.

Isolation—there is often a belief that the brother or sister is the only one in this situation; no-one else has ever had a sibling who has such an impact on the way a family lives their lives.

Fear—will the other kids at school think it's catching? What if they want to come to my house? If they come what'll I do if my sibling acts out? A 'major concern from the teen's perspective is to be accepted by peers; above all, they don't want to be 'different".[3]

Burden—anecdotal evidence from a professional experience demonstrates that there is often an unspoken belief that the non-disabled sibling will assume some responsibility for the sibling with an ID, whether that be in providing a home, financial responsibility, or emotional/social responsibility. Parents often reinforce to the non-disabled sibling their 'duty' to always care for the brother or sister.

Guilt—the concept of 'why wasn't it me?' needs considering in the psychological welfare of the sibling, in particular of the sibling whose brother or sister has acquired their ID after birth. Coupled with the isolation experienced by parents[4] and the guilt of leaving home and starting a life independent of the family of origin.

Loss of childhood—the need always to be the sensible sibling, the one who 'minds' the less able member of the family group. The one who misses out on family days out because one parent has to stay at home with the sibling who reacts badly in crowds or to loud noises.

Resentment—why are they described as special and I am not? It is important to acknowledge that siblings who require support and consideration with the person-centred process are not always children.

Confidence—some siblings develop a clear understanding of their brother's or sister's abilities and needs, and become confident in interacting with them and professionals.

Caring skills—over the years of growing up siblings are often involved in providing day-to-day support, and at times physical and emotional care, to their younger siblings. This can increasingly become the situation for adult siblings.

Increased communication skills—siblings can become very adept at understanding their brother's or sister's non-verbal communication. These skills are often transferable to working with other people, in particular the confidence and ability to communicate with someone who cannot communicate verbally.

Understanding of difference—siblings have often witnessed the range of difficulties in acceptance that their brother or sister had, and how they were treated differently by others. These insights often encourage a recognition of the impact of treating people differently due to a disability and encourage a greater acceptance of the diversity in people.

Remember, just because one sibling has an ID does not mean that the other will like them any more than if they did not; by the same token some siblings remain close and attached for all their lives. The key feature in offering support to siblings has to be that the support is what the individual says they need, not what we believe they want/need, and individuals grow both within and independently of their family of origin. Support should not make the sibling feel different or reinforce negative feelings, it should be personalized and tailor made. How may this be achieved: can you suggest 3 or 4 key points?

So how to support brothers and sisters to have close and proactive relationships? Kate Strohm's work in exploring 'being the other one' highlights the need for all brothers and sisters to be treated as 'special', and while they are unique individuals they are not 'different' in their place in the family.[5]

Further reading

Fender S, Schieffler R (2007). *Brotherly Feelings. Me, My Emotions, and My Brother with Asperger's Syndrome.* Jessica Kingsley Publishing: London.

1 Mitchell D (1998). Learning disability nursing: reflections on history. *Journal of Learning Disabilities* **2**(1), 45–49.

2 Wilson J (2002). *Sleepovers*, Corgi: London.

3 Davis SE, Anderson C, Linkowski D, Berger K, Feinstein C (1991). In: Dell Orto AE and Marinelli R. *The Psychological and Social Impact of Disability.* Springer Publishing: USA.

4 Mencap (2001). *Ordinary Life.* Mencap: London.

5 Strohm K (2005). *Being the Other One: Growing up With a Brother or Sister Who Has Special Needs.* Shambhala Publication: Boston.

People with intellectual disabilities as parents

The ethical dilemma

The idea of adults with an intellectual disability becoming parents often causes us moral and professional difficulties—particularly in our thought process.

- Firstly the historical notion of the individual who has an ID is seen to have a looked after life—for example the Wolfensberger[1] concept of deviancy reinforces the eternal child notion, and therefore the need for that individual to be 'looked after'; in today's climate most modern social policy reinforces the 'label' of vulnerable adult, which most people who have an ID fall into, and therefore have some level of service intervention in the day-to-day running of their lives.
- Secondly we are not always comfortable with the idea of people with an ID having a sexual identity, let alone engaging in consensual sexual activity.
- Thirdly the concept of pregnancy does not feature prominently in health action plans or healthy living programmes; much of the limited literature concentrates on safe sex and therefore avoiding pregnancy.
- Fourthly who is going to be left holding the baby? Not many adults who have an ID get the opportunity to demonstrate that they are *poor parents* let alone the opportunity to learn and demonstrate *good* parenting skills.

The most prolific and supportive writers on adults with ID as parents in Europe are arguably Wendy and Tim Booth; in support of the right to fulfil the role of parents they write "Almost nothing is known about the long-term outcomes for children brought up by parents who have learning difficulties".[2]

Therefore, if little is known about the long-term outcomes of these children surely the starting point should be how to support adults with ID to become 'good enough' parents? After all, there is no model of good parents that is inherent in all theory on family life, this is often the unspoken benchmark of professionals rather than a reality based actual of 'good enough parenting' for each given situation.

"Every child has the right to expect that the professional intervening in their lives will do so on the basis of the best knowledge available. But most interventions in social care are not evaluated before they are introduced. In that sense much of the work done with children is an uncontrolled experiment".[3]

Barnardos describes that the "primary task of health and social care services is to provide parents with learning disabilities with the support they need to care adequately for their children. As with all childcare practice, the welfare of the child remains paramount and must precede any consideration of parental rights. Parent's rights and children's welfare are best supported through a combination of positive attitude and evidence-based practice".[4]

So how is this supported by practice-based evidence?

In discussing the notion of who can and who can't parent Booth & Booth[5] set the scene that for most parents with ID, family life is constantly under threat, yet adequate support services geared to their needs are almost non-existent.

"Parents with learning disabilities often need to overcome preconceived ideas among other people about their ability to parent. For example, there may be a willingness to attribute potential difficulties they may have to parenting to their impairment than to disabling barriers or to other factors that affect the parenting of all parents. This has been described as 'the presumption of incompetence'.[6]

So, how to support (i.e. avoiding system abuse—help that harms)?
- Good, clear, and accessible information for the professionals offering the support—a geographical audit on local support services; holistic assessment of the coping strategies on the individuals; networking across non-traditional boundaries and therefore a willingness to find sustainable solutions grounded in the real world, not just in services
- A commitment from services to discuss conflict and difficulties openly and proactively. Remember that meetings are designed to discuss the way forward not the difficulties a service is having at a macro operational level
- Avoiding crisis-driven services/responses
- Trust—especially between the parents and the multidisciplinary team, and between different agency professional staff
- A recognition of the right to family life that acknowledges parents, children, and grandparents
- Holistic family health being incorporated into healthy living programmes, to include relationship building and preconception care
- A willingness by professionals to acknowledge a trap of 'diagnostic overshadowing' (i.e. blaming everything on the ID)
- Remembering that there is choice involved in becoming a parent, and that choice belongs to that adult, not the 'system'.

1 Wolfensberger W (1991). *A Brief Introduction to Social Role Valorization as a High-order Concept for Structuring Human Services.* Syracuse University Training Inst: USA.

2 Joseph Rowntree Foundation (July 1998). Ref 7108 Advocacy for Parents with Learning Difficulties. ▣ http://www.jrf.org.uk/knowledge/findings/socialcare/scr7108.asp [accessed April 2009]

3 McGraw S (2000). *What Works for Parents with Learning Disabilities.* Barnardo's: Ilford. Summary available at ▣ http://www.barnardos.org.uk/wwparwld.pdf [accessed April 2009]

4 Barnardo's (2000). What Works for Parents with Learning Disabilities—Summary. ▣ http://www.barnardos.org.uk/resources [accessed April 2009]

5 Booth W, Booth T (1994). *Parenting Under Pressure: Mothers and Fathers with Learning Difficulties.* UK Open University Press.

6 SCIE Research briefing (February 2005). *14: Helping Parents with Learning Disabilities in Their Role as Parents.* ▣ http://www.scie.org.uk/publications/briefings/briefing14/index.asp [accessed April 2009]

Family quality of life

It has long been accepted that families experience a higher quality of life both individually and collectively when their needs are met.[1] Recognition of those collective and individual needs being met could include families that enjoy spending time together, alongside being supported to be independent and do things that are important to them. Factors that influence family quality of life are community participation, friendships, family interaction, parenting, emotional well being, alongside access to support mechanisms that promote health, and opportunities for financial well being. This is no different for the family who has a member with ID.

"I was attending Down's syndrome support group meetings and making presentations at local hospitals with mothers of children with Down's syndrome. I also conducted my first research study *Parental responses to the birth of a child with Down's syndrome*. The families I was interviewing now did not sound like other families I had read about. Rather than using words like 'burden', 'tragedy', and 'suffering' to describe their child and the experience of raising a child with Down's syndrome, these parents used words like 'joy', 'challenge', and 'thriving'."[2]

Pillitteri described the key factors of family centred practice:[3]
• The family is the basic unit of society.
• Families represent racial, ethnic, cultural, and socioeconomic diversity.
• Children grow both individually and as part of a family.

So how can family quality of life be measured?

"Parenthood is a major transition",[4] and therefore the way a family forms and views itself relates to that transition. It is important to acknowledge that transitions occur both on and off time; and in relation to the family who has a member with a diagnosed extra special need this is no different (see 📖 The process of family adaptation, p.32). It is very easy for families and professionals to latch on to a notion that everything that happens in a family is related to the ID that one member lives with. However, it is important to acknowledge that systems and services often create 'disabled families' rather than acknowledging that one member of the family has a disability.

It is widely acknowledged (particularly in illness related literature) that the measurement of family quality of life cannot relate solely to the perceived 'burden' of a disability or illness, and that issues of independence, resilience (see 📖 Resilience in families, p.34), and hope have to be taken into consideration.[5] There is no one definitive checklist that the professional can take into an assessment and measure the quality of life a family is experiencing; what is intolerable for one family is an everyday occurrence for another, and when exploring family quality of life the key factor to remember is that families and the individuals who live in them are not part of a homogenous group.

Family quality of life has the same key domains as individual quality of life, which are:
• Physical well-being
• Emotional well-being
• Interpersonal relationships
• Social inclusion

- Personal development
- Material well-being
- Self determination
- Human and legal rights (Schalock 2000).

In seeking to gain an understanding of a family's quality of life it is necessary to consider the degree to which the above domains result in families being able to have meaningful life experiences that they value, and the degree to which life domains contribute to a full and interconnected life.

It is important for professionals to recognize and acknowledge that the way an individual with an ID lives their life within a family is ordinary for them, and our response is not to be judgemental and subjective; we are often the ones that describe that way of living as out of the ordinary, even when families consider they are coping well.

Further reading

Cass H (2006). *The NHS Experience. The Snakes and Ladders Guide for Patients and Professionals.* Routledge: London.

Orr R (2003). *My Right to Play: A Child With Complex Needs.* Oxford University Press: Oxford.

Swain J, French S (2008). *Disability on Equal Terms.* Sage: London.

Turnbull A, Brown I, Rutherford Turnbull H (2004). *Families and Person With Mental Retardation and Quality of Life: International Perspectives.* AAMR: Washington.

1 Schalock RL (2000). *Outcome Based Evaluation* 2nd edn. Kluwer Academic: Norwell, USA

2 Van-Riper M (2004). *What Families Need to Thrive.* ▣ http://www.downsyn.com/thrive.html [accessed March 2009]

3 Pillitteri A (1999). *Child Health Nursing: Care of the Child and Family.* Lippincott Williams & Wilkins: USA.

4 Busfield J (1987). Parenting and parenthood. In: Cohen G, ed. *Policy is Personal: Sex, Gender and Informal Care.* Tavistock: London.

5 Muldoon MF, Barger SD, Flory JD, Marwick SB (1998). What are quality of life measurements measuring? *BMJ* **316**: 542–545.

Respite services for people who have an intellectual disability

This discussion works on the premise that respite is a 'gift of time';[1] it should be planned and have purpose for both the individual in receipt of care and the people left at home, which in turn supports the philosophy that planned care is a right for those who live a looked-after life.

A widely used definition of respite care is provided by Treneman et al. and is commonly used in intellectual disability literature:[2]

"The shared care of a person with learning disabilities and/or physical disabilities, either at home or in a short-term residential setting, in order to give the family a break from the routine care-taking."

For modern 21st century services to people who have an ID, the more traditional idea of what respite is can be considered largely out of date. Oswin described a service of respite for children in long-stay hospitals as something akin to a barren isolated world of existence.[3]

Adults and children who have an ID today receive a far more creative and proactive gift of time.

- Respite in the community for a set period of hours to undertake a specific activity usually related to leisure
- Respite in the home of another—who is an approved carer and registered under a scheme such as 'adults supporting adults'. See 🖳 www.asaorg.co.uk for more information.
- Respite in an approved service for example hospice (for children with a life-limiting diagnosis).

However, the recognition of respite provided by family carers such as grandparents has been acknowledged through the use of individual direct care payments and should no longer remain hidden.

There is often a misconception that all care away from the home of origin for a fixed period of time has to be considered as respite, and with this in mind practitioners need to remain cognisant that assessment and treatment services are not respite facilities (even though this may be an unintended benefit for the person in receipt of such a service).

The Mencap *Breaking Point* campaign illustrated effectively both the need for a 'break from caring' but also the need for respite to have purpose for the individual who receives it.[4] Respite is part of a professional seamless web of care and not just a 'holiday'.

So why is respite offered as, and often considered, the panacea of all 'ills'? It may be useful for the reader to consider respite services that they have knowledge of under the following points:

- What is the purpose of the respite?
- Is the service offered the most appropriate?
- What could be an alternative?
- What has influenced your thoughts?
- Does anyone benefit from this service?
- What is the way forward?

It is also necessary to consider some key differences between the services offered to children and adults. Often respite for children unless they have complex health needs or behaviour, and/or a life-limiting diagnosis, is delivered within generic 'share-the care' schemes (National Children's Home). Children and families become used to relating to one type of service/provider and then the reality of the caring experience at the point of transition to adult orientated services is often very different; perhaps in the advent of such advances in medical technology one of the questions that should have prominence in service planners minds is 'where do we care for the young adult who has outlived their life-limiting diagnosis'? (🖥 http://www.act.org.uk/content/view/59/1/)

There is presently limited robust research and literature that shows respite care is more than a rest period for parents and siblings, or the perspective of the person with ID receiving it. Respite care provided is often for the benefit of the primary carers rather than the individual who is in receipt of the care. Although a break in caring for parents or other family carers is for many carers a major help, further research is required to demonstrate how to maximize the benefit of respite care for the person with ID and their families. Respite needs to be proactive, planned, and have purpose if it truly is to be a 'gift of time'.

Further reading

Cotteril L, Hayes L, Flynn M et al. (1997). Reviewing respite services: some lessons from the literature. *Disability & Society* **12**, 5, 775–788.

Department of Health (2001). *Family Matters: Counting Families In.* Department of Health: London.

Wilkie B, Barr O (2008). *The experiences of parents of children with an intellectual disability who use respite services. Learning Disability Practice* **11**, 5, 30–36.

1 Laverty H, Reet M (2001). *Planning Care in Respite Settings: Hello! This is Me!* Jessica Kingsley: London.

2 Treneman M, Corkery A, Dowdney L et al. (1997). *Respite-care needs—met and unmet: assessment of needs for children with a disability. Developmental Medicine and Child Neurology* **39**, 8, 548–553.

3 Oswin M (1991). *They Keep Going Away: Critical Study of Short-term Residential Care Services for Children with Learning Difficulties.* King Edwards Hospital Fund for London.

4 Mencap (2006). *Breaking Point. A Report on Caring Without a Break for Children and Adults with Severe or Profound Learning Disabilities.* Mencap: London.

Older carers

Older carers, generally but not always parents, are a focus of policy concern for many reasons.

- There is growing awareness that older carers have been neglected or taken for granted and that this should be remedied, both for their own benefit and for the well-being of the person they are supporting
- There is recognition of the cumulative disadvantages that have affected people who have been carers for many years, often with little support. These may be termed 'hidden' or 'invisible' carers
- There is concern at the prospect of replacing the support provided by large numbers of carers by formal or state services and the costs that this will imply
- There is recognition that older carers are very diverse and while 'older' there may be wide variations between them and their experiences and aspirations.

Policy support for older carers was crystallized in the target set by the White Paper *Valuing People*[1] that local authorities should establish a register of older carers to enable them to profile local needs and to commission services that could work in partnership with older carers, rather than being brought in at crisis points, for example, on the death of a parent. Government strategies[2] set out policy goals and commitments.[3]

Older carers may also face problems associated with the premature ageing of the person they are supporting, for example, the increased risk of people with Down syndrome of developing dementia at an earlier age than the general population—as much as 30–40yrs earlier.[4] People with severe disabilities are more likely to have health complications that lead to shorter lives. This means that older carers may face bereavement, and specific support should be offered at such times.

Practice

Older carers are a good source of information about the person and their family, and this information should be used as a current resource but also carefully kept for the future, for example, by compiling a life story book. Their expertise may usefully inform training, services development, service monitoring, and peer support.

Bereavement services and/or counselling may be helpful for older carers, and nurses may enable access to these services from primary care or other routes that may be non-stigmatizing and free of charge.

Older carers many find 'cash for care' or self directed support (Direct Payments and Personal Budgets) enable them to set up tailored and flexible support, with different levels of assistance with their management, reflecting their wishes and capacity. Local councils should be able to provide information on this, or carers' groups and carers' centres should have such details.

Older carers may be unknown or unrecognized to services and may need time, patience and sensitivity in order to undo earlier bad experiences, and to inspire confidence in outside support.

Older carers may have complex needs but they may benefit from relatively simple responses. Listening to what they want is invaluable, and working with them to plan for possible crises, such as their own possible ill health, may be valuable in setting up a safety net of support.

Assessment of older carers should be undertaken in partnership, with recognition of the expertise of the carer. There should be an agreed timescale for review and agreements about what to do if matters change suddenly.[5]

Local carers' networks are good sources of advice and support for older carers, and details of how to contact them should be widely available in community and specialist settings.

Further reading

Carers Northern Ireland (2007). *Involving and Consulting Carers: A Guide to Giving Carers an Effective Voice.* ▣ www.carersuk.org/Policyandpractice/Involvingcarers/

Contact a Family ▣ www.cafamily.org.uk (support groups)

Mencap ▣ www.mencap.org.uk (national support organizations with local branches)

Carers UK ▣ www.carersuk.org (national support organization)

Foundation for People with Learning Disabilities ▣ www.learningdisabilities.org.uk

Carers Scotland ▣ www.carerscotland.org

Carers Northern Ireland ▣ www.carersni.org

Carers Wales ▣ www.carerswales.org

1 Department of Health (2001). *Valuing People.* Department of Health: London (see also accompanying documents on families).

2 Department of Health (2008). *Caring at the Heart of 21st Century Families and Communities: A Caring System on Your Side, A Life of Your Own.* Department of Health: London.

3 Morgan H, Magill D (2005.) *Older Carers Briefing Sheet.* Foundation for People with Learning Disabilities: London.

4 Holland AJ (2000). Ageing and learning disability. *British Journal of Psychiatry* **176**, 26–31.

5 Barr O (2007). Working effectively with families of people with learning disabilities In: Gates B (Ed). *Learning Disabilities: Towards Inclusion.* Churchill Livingstone: London, 567–598.

Cultural, religious, and spiritual impact

Increasingly, healthcare professionals need to be responsive and sensitive to the cultural needs of people with ID from minority ethnic backgrounds. The preferred approach to cultural care is ethnicity, cultural diversity, and nursing practice. This may include spiritual care according to the needs of clients. Spiritual care is distinct from religious needs, but religious care may be part of cultural and spiritual needs. It is important to make no assumptions about people's ethnicity, culture, spirituality, and religion. It is always best to be guided by clients, their next of kin, or their representatives about their individual preferences with regard to above dimensions of care. In the absence of personal preferences for reasons of incapacity to express wish, cultural and religious factfiles are consulted, but these should be used judiciously as many cultural and religious preference may be fixed or permanent.

Ethnicity

Ethnicity is the preferred term to explain race and culture. It is a fluid term that is used by individuals to assert their identity at any point in life. The use of the term 'ethnicity' in nursing and healthcare encourages individuals to exercise their choice to locate themselves in whatever categories they wish to be identified with. Such an approach treats clients as individuals, and invites them to determine their cultural and spiritual preferences. It avoids the essentialist assumption that cultural identities of individuals are fixed and frozen in time. It is important to appreciate and acknowledge that individuals negotiate and move between ethnic, cultural, and spiritual identities and affiliations as part of their life course transitions. Various trajectories in life affect an individual's experience of identity, ethnicity, culture, and spirituality.

Cultural diversity

The literature acknowledges that the UK is regarded as one of the most ethnically diverse countries in Europe. Globalization, communication and internet revolutions, transnational corporations, global migration, asylum seeking, diasporas, international studentships, sports, and European Union ascension and integration have all contributed to the diversity in the UK. It is within this ethnically diverse society that healthcare providers must deliver a service that is culturally sensitive and appropriate to meet specific needs.[1]

Spirituality

Spirituality contains a multiplicity of meanings to an extent that the ambiguity of the concept allows for deep misunderstandings as well as misuse. Spirituality refers to the essence of our being and it gives us meaning and purpose in our lives.[1] Our spirituality gives us a sense of personhood and individuality. It is the guiding force behind our uniqueness and acts as an inner source of power and energy, which makes us 'tick over' as a person. It provides us with a sense of wholeness, stability, wellness, security, hope, and peace. Spirituality can be an important source of wisdom, inspiration, meaning, and purpose. It comes into focus at critical junctures in our lives when we face emotional stress, physical illness or death.[2]

Religion

Religions are often described as to do with a supernatural or divine force, a system of beliefs, a comprehensive code of ethics or philosophy, or a prescribed set of practices to be followed. Religions are also associated with institutional and symbolic things such as places of worship, religious artefacts and so on. Spirituality is much broader than religion. Some people may use religion as a medium to express their spirituality.

Cultural care framework for practice

The **ACCESS** Model derived from Narayanasamy[1] could be used as a framework for delivering culturally sensitive care.

Assessment—focus on cultural aspects of clients' lifestyle, health beliefs, and health practices to create a life story file.

Communication—focus on cultural variations with respect to verbal and non-verbal aspects of client's communication.

Cultural negotiation and compromise—pay special attention to other people's culture.

Establishing respect and rapport—a therapeutic relation that portrays genuine respect for clients' cultural beliefs and values is required.

Sensitivity—deliver diverse culturally sensitive care to culturally diverse groups.

Safety—enable clients to derive a sense of cultural safety. Its strategy is to avert actions that diminish, demean or disempower the cultural identity and well-being of an individual.

Further reading

Narayanasamy A (2001). *Spiritual Care: A Practical Guide for Nurses and Health Care Practitioners*. Quay: London.

1 Narayanasamy A (2006). *Spiritual Care and Transcultural Care Research*. Quay: London.

2 Narayanasamy A (2004). The puzzle of spirituality for nursing: a guide to practice assessment. *British Journal of Nursing* **13**(19), 1140–1144.

Communication

Promoting effective communication

Overview

Human communication can be extremely complex; it is an essential part of our experience of forming and building relationships, making choices, and expressing emotions (including discomfort or pain) and opinions. This consequently affects the control we have over our own life and impacts on mental health. Communication is dynamic, whereby we adapt what we are saying and how we are saying it in response to what another person is saying and how. This negotiation goes on throughout the interaction and when successful, can lead to multifaceted meaning that is understood by both parties. The history of communications between people (what each one knows about the other and about communicating with the other), as well as what is currently happening around us, how we are feeling at that moment, and our reasons for communicating, will all impact on how effective our communication will be.

Communication disabilities

People with ID are highly likely to experience difficulties in communication:[1]

- 50–90% of people with ID have communication difficulties due to the nature of ID and/or associated sensory or physical disabilities
- ~80% of people with severe ID do not acquire effective speech
- ~20% of people with ID have no verbal communication skills but do demonstrate intentional communication. Another 20% have no intentional communication skills (i.e. they are unable to deliberately signal their thoughts to another person) but it is still possible to recognize positive and negative emotions from their behaviour. It must be remembered that all humans communicate, whether or not it is intentional (or conscious).

Communication strengths and needs

Most of us think of speech as fundamental to human communication but many people with ID can learn to communicate well without necessarily relying on speech. They can use objects, photos, pictures, symbols, and signing, as well as or instead of speech. However, they often rely on others to pick up and interpret these signals. They may also need help with using these methods, not least in having reasons and opportunities to communicate provided for them. Their communication partners will also need to amend their way of talking and use augmentative methods in order to promote understanding.

Interaction styles used by communication partners

Those paid to support people who have ID do not always communicate effectively. For instance, we may:

- overestimate the ability of people with ID to understand what we are saying to them (i.e. we pitch our language too high)
- fail to adjust to the comprehension of the person level even where known
- not recognize the person's non-verbal signals
- underestimate the amount and complexity of our own speech

- overly rely on using speech, even when communicating with predominantly non-verbal individuals
- underestimate the level of hearing impairment (40%).

A recent study on communication strategies used by staff nurses in residential care[2] concludes that nurses do not always adopt optimal strategies when communicating with people with ID. Furthermore, hospital staff not recognizing or supporting patients' communication has been highlighted as a major factor in systematic failure in service provision for people with ID by the NHS.[3] Ongoing education in communication is therefore necessary across a range of health and social care services.

Person-centred service provision

Service philosophies in the UK and elsewhere are now expected to promote independence, choice, rights, and inclusion. However, when communication is difficult there are likely to be problems in acting independently, making choices, exercising your rights, and feeling you belong. Effective communication is fundamental to the delivery of person-centred services. To include people with ID in making the important decisions about their lives as well as day-to-day decisions will involve taking care to communicate in ways that make sense to any one individual, as well as recognizing and listening to the different ways people with ID communicate to us. What we can do to support communication should be considered for each person we interact with.

Strategies to promote effective communication

The approach generally taken within ID services to promote effective communication is known as 'inclusive (or total) communication'. This is providing a supportive environment where any and every available means of communication is used to understand and to be understood. This may involve simplifying our language, slowing down, using easier words, and *showing* people what we mean (using pictures, photos, objects, actions) in order to maximize communication potential and therefore participation in everyday life experiences. More about strategies to promote effective communication are given in the following sections.

1 Foundation for People with Learning Disabilities (2000). *Everyday Lives, Everyday Choices: For People with Learning Disabilities and High Support Needs.* Edited by A Wertheimer. The Mental Health Foundation: London.

2 Healy D, Walsh PN (2007). Communication among nurses and adults with severe and profound intellectual disabilities. *Journal of Intellectual Disabilities*, **11**(2), 127–141.

3 Mencap (2007). *Death by Indifference: Following up on the Treat Me Right Report.* Available on: http://www.mencap.org.uk [accessed March 2009]

Verbal communication

What is verbal communication?

The term 'verbal communication' is used here to mean the use of language to send and receive messages. This can involve words written down or spoken. Speech, language, and communication are essentially interlinked yet each can occur in isolation, so that it is possible to have:

• language without speech (sign language or written words)
• speech without language (when words are used without meaning e.g. some people with ID and autistic spectrum disorder may apply rote learned or copied words in certain situations without necessarily understanding them)
• communication without speech or language (i.e. non-verbal communication—see ☐ Adaptive behaviour rating scales, p.82).

What is language?

There are over 3000 languages and major dialects currently spoken around the world. Humans typically start life with an inherent ability to learn any language, and the one(s) they acquire will depend on the culture they are born into. Language consists of socially shared rules that specify:

• the meanings of established words
• how to create new words
• how to string words together to form an infinite variety of sentences.

Most of us are capable of creating language to express anything and everything we may wish to say in any situation. Within the language of the person's culture, difficulties in understanding others (receptive language), or in sharing needs, wants, ideas and emotions (expressive language), is known as a language disorder. This may be developmental or acquired through brain injury.

What is speech?

Speech is the means by which most of us use language to communicate on a daily basis. It consists primarily of:

Articulation—how different speech sounds are made through a coordination of rapid movements of the articulators (primarily the tongue, jaw, soft palate, teeth, and lips). There are a variety of mouth shapes and placements of the articulators, as well as different ways of producing sounds within the human vocal tract. This is done in combination with *voice* and a sustained release of air from the lungs. There are 44 speech sounds in the English language, which are typically acquired in a developmental order.

Voice—use of the vocal folds to produce vibrations in the outgoing airstream, which then reverberate in the oral and nasal (possibly also pharyngeal and thoracic) cavities. The 'voice' can be switched on or off so that sounds are either voiced or voiceless.

Other aspects of speech do not convey language (i.e. what we are saying), rather they add meaning to the words and express notions such as sarcasm, innuendo, humour, and emotions (i.e. how we are saying it).

Fluency—the rhythm of speech (hesitations, blocking, repetitions, stuttering or stammering).

Pitch—how high or low our voice is (women are usually higher pitched than men and pitch tends to go up when we are anxious).

Intonation—how the pitch of speech is altered across a sentence to emphasize certain words or indicate some aspect other of meaning (e.g. going up at the end for a question).

Rate—the speed with which speech is delivered (e.g. fast often means anxious).

Volume—and how loud or quiet we are (e.g. loud often means angry).

Likely problems in verbal communication for people with intellectual disabilities

For many people with ID, difficulties in understanding and producing language can form part of their global developmental disabilities. Some people with ID will never develop language. Others might use a few single words and/or short phrases in combination with non-verbal signals. Some may talk in fluent sentences yet still have difficulty understanding complicated concepts such as emotions, time, and money. They might also need more time to process what someone else is saying and then to formulate a response. Many people (particularly with autistic spectrum disorder) may have difficulty with the rules of how to apply language to interaction with others.

Difficulties with language production may be compounded by hearing impairment or by problems in combining speech sounds to form words due to poor motor sequencing (dyspraxia). Also, as acquisition of the phonological (sounds) system is aligned to cognitive development, some people with ID may not achieve a full range of speech sounds. This may affect the intelligibility of their speech, particularly to people who do not know them well. They may use signs to back up their speech and/or other augmentative means. People with muscle coordination problems (e.g. cerebral palsy) often have a condition known as dysarthria, which leads to difficulties in clearly articulating sounds for speech. They may use alternative or augmentative systems of communication (see 📖 Assessing pain, p.88).

Further reading

Healy D, Walsh PN (2007). Communication among nurses and adults with severe and profound intellectual disabilities. *Journal of Intellectual Disabilities* **11**(2), 127–141.

Non-verbal communication

What is non-verbal communication?

The term 'non-verbal communication' is used here to mean the use of any signals that do not contain language to send and receive messages. This is often referred to as 'body language' but also includes aspects of our speech (how we speak rather than what we say—see 📖 Framework for nursing assessment, p.80) and other sounds we produce that carry meaning (e.g. laughing).

Pre-intentional (or unconscious) communication

Initially, babies are not aware that they can influence other human beings through what they do (they do not understand *cause and effect*). This does not mean that they do not communicate, merely that they have yet to learn to send messages that intentionally signal meaning to another person. For example, a baby may cry in a particular way and the parent interprets this as meaning she is hungry and feed her. Long before the development of speech, she will learn to cry like this on purpose to indicate hunger, and also to signal in different ways to indicate other messages. Some adults with ID may still be at the pre-intentional stage of communication development. They rely on us to interpret their signals and to support them to develop intentional communication, if at all possible. It is important to remember that we all send unconscious signals sometimes (often giving away our thoughts).

The communication ladder

Typically, we progress through developmental stages to learn increasingly more complex means of communication (moving up the ladder).

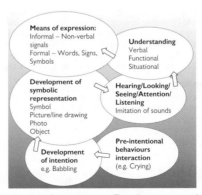

Fig 3.1 The development of communication. Typically, we progress through developmental stages to learn increasingly more complex means of communication. As the diagram shows, we develop recognition of objects before we can recognize photographs.

As Figure 3.1 shows, we develop recognition of objects before we can recognize photographs. Only then can we develop the skill of recognizing pictures, symbols (or icons) that represent a word or idea. Similarly, we develop situational understanding (taking meaning from what is going on around us) and functional understanding (e.g. that a cup is for drinking from) before we go on to understand what words mean. Unless we understand what words mean, we cannot use words to express ourselves. Some people with ID may rely on situational understanding (including others' non-verbal signals) to know what is happening, and these people are likely to express themselves wholly or primarily through non-verbal means.

Even where people are verbal, non-verbal communication plays a significant role in carrying meaning (we certainly tend to believe how people tell us things, rather than what they are saying, should the messages be in any way conflicting).

So what are non-verbal communication signals?

Head signals—eye contact can be essential in effective communication; frequent eye contact can put people at ease, show interest and help maintain the interaction, but staring can be seen as rude or threatening. Facial expressions (e.g. smiling, frowning, grimacing) are very effective in relaying our emotions. Head nods (positive or negative) are an integral way of expressing 'yes' and 'no' and also play a role in maintaining interaction (we move our heads almost constantly during conversation).

Hand signals—gestures are used to describe, emphasize, demonstrate, and to give directions or instructions. Most of us would be lost without use of our hands while talking! Signs (e.g. Makaton) can be used instead of speech or to augment speech. Touch is another important aspect to human communication and can be positive or negative.

Whole body signals
- Posture—e.g. slumped and arms folded (bored)
- Orientation—e.g. facing each other (interest) or turning away
- Distance—how near or far you are from another
- Appearance—clothing (e.g. uniform), personal grooming

Vocal signals—Intonation, rate, volume, fluency of speech (see ☐ Framework for nursing assessment, p.80) adds meaning to what we say. Remember, it is not what you say, it is the way that you say it.

Providing information

Accessing healthcare

It is recognized that health services are generally less accessible for people with ID.[1] This is partly due to problems in physically getting to the doctor's surgery or hospital, and also with reading written health promotion materials or invitations for health screening (and consequently missing appointments). Furthermore, people with communication difficulties may not be able to effectively tell a medical professional what the problem is or be able to understand the advice/treatment options being offered.

The nurse's role and communication

ID services generally attempt to support people to access generic healthcare services wherever possible, although health screening and certain specialist support may also be provided by them. As well as this, nurses within community ID teams may need to provide information about care packages and service plans, and then support the person to make important decisions about what happens in their life. Both roles require nurses to consider how to provide information effectively to people in a format that will assist them to have the best chance of participating in the decisions which affect them.

Assessing capacity to consent—understanding

Understanding the information that has been provided forms a major part of a person's capacity to consent to examination, treatment and care (see 📖 Capacity and consent, p.98). It is our responsibility to ensure that a person's capacity is maximized by providing pertinent information in whatever means appropriate to each individual. Even where 'best interests' are followed, the person deserves to be informed as far as possible as to what is to happen to them. As decisions need to be made about capacity to consent on a daily basis when working with people with ID, care should be taken when note-writing to include not just what was said to the person but *how* it was said (e.g. that gestures, signs or symbols/pictures/photos were used and note which ones, including a copy of any materials used).

Pitching language to match the level of understanding

It can be difficult to know how far to simplify information to help someone with ID to understand, as a person's level of understanding is not always apparent. People with ID have often learned through experience to appear to understand when in fact they are not sure what you mean. Think of yourself in a foreign language situation, where you are catching key words and nodding and smiling, and hoping that you will get the meaning soon or at least the person will appear satisfied with your minimal response and go away. For many people with ID, it may well be a similar experience when you are talking to them, especially if you are using any medical jargon and/or if they are anxious or in pain. Also remember that visual or hearing impairment may not be obvious (see 📖 pp.194–197).

While no one wants to appear patronizing by unnecessarily over-simplifying, there is a real danger in making assumptions about how much language a person can understand. We cannot be effective if we cannot communicate with the person—it is our responsibility to get our message across as far as possible. If you are unsure, assessment of a person's level of understanding and advice regarding strategies to promote under-standing for that individual can be requested from speech and language therapy.

General guidelines

In reality, we make judgements about others' communication all the time —we say something, wait for a response and adjust what we say next. Communication with people with ID is as much trial and error as it is with anyone else. Some general guidelines are:

- Wherever possible, plan how you are going to communicate in advance. Consider which augmentative tools you might need—pictures, photos, signs, written information—see 📖 Principles in using augmentative and alternative communication (AAC), p.66.
- Consider the person's attention span—maybe short bursts of information are better (repeat visits?)
- Make reasonable adjustments to allow for any problems with hearing or vision
- Reduce background noise and other distractions
- Allow processing time—do not talk too quickly
- Use short, straightforward sentences (one or two ideas at a time)
- Use easy words (reduce jargon/long words/abstract ideas)
- Watch the person—be prepared to repeat/rephrase
- Check they have understood—ask them to confirm what has been said.

ASD and communication

An important thing to remember when talking to verbal people with ASD is that they often have a literal understanding of language (see 📖 Autistic spectrum disorders, p.240). They are likely to have difficulties understanding figurative language (e.g. 'cut it out') and also in reading others' non-verbal signals. Providing visual information (pictures, photos, written words as appropriate) along with your spoken words can be helpful (see 📖 TEACCH, p.318). Explaining exactly what is to happen and why will often reduce anxiety about new social situations (or perhaps ones for which there are existing negative emotions), such as visiting the dentist, having injections, having hair cut, meeting new people. Writing Social Stories™ for these can be very effective and are easy to do with a little guidance (🖥 www.thegraycenter.org).

---

1 Equality Commission Northern Ireland (2007). *The Accessibility of Health Information for People with a Learning Disability in Northern Ireland.* ECNI: Belfast.

Active listening

What is active listening?

Active listening is widely promoted in self-help books and websites as a set of techniques to promote empathy and effective communication with people around you, whether in personal or working environments.

The application of active listening principles to people with ID means observing whatever communication signals the person is sending. It is about genuinely hearing the message the person is telling us, rather than merely part of this message, or some version of it that better suits our own needs, and then verifying the message with the person (letting them know they have been heard).

Active listening can be tiring as it takes effort. For nurses, it involves taking the time to develop a rapport with the person before engaging in clinical treatment or social care intervention. We must 'tune into' the person and be sensitive to their communication signals if we are to understand their point of view and so prevent communication breakdowns. This enables us to know how much to do at any one time: when to start, when to take a break, when to encourage someone into doing a little bit more, and when to stop. It is about finding the right balance between listening, hearing, and responding.

An important part of promoting expressive communication for people with ID (so that we can actively listen to them) is to ensure that we maximize their understanding of what is being communicated to them (see 📖 Providing information, p.62). To effectively listen to others, we must recognize and own the communication signals we are sending out.

Strategies to hear what the person is telling us

- Remaining calm and showing patience—putting the person at ease
- Allowing processing time for the person to think about what to say and also to get the message across
- Encouraging the person to say it another way if they get stuck ('Show me?'—see 📖 Principles in using augmentative and alternative communication (AAC), p.66)
- Commenting (providing statements rather than questions) or asking open questions (e.g. 'How are you feeling? rather than closed ones 'Do you feel sad?') to draw out the person's own opinions
- Focusing questions down ('Is it x or y?') if the person is struggling with comments or open questions
- Encouraging elaboration by keeping quiet and indicating that we are listening (head to one side, leaning forward, eye contact, nodding, smiling, 'uh-huh' type vocalizations, words of encouragement, etc)
- Rephrasing what we've understood—checking this with the person.

Barriers to communication

Sometimes what we say or do may have a negative effect on the person's expressive communication capabilities. At times, especially when we are busy and already focusing on what we need to do next, we may all be guilty of:

- not listening (**very** offputting)
- rushing the person
- providing reassuring cliches or stereotyped comments
- giving advice (we do not always know what is best)
- expressing approval/disapproval (making value judgements)
- requesting an explanation (asking why? Just accept what they say)
- defending ('I'm sure he didn't mean that')
- belittling feelings ('Now, now, don't cry! It's not that bad')
- changing the subject (perhaps when the topic is difficult).

Cultural differences

Having English as a second language may exacerbate communication difficulties for some people. Cultural differences in the use of both verbal and non-verbal communication will need to be taken into account if the person comes from a different ethnic background to yourself (you may need to seek advice on this). Active listening occurs when we treat people as they would want to be treated, not as we ourselves would necessarily want to be treated.

Assessing capacity to consent—expression

Cognitive behaviour therapies (📖 p.324) deals with helping people to understand information provided to them about the decision to be made. Once they have weighed this up and retained it, communicating any decision forms a major part of a person's capacity to consent to examination, treatment and care. It is our responsibility to ensure a person's capacity to communicate is maximized by supporting each individual to communicate in whatever means is appropriate to them, and to actively listen to their response.

Sharing information about communication with others

When writing in clinical notes we should include *how* the person communicates, not just was 'said'. Written records should always be clear, concise, and comprehensive, as they provide documentation of the person's status and treatment in order to ensure continuity of care as well as serving as legal documentation. If a person has communication difficulties it is important to share known strategies for listening to and supporting communication for that person with any other potential communication partners. This can be done simply through the use of a Communication Profile and/ or a Communication Passport (see 📖 p.70) for each person.

Further reading

Ellis R, Gates B, Kenworthy N (2003). *Interpersonal Communication in Nursing*. Churchill Livingstone: Edinburgh.

Principles in using augmentative and alternative communication (AAC)

What is AAC?

AAC refers to ways of communicating in addition to speech (augmentative) or instead of speech (alternative), bearing in mind that speech could be in sentences, phrases, single words or parts of words. AAC could just be that the person uses gesture or signs, or it could be a communication pocket book with words/symbols in to point to, or an electronic communication aid that produces speech when the person activates it.

The various levels of communication development outlined in ☐ Non-verbal communication, p.60, should be borne in mind when considering the most appropriate means of communication with and for any one person. Formal assessment may be sought from a speech and language therapist. However, applying basic principles described in this section should promote communication on a day-to-day basis. Used in conjunction with appropriate modifications to the way we provide information (see ☐ p.62) and active listening (see ☐ p.64), AAC should result in *inclusive communication*.

Objects

Objects of reference are used where people are just beginning to understand symbolic representation (see ☐ Objects of reference, p.72). However, we all take meaning from objects quite readily because they are concrete. The other advantage is that we can show people the action associated with the object. Showing someone a cup and miming taking a drink is likely to be more effective than merely using the word 'drink'.

Pictures/drawings

A picture tells a thousand words, or so it is said. Most of us think we are useless at drawing but with a little effort, we can all manage simple line drawings (use 'stick people' and ideas from symbols or pictures you have seen). Having a pad of paper and a pen handy is all that is needed to overcome communication breakdown at times—if we use it to show what we mean, maybe the other person will too. Thinking about how to draw what we are saying will help us to stick to everyday words.

Photographs

The arrival of the digital camera has been a huge boon to AAC. So long as the person is able to take meaning from photos we can use photos of their possessions, of their friends and family, of them actually doing something or to show places they go to. This can make for a truly effective and person-centred communication tool; we can inform them of coming events, explain everyday, service or intervention option, and support the person to make decisions. The person can express opinions and choices, make jokes, tell stories and pass on information. However, do not forget the consent issues surrounding the use of photography.

Symbols

One problem with photos is that they may contain extraneous detail which could distract from the message. For this reason, symbols may be preferred as they tend to be iconic representations of general concepts, rather than of specific people, actions or objects. This is particularly important for people with autistic spectrum disorder. There are a number of symbol sets used around the world; some well-known examples are Picture Communication Symbols,[1] Widgit-Rebus[2] and Makaton.[3] Symbols can be used at an individual or environmental level; for example on signage for buildings, for personalized communication books or communication passports, for schedules, pictorial timetables, choice boards, etc. Symbols may be used with or without words. Talking Mats™ is a very effective but simple visual framework, which uses picture symbols to support effective communication and decision making.[4]

Gestures and signing

Many people with ID will find it easier to understand what you are saying if you back up your speech with gestures and/or by signing key words. Note that this is not the same as using sign languages, which are totally different to spoken languages and based in a different linguistic culture. However, some people with ID may have learnt a sign language such as British Sign Language. Makaton is a language programme integrating speech, manual signs, and symbols. Many people with ID use Makaton to sign key words along with speech. Signing a few keys words helps us to slow our speech down a little and think more carefully about which words we are using.

Voice output communication aids

There is now a huge range of these aids.[5] Pictures, symbols or typed words may be used to generate speech, which may be digitized or recorded:

- Single message output devices (you record and re-record one message at a time and press to play it)
- 4 message, 9 message, 12 message, 32 message devices, etc where there is a message for each keypad and you may be able to switch between overlays to get a separate set of messages
- Hi-tech devices that are multilayered and can be used to produce more complex language.

---

1 Mayer-Johnson - 🖳 http://www.mayer-johnson.com/

2 Widget-Reburs - 🖳 http://www.widgit.com/

3 Makaton - 🖳 http://www.makaton.org

4 Talking Mats - 🖳 http://www.talkingmats.com

5 Inclusive Technology - 🖳 http://www.inclusive.co.uk

Developing accessible information

Why do we need accessible information?

It has been identified that people who have communication difficulties report feelings of disempowerment and extreme anxiety when trying to communicate with healthcare professionals. People with ID have also reported that they often find the experience of accessing healthcare frightening and confusing. It is suggested that providing information in an accessible format will make healthcare journeys for people with ID easier to manage and less frightening.

What is available?

Books Beyond Words

This is a series of picture books that were developed to make communication and discussion easier for people with ID. The titles include: (⌨ www.rcpsych.ac.uk/publications/booksbeyondwords.aspx)
- *Going to the Doctors*
- *Going to Hospital*
- *Going to Outpatients*

The Royal Institute for the Blind (www.rnib.org)

The Royal Institute for the Blind produce both booklets and tapes on:
- *Getting your eyes tested*
- *Getting new glasses*
- *Having a cataract operation*

All of these could be modified for people with ID.

The Guide and Directory to Health and Medicines

Helps people with ID understand their medication and possible side effects. They also enable people to formulate appropriate questions about the medication that they are prescribed.

Talking Mats™

This is an interactive resource that can be used in life planning and decision making. These type of communication ramps can be adapted for use within any healthcare setting.

Pain assessment tools

A variety of pain assessment tools have been developed in individual healthcare settings for assessment of pain. Those developed with smiling and non-smiling faces seem to be particularly successful in assessing the pain of a person with ID (see 📖 Assessing pain, p.88).[1]

Creating accessible information

The patterns of mortality and morbidity of people with ID vary from the general population.[2] Also as the communication ability of people with ID varies it means that often the information required for an individual's personal healthcare journey needs to be created on an individual basis.

Considerations when developing accessible information

It has been suggested that creating individualized information packages is not without its pitfalls. The person who requires the information should be assessed carefully to identify if they would benefit most from simple language, plain English, symbols, pictorial images, or photosymbols. It would be good at this point to liaise and take advice from the speech and language therapist.

Creating your own accessible information

There are now many symbol systems that either substitute for speech or provide help for those with linguistic issues. The common symbol systems that can be accessed and used to create individualized accessible information are:
- Rebus
- Gridmaker and Writing with Symbols
- Picture Communication system
- Boardmaker
- Blissymbols
- Blissymbols for Windows
- Bonnington Symbol System.

Many websites offer free downloads of symbols or photographs, and these could be used to develop individual accessible information

Benefits of accessible information

The development and use of accessible information will lead to:
- Seamless approach to care
- Better communication
- Reduced anxiety and distress
- Increased capacity to consent
- Reduction in risks
- Increased choice
- Increased participation of people in their own care
- Better information.

1 Regnard C, Reynolds J, Watson B, Matthews D, Gibson L, Clarke C. (2007). Understanding distress in people with severe communication difficulties: developing and assessing the Disability Distress Assessment Tool (DisDAT). *Journal of Intellectual Disability Research* **51**(4), 277–292.

2 NHS Scotland (2004). *Health Needs Assessment Report: People with Learning Disabilities in Scotland.* NHS Scotland: Glasgow.

Communication passports

Communication passports provide a special and efficient way of sorting and presenting accessible information about an individual. The information contained within the passport can enable healthcare professionals to communicate with the person with ID, and also to ensure that the person's individual needs, likes, and dislikes are taken into account. They gather important and complex information about the person and make this accessible to others.

Types of communication passports

Type 1—Personal communication passports

This type of passport contains information about all aspects of the person's life and is used as a tool in enabling the person to have a say and to make choices.

Type 2—Personal communication passports

This type of passport is used to facilitate and support access between different services. It is a snapshot of the person's life and individual needs at the time of access. This type of passport tends to concentrate on the health needs or health profile of the person at a particular point in time and therefore they will require review and updating at each point of access.

Type 3—Combination of Type 1 and 2

This type of passport is a combination of type 1 and 2. This type then includes all the personal information of a type 1 passport plus the health profile information of the type 2 passport.

Features of passports

All types of passports present highly personal information, in an empowering and positive manner. They usually contain information on:
- Personal contact details
- Professional contact details (e.g. social worker, community nurse)
- Medical history
- Communication details
- Language
- Spirituality
- Likes and dislikes
- Current medication
- Allergies
- Issues around capacity and consent.

Depending on the individual's level of communication, the passports may use plain English, symbols or photographs. They should be bright, attractive and easy to use.

Benefits of passports

Passports are a positive way of supporting, enabling, and empowering people with ID who have communication problems. The benefits include:

- Ensuring continuity of care
- Supporting the person
- Orientating new staff more quickly
- Empowering the person
- Enabling more competent observation
- Valuing all contributions to the person's care
- Enhancing relationships
- Providing a focus for discussion
- Enabling rapid access to care
- Responding to the person's individual need
- Improving treatment and care.

Constraints of passports

Passports do not have any legal status although their use is recommended. This could pose some ethical problems for healthcare professionals. They contain highly personalized information about the person and their health needs. It is suggested that healthcare professionals use the passports to make decisions about future treatment and care; however, this can be problematic if the information in the passport is flawed or out of date. It is important, therefore, that healthcare professionals check out the information contained within the passports with the individual and relevant others. All passports and updated information within these should also be dated and signed.

Further reading

Harrison S, Berry L (2005). Improving primary care services for people with a learning disability, *Nursing Times* **101**(1), 38–40.

Millar S (2003). *Personal Communication Passports: Guidelines for Good Practice*. CALL Publications: Edinburgh.

Objects of reference

People with ID have a wide range of communication abilities. Some will be able to communicate verbally while others may learn how to use symbols or photos. Others will not be able to grasp that a symbol means something. In these cases objects of reference may be useful.

Definition

The term 'objects of reference' refers to the use of tangible objects as a method of communication with children and adults who have an ID.

Using objects of reference

Objects of reference are tangible items that are used in a systematic way with people with ID and additional communication difficulties. The objects are items that have meaning for the individual and they help with identifying what is going to happen next or in making choices between two different activities. The objects are real items that are used everyday by the person. So a toothbrush may be used to signify teeth cleaning, or a spoon to indicate eating.

Much of the literature identifies that each individual should have their own unique objects of reference. This can be time consuming for professionals, however, and may also be confusing. Studies where the same objects of reference are used in a group rather than an individual basis suggest that using objects in this way is beneficial both for the people with ID, who mostly progressed in the use of objects as a means of communication, and for the care staff, in that they could use the same objects for a number of people.

Constraints of using objects of reference

It should be noted that the objects themselves are representations of activities and they tend to be chosen by the healthcare professional or the educationalist. Park suggests that this may be problematic, because the object chosen may be a commonsense choice to the professional but may be meaningless to the person with ID.[1] He goes on to suggest that a spoon is part of the activity of eating rather than being an object of reference that represents eating.

It is also identified that objects of reference are only used to order or represent utilitarian activities of daily routine like eating or having a bath, and are not used for ordinary social communication. Thus Park argues that objects of reference are rarely used for activities such as play.[1]

How is success achieved?

It is argued by Hengst that in order to be successful, referencing is dependent on the collaboration between the speaker and the listener.[2] She identifies that analysis of the discourse of interaction shows that both verbal and non-verbal communication is actively negotiated across the referencing task. These findings have implications for professionals in that they are suggesting that successful use of objects of reference is best achieved through close relationships.

Interactive storytelling

Park explores success and use of objects of reference in more detail.[3] He suggests that the use of interactive story telling enables people with ID to share experiences in which they choose or negotiate the object of reference. He believes that this empowers the individual at the same time as enhancing their early communication skills.

Further reading

Jones F, Pring T, Grove N (2002). Developing communication in adults with profound and mutiple learning difficulties using objects of reference. *International Journal of Language and Communication Disorders* **37**(2), 173–184.

1 Park K (2001). Oliver Twist: An exploration of interactive storytelling and object use in communication. *British Journal of Special Education* **28**(1), 18–23.

2 Hengst JA (2003). Collaborative referencing between individuals with aphasia and routine communication partners. *Journal of Speech, Language and Hearing Research* **46**(4), 831–848.

3 Park K (2002). Macbeth: A poetry workshop on stage at Shakespeare's Globe Theatre. *British Journal of Special Education* **29**(1), 14–19.

Compiling life stories

People with ID are not a homogenous group. Even people with a similar diagnosis, for example Down syndrome, have different abilities and capabilities. Enabling individual people to compile their individual life story can be empowering for the individual but it also give the healthcare, social care, or educational professional opportunities to glimpse the cultural and social aspects of the lived experience of the person.

Life stories provide sensitive individual accounts of the person with a disability and are contextualized by the environment the person lives within, the community the person is part of, and wider society.

Recording personal histories

Facilitating people with ID to record their life stories can be challenging. Some people will have the ability to recall and record their own narrative, whereas others will need communication aids, which will make this process more accessible for them. It is suggested that Talking Mats™ could be a useful tool. This is an interactive resource that concentrates on thirteen life-planning topics (see 📖 Developing accessible information, p.68). Other life-planning tools may also be of use in this process (see 📖 Person-centred planning, p.250). These would include all of the following:

- Person-centred planning
- Personal futures planning
- Essential lifestyles planning
- Planning Alternative Tomorrows with Hope (PATH)
- Making action plans (MAPS).

Many people with ID have been empowered to develop their life stories by becoming involved in an advocacy group or by having an individual advocate.

Benefits of compiling life stories alongside the person with intellectual disability

- Empowerment
- Participation
- Emancipation
- Coming to terms with the past
- Understanding the present
- Looking to the future
- Increasing self identity
- Increasing the capacity to consent.

Benefits of compiling life stories for healthcare professionals

- Better understanding of patterns of behavioural distress
- Better understanding of the effects of service redesign
- Limiting possibilities of past mistakes being replicated
- Increasing empathy
- Creating a basis for communication
- Creating a basis for future person centered planning.

Further reading

Cameron L, Murphy J (2002). Enabling young people with a learning disability to make choices at the time of transition. *British Journal of Learning Disabilities* **30**(3), 105.

Jennings C, Courell D, Gallagher DW (2006). Life planning. In: Gates B, (Ed). *Care Planning and Delivery in Intellectual Disability Nursing*. Blackwell Publishing: London.

Further reading

Assessment

Purpose and principles of assessment

The purpose of assessment is to 'gain a picture' of the needs of a person. Assessment begins the systematic process of developing plans of care by gathering relevant information and facts about the individual. In pure nursing terms, assessment should gather two main kinds of information:

- Objective—valid and reliable measurable data, such as body weight, temperature etc.
- Subjective—how the service user feels and what they think about things.

A nursing assessment should follow a structured holistic framework, and is an ongoing process that can be used to enhance existing skills as well as promoting the growth of new skills. Effective communication is an integral part of the assessment process; you cannot assess a person's needs or wants effectively if you cannot communicate effectively with them.

Overall purposes (dependent on need)

- Health screening
- Physical and mental health assessment
- Assessment of specific symptoms, such as pain or anxiety
- Assessment of independence and social functioning
- Holistic nursing assessment of bio-psycho-social needs
- Behavioural and risk assessment
- Assessment of cognitive ability and capacity to consent.

Information from these assessments can be used to inform and develop:

- Health Action Plans (HAPs)
- Person-centred nursing care plans and support plans
- Person-centred plans (e.g. Essential Life Plans, MAPS, PATH etc.).

Sources of information

Information can be gathered from a range of relevant sources:

- Interviewing the person who is the focus of the assessment
  if possible, using enhanced verbal and non-verbal communication skills (see 📖 Chapter 3, pp.55–76)
- Interviewing family members, carers, advocates, and 'significant others', including members of the service user's support network
- Observing the person's behaviour and body language
- Observing other peoples' behaviour and interactions
- Observing the physical setting, context, and environmental factors
- Physical examination, using objective measurements and tools
- Using written records and establishing a health history.

However, it is important to 'triangulate' the picture by comparing information from the different sources. If there is not close agreement, you will need to check the reliability and validity of some data.

The principles of person-centred assessment

In ID nursing, the basic principles of nursing assessments need to be undertaken within the principles of person-centred processes, in which assessment is oriented around the service user, who is in control of what is happening. A person-centred assessment would incorporate the following elements:

The person is at the centre

- Remember that the assessment belongs to the service user. Think about whom the assessment is being done for
- The service user should be as actively involved as possible
- Use language that the service user understands, and use communication and visual aids if necessary
- Give the service user choice about who carries out the assessment and when and where it is done.

Family members and friends are full partners

- Look at the service user in the context of people who are important to them. Encourage family and friends to be involved, while recognizing the views of the person with ID
- Use the knowledge, concerns and skills of the support circle but remember that the final say should rest with the service user.

Person-centred assessment reflects what is important to the person, their capacities, and what support they require

- Work with the person to choose what and how to assess. Explore their perspective on issues
- Behavioural and risk assessment might be about other peoples' concerns.

Person-centred assessment results in actions that are about life, not just services, and reflects what is possible, not just what is available

- The assessment is about identifying the person's abilities and needs, rather than how the person can be accommodated in existing systems
- Think about 'what it would take' to meet the person's needs
- Use creative thinking to think outside existing approaches and possibilities.

Person-centred planning leads to continual listening, learning and action, and helps the person get what they want out of life

- Assessment is about *listening* to the service user and finding out what *they* think and feel about things
- Assessment is an ongoing process, rather than a one-off event. It will probably take quite some time to work with the service user to develop a relationship that will facilitate a clear holistic assessment
- Assessment is about learning through shared action, reflecting and refining—it is a team effort, with the service user as a major player wherever possible.

Professional assessments and support plans are part of a person-centred plan, rather than being separate to it

- A nursing assessment can contribute to the person's HAP and help the person with this aspect of their person-centred plan
- Professional assessments should be an integral part of the service user's overall life plan.

Framework for nursing assessment

Although there are many conceptual frameworks for holistic nursing assessment, most of these have been developed in the context of medical surgical nursing. Although a number (e.g. Roper, Logan & Tierney; Orem) have been adapted, they often still lack a theoretical grounding in ID. One conceptual framework specifically designed for ID nursing is the Ecology of Health Framework,[1] which is briefly described below.

The framework uses the concept of the person's health and independence as an ecological system. A range of 'internal' and 'external' factors interacts with independence skills in a complex way to produce an individual dynamic of health. The framework prompts the nurse to look more deeply than mere description, and to search for the causative and maintaining factors that affect the individual's health. The framework should be used as a menu of potential assessment factors, rather than slavishly as a 'tick list' assessment.

Table 4.1 Skills for independence

• Being a parent (if appropriate)	• Getting around
• Being a woman/being a man	• Having a home of my own
• Being happy—having good mental health	(including looking after my home)
• Being part of my family	• Having fun with friends
• Being part of my neighbourhood	• Learning new things
• Being part of my religion and culture	• Looking good and keeping clean
• Being well—having good physical health	• Managing money
• Choosing what I want	• People in my life
• Doing a job	• Saying how I feel
• Eating and drinking	• Sleeping, resting and relaxing
• Feeling safe	• Talking to people

Table 4.2 Internal factors

The physical self

• Blood, circulation and breathing	• Healthy body temperature
• Dental and oral health	• Healthy bones, joints and muscles
• Effects of medication on physical health	• Healthy skin, hair and nails
• Endocrine health	• Neurological health
• Excretory health	• Nutrition and gastrointestinal health
• Pain and discomfort	• Sensory health
• General pattern of physical health, wellness and fitness	• Womens' and mens' sexual health

Table 4.2 Internal factors (continued)

The thinking self

- Cognitive maturity
- Attention and concentration
- Memory
- Moral reasoning
- Knowledge, beliefs and understanding
- Effects of medication on cognitive processes

The emotional self

- Confidence, anxiety and the need for reassurance
- The individual's mood and range of emotions
- Stability of mood
- Emotional response to stressors
- Emotional awareness, communicating feelings
- Effects of medication on emotional processes

The personal and spiritual self

- Religious, cultural and ethnic self
- Locus of control, self-confidence
- Self-concept and self-knowledge
- Self-esteem and self-regard
- Self-expression and communication
- Mental health

The effects of the person's disabling condition

- Risk factors for physical and mental health
- Prognosis and development of their health and disabling condition

Table 4.3 External factors

The social environment of health

- Cultural, ethnic and religious environment
- Neighbourhood and housing, living conditions and circumstances
- Socioeconomic status, financial status and stability
- Family membership and dynamics
- Social and friendship networks
- Formal support networks, involvement of professionals

The effects of time and personal history

- The past
- The present
- The future
- These are seen as 'slices' that run through all the other elements

1 A full version of the Ecology of Health Framework (Version 3) is available as part of the *Assessment Frameworks for Learning Disability Practice* package from John Aldridge, The University of Northampton. Email john.aldridge@northampton.ac.uk

Adaptive behaviour rating scales

Measurement of IQ (see 📖 p.96) indicates that a diagnosis of an ID cannot be made on an IQ score alone, it must also be assessed by significant deficits in adaptive functioning. Adaptive functioning relates to the skills required for a person to cope successfully with the daily tasks involved in living from day to day, linked to a person's chronological age. These adaptive functioning skills include: communication, self-care, home living, social, community use, self-direction, health and safety, leisure, and work.

Purpose of adaptive behaviour rating scales

Adaptive behaviour rating scales will help nurses and professionals to:
- obtain a prompt and accurate picture of the level of ability in people with ID, and who also have autism, communication deficits and other developmental delay (i.e. functional skills impairment)
- aid in determining the person's eligibility for the appropriate supports
- plan a socially valid and effective intervention package of care
- evaluate intervention outcome and demonstrate if the person has returned to their optimal level of functioning as they were before they became ill.

Measurement of adaptive functioning

Adaptive behaviour rating scales are standardized tests based upon measurement from large samples of populations. There are a number of adaptive behaviour rating scales commercially available for nurses and other professionals to use to measure a person's adaptive functioning. Some of these include:
- Developmental Profile II (DPII)
- Early Coping Inventory (ECI)
- Bayley Scales of Infant Development (BSID)
- Scales of Independent Behaviour: Revised (SIB-R)
- Adaptive Behaviour Scales (ABS)
- Vineland Adaptive Behaviour Scales (VABS).

Vineland Adaptive Behaviour Scale

The most widely used tool within the field of ID is the Vineland Adaptive Behaviour Scale (VABS).[1] This scale measures the personal and social skills of a person from birth to adulthood. It can be used in clinical settings, for education, and in home settings. It uses a questionnaire format and has 213 questions/items. A teacher, parent or nurse who knows the person well indicates whether the individual has mastered the skill in question.

The VABS assesses a wide range of adaptive behaviours:
- *Communication*—receptive, expression, written, and the ability to listen.
- *Daily living skills*—personal, domestic, and community.
- *Socialization*—interpersonal relationships, play and leisure time, and coping skills.
- *Motor skills*—gross and fine motor skills.

With the VABS there is standardized and normative scores, where the person's scores can be compared based upon age and gender. This scale has very strong internal consistency, test–retest reliability, and inter-rater reliabilities.

Vineland Adaptive Behaviour Scale-II

More recently the VABS has been redeveloped and now called VABS-II.[3] Along with the earlier benefits of the VABS (1st edition) it has been updated with new norms, expanded age ranges, and improved items. In addition to assessing the four areas above within the original VABS, the latest edition has a fifth category of assessment: Maladaptive Behaviour Index: Internalizing, Externalizing, and Other. The VABS-II can now measure adaptive behaviour of people with:

- ID
- ASD
- ADHD
- Post-traumatic brain injury
- Hearing impairment
- Dementia/Alzheimer's disease.

Using the adaptive behaviour rating scales

Learning more about the person's adaptive behaviours will help nurses to gain a broader picture of the individual—of what they can and cannot do. When completing an assessment on an individual with an ID, you should identify an informant who knows the person well (i.e. parent or teacher). If there is not sufficient information to score the form, return again and continue with the assessment and/or seek information from other members of the multidisciplinary team. Also ensure the person is offered a range of opportunities to demonstrate the skills that are required to achieve a score on the form.

Ensure the person is physically and emotionally well, and performing at their best. If the person is unwell it may be better to return another day to complete the assessment. Be confident and competent in scoring and interpreting the behaviour rating scale, as these scores will be compared with similar people of age and gender, which will then be used to develop an appropriate care plan for this person.

1 Sparrow SS, Cicchetti DV, Balla DA (1993). *Vineland Adaptive Behaviour Scale*. Pearson Assessments: Minneapolis. Available at 🖳 http://pearsonassessments.com/vinelandadapt.aspx

2 Sparrow SS, Cicchetti DV, Balla DA (2008). *2nd Ed: Vineland Adaptive Behaviour Scale - 2.* Available at 🖳 http://pearsonassessments.com/vinelandadapt.aspx

3 Vineland Adaptive Behavior Scales, Second Edition (Vineland-II). A measure of adaptive behavior from birth to adulthood. Published by Pearson (🖳 http://ags.pearsonassessments.com/Group. asp?nGroupInfoID=aVineland)

Health checks

The term 'health checks' refers to an important service that people with ID are eligible to access, which is provided by their own GP. It is the information that comes from health checks that forms the basis of the individual's HAP (see 📖 Health action plans and health facilitation, p.276). The development of health checks is in response to the considerable research-based evidence identifying that, relative to the general population, people with ID have higher rates of unmet health needs, yet access health services less often. Research has shown that such checks do result in previously unrecognized health needs being identified.

An annual health check is likely to include certain core areas as a matter of routine, such as:

- History of illness in the individual's family and associated health risks
- Review of current medication
- Immunization history and current status
- Height, weight, blood pressure
- Assessing levels of fitness and advice about exercise
- Take up of health screening services available to members of the general public such as mammography (breast screening—see 📖 Screening of physical health, p.86)
- Access to health promotion messages, such as those concerning healthy eating.

Where necessary the following health checks may also be undertaken:

- Eye test (optometry)
- Hearing test (audiometry)
- Monitoring long-term conditions such as epilepsy, asthma, and coronary heart disease
- Sexual health
- Guidance where necessary regarding drugs and alcohol
- Elimination and continence
- Investigating any reports of behaviour that other people find difficult (e.g. sometimes called challenging behaviour)
- Assessing mental health and emotional needs
- Assessing mobility and posture
- Oral and dental health.

A GP or senior nurse (such as a practice nurse) should take responsibility for implementing the programme of health checking, ensuring that accurate records are kept and any health action plans completed. Depending on the need of the individual concerned, other professionals (such as ID nurses) or carers will be required to assist with aspects of the process. For example, community nurses in ID services may assist the practice to identify which of their patients are priorities for health checking for example as follows:

- Individuals with severe or profound impairments
- Individuals in transition from young person to adult services
- Individuals who have complex health needs
- Individuals at risk of developing health needs (for example those who are missing important health promotion or health education messages)
- Individuals named on the local authority register of persons with ID.

It is now considered good practice to name a registered nurse in ID from the local community team to link with the practice to support the health check process. ID nurses are well placed to alert healthcare professionals to the particular needs of people with ID (for example with regards to communication), and to support individuals to understand their right to a health check. They can also have a role in encouraging and advising people who may be reluctant to attend. ID nurses may also take the role of health facilitator (see 📖 Health action plans and health facilitation, p.278) as this is fundamental to ensuring that the health action plan is implemented.

It is important to remember that ID service providers share a responsibility for the health and well-being of people in their care. If health checking is not happening automatically as it should (i.e. that people are being invited annually) it may sometimes be necessary to prompt a local GP to provide the health check as required. This advocacy can be fundamental in ensuring that health needs are met. Sometimes advocacy will also be needed to ensure an individual gains access to the healthcare intervention identified as required, especially when resources are limited (e.g. dialysis). ID service providers who see people on a day-to-day basis must be vigilant in their observation of those they have contact with. The early reporting of any signs or symptoms of ill health or change in health status of people with ID can result in earlier health interventions, and as a result an improved prognosis.

For more information see:
🖥 www.primarycarecontracting.nhs.uk/204.php

The *Choosing Health: Making Healthier Choice Easy* White Paper[1] introduced the target of health checks. Later the Primary Care Service Framework[2] stipulated that it should be the role of GPs to develop and deliver a routine, comprehensive, and individualized annual health check to their patients who have an ID.

---

1 Department of Health (2004). *Choosing Health: Making Healthier Choice Easy*. Department of Health: London.

2 Primary Care Service Framework (2007). *Management of Health for People with Learning Disabilities in Primary Care*. NHS Primary Care Service Frameworks: London.

Screening of physical health

Physical health screening is a proactive intervention, which seeks to detect any possible sign of ill health before it has fully developed. An example of this is a smear test to screen for cervical cancer. Health screening is a central tenet of health promotion activity as its aim is that ill health is prevented. All people with ID who use NHS services should be offered health screening in the same way as other citizens. For example, routine invitations to women 50yrs and over to have breast screening (mammography) should include women with ID. However, in practice this has not always happened. For example women with ID are about 4 times less likely to be offered a cervical smear test than are women who do not have an ID (~24% vs 82%).

In recent years there has been a growing concern about the unmet health needs of people with ID. Screening (and health checking—see 📖 Health checks, p.84) can help to identify otherwise undetected conditions, which may have remained hidden for various reasons for example:

- The signs and symptoms of ill health may be masked by the ID. This is sometimes referred to as diagnostic overshadowing
- Low rates of self-reporting health problems by people with ID
- Polypharmacy can mask signs and symptoms of ill health.

Additional obstacles to people with ID accessing physical health screening have included (see 📖 Chapter 10, pp.333–398):

- Ineffective means of communicating health screening information to this client group
- The knowledge and attitude of staff who support people with ID
- Lack of time and specialist equipment
- Concerns about a person's ability to consent to treatment
- Lack of confidence and experience of medical professionals to work with 'difficult clients'
- Anxiety and fear of individuals based on previous negative experiences of the NHS.

The Disability Discrimination Act (2005) and the Public Sector Disability Equality Duty (DED) effective from December 2006 require that disabled people have equal access to health services, and this includes the right to have physical health screening. For example, the care standards outlined in national standards such as the National Service Frameworks (NSFs) in England or equivalent in other countries within the UK and the Republic of Ireland for cancer, coronary heart disease, older people, renal, and diabetes apply equally to people with ID as they do to the rest of the population.

Where service users themselves are unable to do so, staff working with people with ID will need to ensure appointments for health screening are made when necessary. A requirement for these may be prompted via the routine annual health check conducted by the person's GP, practice nurse or health facilitator (see 📖 Health action plans and health facilitation, p.276). People may access current national screening programmes (as referred to above). Others may be referred for non-routine screening as their health needs determine.

This may include:
- Faecal occult blood (for colorectal health)
- Bone density scan
- Urinalysis
- ECG
- Blood tests for thyroid function, cholesterol levels, diabetes etc
- Eye and hearing tests.

It may be necessary to advocate on behalf of people you support to ensure that they receive the screening to which they are entitled. Once the appointment has been made it is advisable also to plan ahead and allow enough time to ensure the person understands the process and are able to give informed consent. Double-time appointments may be necessary, and good liaison beforehand with the service providers should ensure that the experience for the person is more positive.

There is also now a wide range of accessible teaching and advice materials which have been developed to help prepare people with ID understand the benefit to them of health screening. These also help explain the process that the person will need to go through and can be used effectively to prepare people for screening well in advance of the appointment. A useful contact for such information is the UK learning disability health network (ldhealthnetwork@ldhealthnetwork.org.uk)

Further reading
See www.easyhealth.org.uk to find accessible health information on the internet.

Assessing pain

Pain is considered to be a subjective experience, which is multidimensional, presenting itself in many ways. The pain experience and an individual's reaction to it are influenced by the individual's developmental stage, cognitive ability, and cultural factors. Assessment and management of pain is challenging, and is further complicated if the individual is a young child, has cognitive impairment, or has communication difficulties.[1]

People with ID are at increased risk of experiencing more pain than others and of not having this pain recognized or appropriately managed. Evidence shows that people with cognitive impairment are prescribed less analgesia than those with no cognitive impairment. A poor recognition of pain in this group of people may increase the risk of harm, or delayed diagnosis of serious medical conditions, which can have devastating consequences.[2]

Challenges in assessing pain

Cook et al. suggest that poor pain assessment and inappropriate management for people with ID is associated with 4 key factors:[3]
- Under-reporting of pain, which is often associated with the individual's inability to articulate the experience of pain
- Even when pain is communicated, there is evidence that this information may not be accepted by others
- Carers may not recognize signs that the individual is experiencing pain
- Poor use of pain assessment tools or indeed a lack of appropriate assessment tools for use with people with cognitive impairment.

Expressions of pain

Pain is expressed in various ways in people with ID, in addition to the physiological signs of pain, it may be demonstrated through unusual or 'odd' behaviours, and an understanding by nurses of the various ways in which pain is expressed can facilitate its appropriate assessment and subsequent management. Collacott and Cooper identify vocalizations, inappropriate laughing, grimacing, withdrawal, self-injurious behaviour, holding of a body part, reduced mobility, and sweating as some of the ways in which pain is communicated.[4]

Assessing pain

The assessment is informed by perceptive observation and interpretation of the individual's communicative behaviour, evidence from carers, followed by sound clinical judgements. Vital to the assessment is the nurse's recognition that challenging behaviour does have a communicative function and nurses must assess if the behaviour is an individual's way of communicating 'I am in pain'.

By using a comprehensive holistic approach, pain can be detected and treated appropriately in people with ID. This holistic approach is informed by the nurse's ability to:
- understand that a nurse's attitude to pain can influence appropriate assessment and subsequent management of pain
- understand that factors such as the environment, situations and emotions can influence both perception and response to pain

- understand the risks and causes of pain in this population and the potential consequences of under diagnosis and treatment
- recognize that pain is often under recognized and therefore under treated in this population
- observe the patient for pain by having an awareness of how the perception of pain is verbalized and demonstrated in people with ID
- have a comprehensive understanding of the various pain assessment tools available and their use, and select the tool that will be most useful in the care of the individual
- participate in frequent pain assessment for people with communication difficulties
- respect the role of the family and other carers who are familiar with how the person normally behaves or has previously expressed pain during the assessment process.[5]

Pain assessment tools
- Pain and Discomfort Scale (PADS)
- Heat–Pain Threshold (HPT)
- Non-Communicating Children's Pain Checklist—revised
- Non-verbal facial expressions as a research tool for assessing pain in persons with ID
- Disability Distress Assessment Tool (DisDaT).

1 Defrin R, Lotan M, Pick CG (2006). The evaluation of acute pain in individuals with cognitive impairment. A differential effect of the level of impairment. *Pain* **134**(3), 312–320.

2 National Patient Safety Agency (2004). *Understanding the Patient Safety Issues for People with Learning Disabilities*. NHS: London.

3 Cook AKR, Niven CA, Downs MG (1999). Assessing the pain of people with cognitive impairment. *International Journal of Geriatric Psychiatry* **14**, 421–425.

4 Collacott RA, Cooper SA (1998). Epidemiology of self-injurious behaviour in adults with learning disabilities. *The British Journal of Psychiatry* **173**: 428–432.

5 Charlton JE (2005). *Pain Issues in Individuals with Little Ability to Communicate Due to Cognitive Impairment. Core curriculum for professional education in pain*. IASP Press: Seattle.

Assessing distress

Distress, pain, and suffering are descriptions of unpleasant experiences that individuals perceive and experience. Like pain and suffering, distress is perceived and experienced differently in individuals and may be felt as emotional, psychological or physical in nature, and just like pain and suffering its impact on the individual needs to be recognized and validated.

Definition

Defining distress is not easy, yet it is used frequently within nursing and is associated with the term discomfort, which can be physical, emotional or psychological in nature. Ridner describes distress as 'a nonspecific, biological or emotional response to a demand or stressor that is harmful to the individual'.[1] With this in mind it is essential that nurses identify the signs of distress, validate its existence, identify possible causes, and deal appropriately with it. Early recognition of distress can help alleviate some of the unpleasant feelings associated with it, avoiding potential crisis.

Increased experience of distress

Many people with ID are more likely to experience distress than others, as they are more likely to experience:

- a lack of response to their rights to inclusion/choice/friends/freedom
- increased incidence of communication difficulties, which increases the risk of their needs not being understood, therefore inadequately addressed
- a greater incidence of both acute and chronic illness
- greater risk of both accidental and non-accidental injury[2]
- more episodes of pain as a result of comorbidities that increase risk of pain, such as contractures, motor impairments, sensory impairments, postural problems (e.g. associated with gastro-oesophageal reflux)
- expressions of pain not being recognized or validated, thus left untreated.

Expressing distress

For people with ID the ability to express distress can be reduced because of their experience of communication difficulties. 40–50% of people with ID have communication difficulties; the degree of difficulty increases with the severity of the ID. Consequently, communicating perceptions or experiences of distress are often expressed through behavioural cues, posture, expressions, or vocalizations. These are often recognized by the families, but this information is often poorly communicated to others, or when communicated is not validated by healthcare professionals, which increases the risk of needs not being identified or addressed.[3]

Assessing distress

Although distress and pain are often used synonymously, Regnard et al. noted that the experience of distress may not include physical pain,[3] and while there are a number of pain assessment tools that may be used with people with ID, distress, which can caused by various factors and is as disturbing as pain, unfortunately is not assessed (see Assessing pain, p.88).

DisDaT is a comprehensive distress assessment tool (not a scoring tool) that seeks to present an accurate representation of an individual's language that 'denotes distress'. Regnard *et al.* found that 'distress signs and behaviours are not specific to the cause and each person has their own 'vocabulary' of distress signs and behaviours'.[3] In addition it is reported to be easy for carers to use, although it is also recognized that interdisciplinary teams using this tool are more likely to pick up distress signals than an individual who uses the tool.

This assessment tool helps to:

- identify distress in people with cognitive impairment and communication difficulties
- record changes in behaviour and other signs that are demonstrated by the person when they were seen to be content, so that changes in behaviour indicating distress would be more easily recognized
- provide a checklist of the possible causes for the distress, while taking account of the context in which the behaviour was demonstrated
- provide an accurate outline of the signs and behaviours of the individual, so that other carers, within different environments, have a clear understanding of the meaning of these, which can help guide their plan of individualized care.[3]

When to use DisDaT:[3]

- When the individual with ID is not distressed, in order to get a baseline
- When the person is known or new to the team to gain understanding of their usual behaviours and meanings of other behaviours
- To provide a record that can be transferred to other environments/teams, enhancing their understanding of the individual and the quality of care.

1 Ridner SH (2004). Nursing theory and concept. Development or analysis. Psychological distress: concept analysis. *Journal of Advanced Nursing* **45**(5), 536–545.

2 Hsieh K, Heller T, Millar AB (2001). Risk factors for injuries and falls among adults with developmental disabilities. *Journal of Intellectual Disability Research* **45**, 76–82.

3 Regnard C, Reynolds J, Watson B, Matthews D, Gibson L, Clarke C (2007). Understanding distress in people with severe communication difficulties: developing and assessing the Disability Distress Assessment Tool (DisDAT). *Journal of Intellectual Disability Research* **51**(4), 277–292.

Screening of mental health problems

Aims of assessment

According to Taggart and Slevin, assessment is a core role of the nurse and has a number of important functions:[1]

• To identify the underlying reason(s) for the person's behaviours
• To identify patterns of normative behaviours and the changes in these behaviours (baseline distortion)
• To clearly describe the person's explicit behaviours in terms of quality of life, life events, gender, and social mores
• To diminish any other explanations for the presenting behaviours thereby formulating a 'working hypothesis' or suspected reasons for the behaviour(s)
• To develop a socially valid and effective intervention programme
• To determine whether the person is eligible for particular supports and who will provide these supports
• To provide a basis so the implemented care can be evaluated/re-assessed.

Structured frameworks

In undertaking a comprehensive assessment based upon a bio-psycho-social-model as proposed by IASSID,[2] it is important that a structured approach to assessment is used, as highlighted by Aman et al.[3] and Deb et al.[4] Some of the key areas to assess are:

• Interview with carers to seek information on the person's baseline behaviours, developmental history, social history (i.e. employment/education status, friends/relationships, routines, likes/dislikes, quality of life), forensic history, family functioning and how they manage the person's behaviours, and also presenting behaviours
• Interviews with other professionals within the person's life
• Direct observation of the person, and also a functional behavioural analysis of his/her behaviours
• Via GP or Medical Officer to obtain a medical history, physical examination, list of medications and side effects. Also, if needed, laboratory tests such as blood levels of medication and toxicology levels
• Unstructured psychiatric interview aided by standardized mental health screening scales (i.e. PAS-ADD, PRIMA, REISS, DASH).

Use of screening tools

Within general psychiatry a number of screening tools have been developed to help nurses to recognize mental health signs and symptoms, thereby aiding in the assessment process. Some of these screening tools include Beck's Depression Inventory and Hamilton Anxiety Inventory. People with borderline to mild ID, with good reading ability, may be able to complete these tools with assistance; however, many more people with ID will be unable to score these and subsequently rely upon third-party informants or their carers to inform professionals about the person's behaviours. Recent developments have seen the introduction of the PAS-ADD schedules.

• *The PAS-ADD Checklist*[5] is a 27-item screening instrument examining 3 affective/neurotic disorders, organic conditions and psychotic disorders.

No formal training is required to use this tool, although knowledge and awareness of mental health in people with ID is an important benefit

- **The Mini PAS-ADD Interview**[5] is a 66-item screening instrument that probes a wider range of mental health symptoms (i.e. depression, anxiety and phobias, hypomania, obsessive–compulsive disorder, psychosis, and unspecified) using a glossary. Specific training of half a day is required for the practitioner to effectively use this tool
- **The PAS-ADD 10 Interview**[5] is a more detailed semi-structured clinical interview designed for the person with an ID and/or informants. Specific training of 1 day is required to use this tool
- **The ChA-PAS (Child and Adolescent Psychiatric Assessment Schedule Interview)**[5] is a 97-item screening instrument that assesses mental health problems in children and adolescents with ID. This tool examines depression, anxiety, ADHD, compulsions, conduct issues, psychotic disorders and ASD. Specific training of 1 day is required to use this tool.

Other mental health tools, specifically developed for people with ID, include:
- PIMRA[6]
- The REISS Screen[7]
- DASH[8]

For information on screening in relation to dementia among people with ID see 📖 Dementia (in people with intellectual disability), p.236.

As medical officers and psychiatrists draw significantly on reports from nurses in making a diagnosis, it is important that nurses are skilled in identifying and reporting the typical and atypical signs and symptoms displayed by this population, as well as the shift from the person's usual pattern of behaviour (baseline).

1 Taggart L, Slevin E (2006). Care planning in mental health settings. In: Gates B (Ed.) *Care Planning and Delivery in Intellectual Disability Nursing.* Chapter 8. Blackwell Science: London.

2 IASSID (2001) *International Association for the Scientific Study of Intellectual Disability Mental Health and Intellectual Disabilities: Addressing the mental health needs of people with intellectual disabilities.* IASSID. Available at 🖥 http://www.iassid.org/

3 Aman MG, Alvarez N, Benefield W, *et al* (2000). Special issue, Expert consensus guideline series: Treatment of psychiatric and behavioural problems in mental retardation. *American Journal on Mental Retardation*, **105**, 159–228.

4 Deb S, Matthews T, Holt G, Bouras N. (2001). *Practice guidelines for the assessment and diagnosis of mental health problems in adults with intellectual disability.* Pavilion Press: Brighton.

5 Moss S (2002). *PAS-ADD Schedules.* Pavilion Press: Brighton.

6 Matson JL, Kazdin AE, Senatore V (1984). Psychometric properties of the psychopathology instrument for mental retarded adults (PIMRA). *American Journal on Mental Retardation*, **5**, 881–889.

7 Reiss S (1988). *Reiss Screen for maladaptive behaviours.* IDS: Worthington, OH.

8 Matson JL, Gardner WI, Coe DA, Sovner RR (1991). A scale for evaluating emotional disorders in severely and profoundly mentally retarded persons: development of the Diagnostic Assessment for the Severely Handicapped (DASH) scale. *British Journal of Psychiatry*, **159**, 404–409.

Assessment of independence and social functioning

The need to assess independence and social functioning

Social competence and social functioning have long been used as a functional means of deciding whether a person has an ID. These concepts relate to peoples' ability to develop skills of independence, and living as a member of society. However, impairments in social competence are not exclusively shown by people with ID, and may be due as much to lack of opportunity as to intellectual functioning. More recently, *Valuing People*[1] reinforced the need for people with ID to develop independence as an entitlement.

In order to help service users identify their independence learning needs it is sometimes helpful to use a skills assessment checklist. A number of these were developed in the 1980s (e.g. Bereweeke Skills Teaching Checklist, Hampshire Assessment for Living with Others [HALO], Pathways to Independence) but, at the time of writing, now seem to be unavailable. Those that are currently available are described below.

Vineland Adaptive Behaviour Scale-II

VABS-II is a comprehensive assessment scale of US origin, and covers personal and social skills from birth to adulthood. These are broken down into the following domains and subdomains:
• Communication—receptive, expressive and written
• Daily living skills—personal, domestic and community
• Socialization—interpersonal relationships, play and leisure time, coping skills
• Motor skills—fine motor, gross motor
• Maladaptive behaviour index (optional)—internalizing, externalizing, other.

A range of assessment forms are available:
• Survey Interview Form and Expanded Interview Form—assessment using a semi-structured interview format
• Parent/Caregiver Rating Form—assessment using a rating scale format
• Teacher Rating Form—assessment in school or day-care setting using a questionnaire format.

VABS-II Survey Forms ASSIST is a computer software program designed to calculate scores and print report forms.

Ordering or more information on VABS-II is available from:
🖳 http://ags.pearsonassessments.com

The American Association of Mental Retardation Adaptive Behaviour Scale (2nd edition)

ABS-RC:2 is of US origin and is perhaps better known for the assessment of challenging behaviour. However, the Part One Domain Scores cover a basic list of independence skills in checklist form under the following areas:
• Independent functioning—self-care and community mobility
• Physical development—vision, hearing, gross and fine motor skills

- Economic activity—money, budgeting and purchasing
- Language development—writing, reading, speech, comprehension
- Numbers and time—basic numeracy and understanding of time
- Domestic activity—cleaning, laundry and food preparation
- Prevocational/vocational activity—job complexity, work performance, work habits
- Self-direction—initiative, passivity, attention span, persistence
- Responsibility—personal belongings, general and personal responsibility
- Socialization—cooperation, social skills, social maturity.

Ordering or more information on ABS-RC:2 materials is available from 🖳 http://www.proedinc.com

The Ordinary Living Framework

This framework is part of the *Assessment Frameworks for Learning Disability Practice* and is comprised of a number of skills for independence using a menu of assessment questions, rather than a checklist. The framework is designed to be person-centred, and encourages the nurse to explore 'things I can do for myself' together with 'things I need to learn' under the following headings:

- Being a parent (if appropriate)
- Being a woman/being a man
- Being happy—having good mental health
- Being part of my family
- Being part of my neighbourhood
- Being part of my religion and culture
- Being well—having good physical health
- Choosing what I want
- Doing a job
- Eating and drinking
- Feeling safe
- Getting around
- Having a home of my own (including looking after my home)
- Having fun with friends
- Learning new things
- Looking good and keeping clean
- Managing money
- People in my life
- Saying how I feel
- Sleeping, resting and relaxing
- Talking to people

A full version of the Ordinary Living Framework (Version 5) is available as part of the *Assessment Frameworks for Learning Disability Practice* package from John Aldridge, The University of Northampton. Email john.aldridge@northampton.ac.uk

1 Department of Health (2001). *Valuing People: a New Strategy for Learning Disability in the 21st Century.* Cmnd 5086. HMSO: London.

Measurement of IQ

The IQ test is the main method used today for measuring a person's intelligence or mental ability. It measures a variety of different types of ability such as:
- Verbal
- Mathematical
- Spatial
- Memory
- Reasoning.

In 1905, a French psychologist by the name of Alfred Binet, working with a physician associate, Theodore Simon, developed the Binet Simon Test designed to measure intelligence. Debate surrounds the validity of the IQ test, as well as the cultural and linguistic problems in developing and completing such a test.

Many see IQ tests as an assessment of a person's problem-solving ability rather than general intelligence. However, IQ tests are not even a comprehensive test of someone's mental ability. Although they may assess analytical and verbal aptitude well, they are not an accurate test of creativity, practical knowledge, and other skills involved in mental ability. Despite this, IQ tests today are still widely used to assess people's intelligence.

Obtaining IQ scores

The IQ test has been conducted on a large sample that is representative of the wider population. The average or mean score of the population has been found to be approximately 100. This indicates that about half of the population's IQ scores fall below the mean, likewise half of the population's IQ scores fall above the mean.

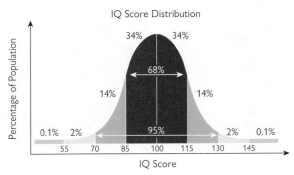

Fig. 4.1 Normal distribution of IQ scores. From www.iqscorenow.com, with permission from Alexander Roulinski.

When the IQ scores of a representative population are pictorially drawn, this graph takes on a 'bell shape' appearance—known as the 'bell shape curve'. You can see from Fig. 4.1 that most people are distributed around the mean, indicating average intelligence, and few people are at the extreme ends of the curve. This is also known as the 'normal distribution curve'.

As previously identified that the mean IQ score is 100, variations from the mean are measured in standard deviations (SD). There are 3 SD below the mean and 3 SD above the mean. 1 SD equals 15 points.

Classification of intellectual disability

In addition to IQ, ID must also be assessed by significant deficits in adaptive functioning. The concept of these adaptive/social functioning competencies relates to everyday life and how the person copes with the demands of his/her own environment (see 📖 Adaptive behaviour rating scales, p.82). This assessment identifies the degree of assistance required by the person in providing the appropriate care and support to live in his/her own social environment. Consequently, classification systems universally agree that three core criteria should be used in making a diagnosis of an ID. These are:

- Significant impairment of intellectual functioning
- Significant impairment of adaptive/social functioning (of at least 2 or more adaptive skills (i.e. communication, self-care, home living, social skills, community use, health and safety, leisure, work)
- Age of onset before 18yrs.

Levels of intellectual disability

According to ICD-10 and DSM-4, there are 4 levels of ID; these are based on standardized IQ scores (i.e. at least 2 SD below the mean).[1,2] Adaptive behaviour should also be included in making the classification.

- Mild ID—IQ 50–70
- Moderate ID—IQ 35–49
- Severe ID—IQ 20–34
- Profound ID—IQ <20.

It is important to remember, however, that the level of one's intelligence does not decide what a person can learn, but may give an indication of how fast they may learn it. It is largely the opportunities for learning presented to people that determine what they will learn.

Further reading

Emerson E, Hatton C, Bromley J, Caine A (1998). *Clinical Psychology and people with Intellectual Disabilities*. Wiley Publications: Chichester.

1 World Health Organization (1992). *ICD-10 Classification of Mental and Behavioural Disorders: Clinical descriptions and diagnostic guidelines*. WHO: Geneva.

2 American Psychiatric Association (1994). *Diagnostic and Statistical Manual of Mental Disorders*, 4th edn. APA: Arlington.

Capacity and consent

'Mental capacity' (often referred to as 'capacity') refers to the legal competence of adults (those 16yrs or over) to make their own major decisions. It is not generally concerned with the important (but more simple) day-to-day choices, such as what to wear or what to eat. Some people lack capacity as a result of an illness or disability e.g. resulting from a mental health need, a cardiovascular accident (stroke), or Alzheimer's disease or dementia.

It is important to understand that a lack of capacity may be a permanent or a temporary state. It also varies according to the level of the decision being made. Formal (usually written) consent is required to indicate a willingness to have surgery, whereas other interventions (e.g. blood pressure monitoring) do not require formal consent. Some people with ID may lack capacity, but many do not.

It is a requirement to assume that all people have capacity, and only where there is doubt to assess; it is important that incapacity is never just assumed. Presenting information in a format and manner that it is understood is essential to this process. Assessments of capacity should be 'decision specific'. This means that the test should be undertaken at the time an important decision needs to be made. If there is doubt about a person's capacity (for example if, even after support with making the decision, the person presents as confused or disorientated) then a judgement must be made as to whether their current condition is affecting their ability to make the decision. At this point a test for capacity would be undertaken to assess the following:

• Does the person understand the information and the implications of making or not making a decision, and can they retain this information?
• Are they able to use information given to weigh up the benefits or disbenefits of making or not making a particular decision?
• Can they (possibly with the use of technology or alternative methods) communicate their decision?

Once a person has been assessed as lacking capacity then any decisions taken on their behalf must be informed by 'best interest' principles. Best interests will always depend on the individual and so will vary from one person to the next. The Mental Capacity Act (2005) gives a checklist of key factors that must be taken into consideration at such times (for example to consider what the person might decide for him/herself if he or she was able). A 'decision-maker' will be nominated (possibly the main care giver or professional involved). This individual must keep records to show how they came to the decision they did having weighed up the (possibly competing) views of others involved. The Independent Mental Capacity Advocate Service (IMCA) now exists to intervene where there are disputes regarding best interests, or if there is no one available to support the person.

Consent

To give consent means to give permission for something to happen or to agree to do something. 'Informed consent' implies that this permission is given by the person with the knowledge of any likely consequences.

Sometimes consent needs to be ascertained and recorded formally (such as when in hospital giving consent for surgery). At other times consent can be implied. For example, consenting to a sexual act can be inferred from manifesting behaviour that encourages rather than discourages the advance. Sometimes people with ID who lack capacity also lack the ability to give consent.

A person has the right under common law to give or withhold consent for medical examination, or treatment, or for any other matter that is important to them (e.g. to decide where to live and who to live with). A person who has capacity has the right to make their own decision irrespective of whether this is the course of action that a health or social care professional would advocate for them. (For example: A doctor recommends to a patient that they have a course of chemotherapy for treatment of a cancerous tumour, and outlines the likely side effects. Having considered the information given the patient refuses treatment. In such a scenario the patient's right is sacrosanct.)

Where a patient who requires treatment lacks the ability to give or withhold consent then the best interest principles must apply. It is essential that where any intervention is reliant on the giving of consent those who are incapacitated are not disadvantaged. So any procedure, treatment or medical intervention must be considered to be in the best interests of the person, and recorded on a consent form particularly designed to record decisions about adults who are unable to consent. In complex cases, or where there may be a dispute regarding the best course of action, it may be advisable to seek a second medical opinion or the involvement of the IMCA.

When working with vulnerable people, it is most important that professionals (including doctors) are alert to the possibility of acquiescence. This differs from consent and suggests permission may be uninformed and given reluctantly yet without protest.

Further reading

England: www.dh.gov.uk

                                  http://www.justice.gov.uk/

Scotland: The Mental Health (Care & Treatment) Act Scotland, 2003

Northern Ireland: www.dhsspsni.gov.uk/public_health_consent

Republic of Ireland: The Irish Mental Health Act, 2001

Risk assessment

Context

Alberg et al have described risk as 'possibility of beneficial and harmful consequences likely to occur'.[1] This is an important definition as it highlights that exposure to risk may also bring about beneficial benefits to an individual with ID. However, exposure to risk will only benefit those where there is a systematic approach to identifying through assessment and managing any harmful risks within a person-centred way. For many years some people with ID have not been supported to grow and develop into independent individuals, as some people and services have adopted a risk-averse approach to care.

The recent publication *A Life Like No Other*[2] highlighted a number of concerns around the way people were supported, such as the use of locked doors, restrictive practices, lack of choice, and lack of understanding in safeguarding people's rights. The authors made a number of recommendations, including the promotion of the use of risk assessments to ensure a personalized approach to care.

Key perspectives in risk assessment

- Duty of care
- Balancing the risks of everyday living
- Least restrictive approaches
- Not being unduly risk averse
- Partnership in identifying
- Using a systematic approach
- Balancing risk and quality of life
- Leadership and training
- Ensuring people's rights are maintained
- Exploring ethical issues.

Key principles of risk assessment

- Organizations should have procedures for assessing and managing risk
- Training should be provided to enable those supporting people to be competent and practice safely when assessing risk
- Those supporting people need to be able to identify possible risks
- Individuals needs to be supported in making decisions about risks in their lives involving family, carers, and partners when necessary
- Risk assessment should be incorporated within the person-centred planning processes
- We should always consider that the person has capacity until demonstrated otherwise
- We should always consider less restrictive options
- People are entitled to make decisions that we may not agree with or make ourselves, and the role of the ID nurse would be to ensure the individual has the capacity to understand the consequences of their actions and the impact upon others
- We should always clearly document all discussions and decisions when assessing and managing risk.

Risk assessment

When undertaking a risk assessment, individual organizations may have their own assessment criteria/assessment tool to support the risk assessment process. There are a number of recognized assessment tools being used; e.g. FACE[3] tools associated with CPA, and Modified Sainsbury Tool.[4]

ID nurses could easily align the process for supporting people with assessing and managing risk within the stages of the nursing process. The key principle must be that this is conducted in a person-centred way.

People involved in working with people with ID may encounter varying degrees of risks for the people who they support. This may include:

• Risks of everyday living (road safety, access to kitchens/bathrooms, lifestyles)
• Health conditions (epilepsy, dysphagia)
• Relationships
• Mental health or offending behaviours
• Vulnerability
• Inequalities in accessing services.

Therefore, the consequences will also vary in degree according to the identified risk. We should never start from the point that the identified activity poses too many risks and therefore will not be considered. People's lives should not necessarily be restricted, as we all take risks as part of everyday living; a life without risk may be impoverished and may prevent a person from living an ordinary life. However, when supporting someone, we cannot ignore identified risks that may cause harm to the individual or others, but need to support them in determining the associated risks in order for them to explore new opportunities. Risk assessment would be a key tool in achieving this.

Further reading

Vallenga D, Grypdonck MH, Tan FI, Lendemeijer BH, Boon PA (2006). Decision making about risk in people with epilepsy and intellectual disability. *Journal of Advanced Nursing.* **54**(5): 602–11.

1 Alberg C, Bingley W, Brown L, Ferguson G, Hatfield B, Hoban A, Maden A (1996). *Learning Materials on Mental Health Risk Assessment.* University of Manchester: Manchester.

2 Healthcare Commission (2007). *A Life Like No Other: a national audit of specialist inpatient health-care services for people with learning difficulties in England.* Healthcare Commission: London.

3 Functional Analysis in the Care Environment (FACE) (2006). 🖳 www.face.eu.com [accessed April 2009]

4 Stein W (2005). Modified Sainsbury tool: an initial risk assessment tool for primary care mental health and learning disability services. *Journal of Psychiatric and Mental Health Nursing* **12**, 620–633.

Quality of life

Context

The past 25 years have seen many significant changes in the way that people with ID receive care and support. The White Paper *Valuing People* in England focused on four key principles; these are rights, choice, independence, and inclusion.[1] The other countries of the UK have also published their own policy documents, which have an impact on the direction on the quality of life for people with ID. The recurring principles within these policy documents across the UK and Ireland highlight the need to promote a high quality of life for people with ID, with an emphasis on inclusion in decision and society.

Autonomy

When considering assessing quality of life for people with ID, the indicators produced by BILD could be used as a framework (Table 4.1). These focus on individual autonomy, and giving control on choices of how to lead their life.

It is important when using these indicators that risk issues are contextualized within the assessment, and people are supported to experience new things in a safe way.

Communication

A key challenge when thinking about assessing quality of life issues through person-centred planning is how we communicate with the individual. Good communication depends on a number of factors (Table 4.2).

Evidence-based approach

A thorough assessment and understanding of the communication needs of the individual will enhance the outcomes for them.

When considering tools to assess a person's quality of life it is important that the nurse adopts an evidence-based approach, and also involving families, friends, other professionals, and agencies. When adopting a person-centred approach, the nurse should be aware of the evidence available that supports this.[4] When identifying quality of life outcomes for people it is essential that possible resource implications are identified and costed. In relation to health needs, with the advent of the Disability Discrimination Act (2005) it is clear that there should be no discrimination for people in terms of rationing health resources for people with ID on the basis of quality of life judgements. If nurses witness this or are unhappy about decisions being made about quality of life measurements, then they have a duty of care to challenge this.

It is recognized that for a good quality of life, the individual's health is a key component. *Valuing People Now*[5] has identified better health as a key priority. *A Life Like No Other*[6] (report of national audit of ID services) identified that for some people, the results of a good health action plan can singularly transform their quality of life. While some people may continue to have long-term health conditions, providing the appropriate health interventions and support are available to the individual, this should not impact on the quality of life for those individuals.

Table 4.4 Assessing quality of life for people with intellectual disabilities. From Hatton.[2] Adapted from the findings in the Healthcare Commission Report, *A Life Like No Other* (2007).

Access	I have full access with support if necessary within my environment
Advocacy	If I need support from someone independent I can access this and we are listened to
Day to day life	I have choices in the activities that i undertake
Finance	I have access to my money
Friends and family	I have supported to keep contact with family and friends and to develop new friendships
Independence and choice	I am supported to make choices and these are presented in a way that I can understand
Person Centred Approach	I have developed my person centred plan which includes my health needs which supports me in living my life
Safety	I feel safe in my environment

Table 4.5 Communication for person-centred planning. From Grove.[3]

How well can you hear?
How well can you see?
How comfortable are you feeling?
How alert and attentive are you?
How well can you understand what is happening?
How well can you express yourself to someone else?
How interested and motivated are you to communicate?

Further reading

Brown I and Brown RI (2003) *Quality of life and disability: an approach for community practitioners.* Jessica Kingsley: London.

1 Department of Health (2001). *Valuing People: a New Strategy for Learning Disability in the 21st Century.* Cmnd 5086. HMSO: London.

2 Hatton C, Ager A (2002). Quality of life measurement and people with intellectual disabilities: a reply to Cummins. *Journal of Applied Research in Intellectual Disabilities* **15**(3), 254–260.

3 Grove N (2005). *Communication for Person-Centred Planning.* Foundation for People with Learning Disabilities. ▣ www.learningdisabilities.org.uk

4 Holborn S, Jacobson J, Schwartz A, Flory M, Vietze P (2004). The Willowbrook Futures Project: A longitudinal analysis of person-centered planning. *American Journal on Mental Retardation* **109**: 63–76.

5 Department of Health (2007) *Valuing People Now. From Progress to Transformation.* Department of Health: London.

6 Healthcare Commission (2007). *A Life Like No Other: a national audit of specialist in patient healthcare services for people with learning difficulties in England.* Healthcare Commission: London.

Life experiences

The focus of ID policy is on the individuals' rights and inclusion in the UK and Ireland. Inclusion should be linked to opportunities for greater range of life experiences, including positive health, social activities, and meaningful activities.

An obstacle to enhancing the life experiences of people with ID can be the perceived risks associated with ordinary living and the opportunity to experience new things. A key finding of the recent Healthcare Commission report *A Life Like No Other*[1] found that there was little evidence suggesting that people's independence is being promoted, and that a number of people were having restrictions placed on them within their homes, in some cases with no access to drinks or snacks without requesting them from staff. It is important to ensure that risk plans in these circumstances should facilitate enhancing life experiences and reducing any restrictions.

Putting people in control

Poll et al. identified one of the main complaints of people who receive services was that they have little, if any control over what services they are to receive and how these services are to be delivered, with a prevailing attitude that the professional or public servant knows best.[2] The report illustrated that being in control is truly life enhancing for the individual concerned, and we all have a responsibility to explore how people can be given real choice and control over the services they receive and how they live their lives.

Person-centred approaches

The key guiding principle for nurses supporting individuals is to approach their care with the central aim of ensuring that the individual is in control of all that happens for them and to them. A key model to facilitate this should be the use of person-centred approaches.

When assessing a person's abilities and needs, the nurse should ensure that all aspects of the individual's life are included. For example, there have been a number of publications which have identified that people with ID have poor life experiences in relation to the health and care they receive (Disability Rights Commission,[3] Mencap[4]). Also, they encounter hate-crime and difficulties with getting a job, as identified within the *Learning Disability Task Force Annual Report* 2006–7.[5]

Enhancing people's life experiences brings with it the risks of people being financially, physically, or sexually exploited. It is important to ensure that risk assessment addresses these issues in a non-paternalistic way, and that local safeguarding policies and procedures are respected, and communicated to the person with ID, and staff.

There are a number of models and guiding principles in supporting nurses to ensure that they take a person-centred approach to assessing people's life experiences (see Table 4.1).

Nurses can demonstrate that they can make a real difference in moving from the headline of the Healthcare Commission Report, *A Life Like No Other*, to enable people to live an equal life *like others*.

Table 4.6 Guiding principles to support people in their life experiences.

Human Rights Act (1998)	Person-centred planning (BILD 2002)
• Make choices about my life • Expect people to listen • Get information about rights • Speak out and complain if something is wrong • Be safe • Choose the people I want to see and who my friends are • Get married (and civil partnership) and have children • Live with people I get on with • Decide what I spend my money on and get paid for the work I do	• I am the centre—person-centred planning is rooted in the principles of rights, independence, inclusion, and choice • My family members and friends are full partners—Person-centred planning puts people in context of their family and communities • Person-centred planning reflects my capacities, what is important to me • Person-centred planning builds a shared commitment to action that recognizes a person's rights • Person-centred planning leads to continual listening, learning and action, and helps the person get what they want out of life
Valuing People Now (2007)[6]	Adapted from *In Control (2006)*[2]
• People have more choice and control over their lives and services (personalisation) • What people do in the days and evening—including getting a paid job • People being healthy and getting a good service from the NHS • People having more choices about where they live • Make sure that *Valuing People* happens for everyone	• I know how much money I am able to receive in a personalised budget • I can use the money in the way that suits me best • I have a person centred assessment and support plan • I can decide how to spend my money • I can arrange personal support to help me do the things I choose • I can live my life to the full • I can change things when I need to

1 Healthcare Commission (2007). *A Life Like No Other: a national audit of specialist inpatient health-care services for people with learning difficulties in England*. Healthcare Commission: London.

2 Poll C, Duffy S, Hatton C, Sanderson H, Routledge M (2006). *A report on In Control's first phase*. In Control Publications: London.

3 Disability Rights Commission (DRC) (2006). *Equal Treatment: Closing the Gap. A formal investigation into physical health inequalities experienced by people with learning disabilities and/or mental health problems*. DRC: London.

4 Mencap (2007). *Death by indifference*. Mencap: London.

5 Learning Disability Task Force (2007). *Learning Disability Task Force Annual Report 2006–7*. Learning Disability Task Force.

6 Department of Health (2007). *Valuing People Now. From Progress to Transformation*. Department of Health: London.

Diagnostic overshadowing

The risks of 'diagnostic overshadowing'[1] is used to describe instances when a healthcare professional makes an association of presenting signs to a previously diagnosed major condition. Thus, there is the potential for failure to recognize and treat another new condition.[2]

For a person with ID, diagnostic overshadowing is seen to occur when a healthcare professional makes an assumption that the presenting signs and symptoms are associated with the already diagnosed condition of ID. Holland suggests that "the problem of diagnostic overshadowing, and of diminishing changes in behaviour, personality or ability that would be taken very seriously in a person without a learning disability are particularly relevant with dementia".

Factors influencing diagnostic overshadowing

People with ID experience greater ill health with regards to both acute and chronic illness, and their attendance at acute general hospitals is greater than that of the general population, though their actual periods spent within hospitals is less. Even though people with ID are high users of health services, evidence shows that many healthcare professionals within acute hospitals have neither been educated in nor have experience working with people with ID.

A lack of knowledge and understanding of the nature of ID, their healthcare, needs assessment, and poor recognition that the presentation of illness may be different in this population, increases this risk. Indeed a diagnosis of ID in itself can result in staff failing to notice fundamental reasons for the signs and symptoms presented.

Up to 50% of people with ID experience problems communicating, increasing their difficulties expressing their health need/s, and healthcare professionals experience challenges communicating effectively with individuals who have communication difficulties. For those with severe or profound ID, their main means of communicating may be through vocalizations, facial expressions, postural movements, or other behaviours. Families and close carers often recognize these as signs of distress, though they experience difficulty in getting their voice heard when advocating for the person.

Consequences of diagnostic overshadowing

Unrecognized health problems remain untreated and the potential consequences of diagnostic overshadowing could be very serious, even fatal for some people with ID.[4] If signs of distress are not recognized, or signs and symptoms are unrecognized or not validated and attributed to the ID, then the risk of harm to the person is increased.

In addition, the term 'differential diagnosis' is the term used to describe the range of possible clinical diagnoses that may result from the person's history; if the full range of potential causes is not investigated then there is a risk of wrong diagnosis, which may also have serious consequences for the individual.

Reducing the risk of diagnostic overshadowing

- See the individual first, before the ID
- Understand that all behaviour is communicative and is telling us something
- Understand that the presentation of illness may be different in a person with ID
- Seek various ways in which to communicate, and communicate with the individual in the first instance
- Understand the role of the family and carers in helping with the assessment
- If a person is presenting with a new behaviour, or an existing behaviour has intensified consider:
  - Physical problems—pain or discomfort, people with ID experience the same range of health problems as the general population, from toothache to oesophagitis
  - Psychiatric cause—mental health problems may be present
  - Social cause—change in carers, bereavement, abuse.
- Be aware of the assessment tools to gain understanding, such as pain scales and distress assessment tools
- Seek consent for examination, treatment, and care, using appropriate guidelines to aid decision making
- Recognize that people with ID are at risk of over investigation, due to poor communication, which can impact on their safety
- However, decisions to withhold investigation or treatments due to poor communication can compromise the individual's health.[5,6]

1 Reiss S, Syzszko J (1983). Diagnostic overshadowing and professional experience with mentally retarded persons. *American Journal of Mental Deficiency* **87**: 396–402.

2 Sudheim TP, Ryan RM (1999). Amnesic syndrome presenting as malingering in a man with developmental disability. *Psychiatric Service* **50**: 966–988.

3 Holland AJ (2000). Ageing and Learning Diability. *British Journal of Psychiatry* **176**:26–31.

4 Sowney M, Brown M (2007). People with learning disabilities: issues for accident and emergency practitioners. In: Dolan B and Holt L. *Accident and Emergency. Theory into Practice.* Baillière Tindall: London.

5 Mencap (2007). *Death by Indifference.* Mencap: London.

6 National Patient Safety Agency (2004). *Understanding the Patient Safety Issues for People with Learning Disabilities.* National Health Service: London.

Changes across the lifespan

Antenatal screening and diagnosis

Prenatal programmes aimed at the general population use ultrasound scanning and biochemical analysis as screening tools to identify pregnancies at high risk of chromosomal disorders or polygenic disorders, such as neural tube defects. There have been many developments in screening for genetic disorders in pregnancy. Whether such screening programmes are deemed successful or not depends on consideration of the appropriate aims and outcomes of these programmes. If the primary aim is to reduce the birth frequency of a serious medical disorder, then some can be considered to have been a 'success', but if the aim is to provide maximum choice, information, and support to women, couples and/or their families, then outcomes are perhaps more questionable.[1]

In any form of ID associated with a genetic condition or disorder, unless a specific diagnosis has been made for the cause of ID no specific prenatal diagnostic testing for the condition will be available. If laboratory-based genetic diagnosis in the presenting affected family member or a known carrier of the disorder has identified the causative gene change or alteration (gene mutation) for the condition, specific prenatal diagnostic tests are likely to be available to the family. If the causative gene mutation in the family has been found and identified, prenatal diagnosis by CVS or amniocentesis is possible. However, both CVS and amniocentesis are invasive procedures with an associated risk of miscarriage of 1–3% regardless of whether the pregnancy is affected or unaffected.

In the case of X-linked ID, where no mutation has been identified, if precise prenatal testing is not available it may be possible to offer sex selection, by CVS or amniocentesis, and termination of male offspring. However, the fact that such testing cannot distinguish between affected and unaffected males, and the possible risks of an affected female child should be explained carefully to individuals seeking testing for sex selection.[2] Parents should also have the opportunity, through effective genetic counselling, to explore ethical aspects that may be relevant to them in relation to sex selection and other decisions, including the continuation of pregnancy.

Further reading

Further information for parents considering or having another pregnancy can be sought by contacting local Genetic or Obstetric Centres, or consulting online resources such as:

AnSWer (Antenatal Screening Web Resource)
www.antenataltesting.info

Antenatal Results and Choices (ARC)
www.arc-uk.org

BDF Newlife (formerly Birth Defects Foundation)
www.bdfnewlife.co.uk

1 Harper P (2004). *Practical Genetic Counselling*. 6th Edn. Arnold: London.

2 Firth HV, Hurst JA (2005). *Oxford Desk Reference: Clinical Genetics*. Oxford University Press: Oxford.

Supporting people during transition

Transition is normal and happens to everyone, not just people with ID, although there may be additional challenges and difficulties in successfully achieving this process. Transition may be defined as a passage or change from one state or set of circumstances to another. Life events, including forming and dissolving relationships, and changes in health status or physical appearance (e.g. puberty) result in external changes that may require major internal adjustment. Change is an inevitable part of living, is often stressful, and can have both positive and negative effects.

Adopting a life cycle approach to ID services and interventions highlights transition as a key theme for the individual, their parents, and paid or informal supporters.

Examples of transitional events
- Recognition of difficulties leading to diagnosis
- Accessing or changing services
- Moving home.

Such transitions may be recurring rather than discrete issues. Recognizing this can help anticipate and understand physical and psychological responses at transitional points. For example, while the safe arrival of a first grandchild into a family is generally joyous, it may simultaneously trigger longing in the individual with ID for a relationship, partner or child, painful memories for their parents, and feelings of guilt or sadness for siblings. Transitions often involve loss, and the potential for successive losses to accumulate and multiply should be acknowledged. There may also be conflict between the right of the individual, for example to greater independence, and parental wishes or fears.

In recent years, discussion of transition has increasingly focused on the particular journey between child and adulthood for people with ID, their families and services (see 📖 School-aged children, p.116).

Transition has been highlighted by successive UK government policy as worthy of targeting for these groups.

Transitional issues for people with intellectual disabilities
- Difficulty understanding the need for change and ability to visualize abstract alternatives
- Barriers to articulating or otherwise communicating views and feelings to others
- Limited information and involvement in planned changes
- Increased likelihood of spending time in shared settings
  - Changes designed for benefit of some may have adverse effects on others
  - Staff turnover.

Some transitions may involve giving bad news, and this is never easy, but withholding information on the basis that it is upsetting (e.g. bereavement) may amount to overprotection that denies personhood. People with ID can be helped to express normal grief. Supporters should also be alert to changes in physical or emotional health that suggest potentially maladaptive responses to transitions, and take appropriate action.

People with ID have a right to be involved in decisions affecting their lives and to make choices. Some conditions associated with ID, e.g. ASDs (see 📖 Chapter 8, pp.249–292), may lead to particular family and staff concerns, which should be explored. Timely introduction of planned change can allow for anticipatory grief reactions and promote adjustment. Provision of accessible and concrete information, constant support, reassurance and empathy are important components of supporting people with ID during transition.

Further reading

Department of Health (2001). *Valuing People: A New Strategy for Learning Disability for the 21st Century*. Cm 5086 HMSO: London.

Department of Health and Social Services and Public Safety (2005). *Equal Lives: Review of Policies and Services for People with Learning Disability in Northern Ireland*. DHSSPS: Belfast.

National Assembly for Wales (2001). *Fulfilling the Promises: Proposal for a Framework for Services for People with Learning Disabilities*. Learning Disability Advisory Group: Cardiff.

Scottish Executive (2000). *The Same as You? A Review of Services for People with Learning Disabilities*. Scottish Executive: Edinburgh.

Preschool children

The preschool years (0–5yrs) are generally characterized by major physical, social, and emotional growth; subsequently an understanding of child development is beneficial to those working in services supporting children and their families. This not only promotes early recognition of developmental difficulties in order that appropriate support can be offered, but also potentially enhances a practitioner's understanding of the psychosocial family adaptations that may be required as a result. Timely interventions that target primary conditions can also prevent or inhibit development of secondary disabilities.

Prenatal, perinatal, and postnatal periods

Where a chromosomal or genetic condition with a degree of inherent ID (see 📖 Common conditions among people with intellectual disability, p.16) is identified during pregnancy, or suspected following delivery, diagnosis should be confirmed in infancy. Children for whom there were no developmental concerns during the pregnancy, but who were born prematurely or experienced difficulties during the labour or delivery should be monitored for early indications in case they are not progressing to achieve the normal milestones. Identification of hypothyroidism or PKU as a result of taking blood from the baby's heel in the first few days of life should ensure that action can be taken in the form of medication or diet to reduce the risk of ID. Babies born to women who have misused substances (such as opiates) during pregnancy also require follow-up after possible withdrawal treatment.

Building relationships with adults to support preschool children amid chaotic lifestyles can be particularly challenging for practitioners. Although ID may imply added vulnerability, preschool children with ID are children first; their welfare remains paramount, and action may be needed to safeguard them (see 📖 Child protection, p.268).

Preschool children with no preceding reason to be alert to their development will be offered routine surveillance from primary health services, for example health visitors (see 📖 Health visitors, p.336), and parents should feel able to explore concerns with their family doctor without fear of being labeled over-anxious. Where potential problems are identified, referral for more specialized assessment (e.g. Griffiths Developmental Scales), should be made.

Possible outcomes

- Global delay
- Delays in areas which may be associated with ID, but not necessarily indicative of (e.g. language or motor skills)
  - Action to exclude other explanations should be taken, e.g. hearing tests in relation to delayed language or unusual behaviour.

Ultimately, ID may be suspected, but not confirmed, in the preschool period. Alternatively, a different diagnosis may be offered, for example cerebral palsy or ASD, where ID may emerge, or not.

Table 5.1 Examples of alerts to the potential for intellectual disability

Period	Alert	Action
Prenatal	Chromosomal or genetic condition suspected via blood tests, ultrasound scanning or identified via chorionic villous sampling (CVS), amniocentesis	Offer information including support groups, e.g. Down's Syndrome Association (DSA), seek early confirmation after birth, follow-up
Perinatal	Premature or difficult birth	Offer information, support, treatment as appropriate, follow-up
Postnatal	Acute illness where inflammation of the brain or dehydration may occur; accident, e.g. road traffic, fall from height	Treat as indicated, follow-up

Involvement with a maze of professionals and services, either to reach diagnosis or consequent to diagnosis, can be bewildering, even without the emotion likely to accompany such a journey. For this reason the use of shared assessments and the appointment of a key-worker or link-worker (acting as co-coordinator and single point of contact) to preschool children with ID and their families, has for some time been advocated. Practitioners should be aware that any solutions they may offer at this stage may have hidden implications for the future. Short break services away from home may provide a real lifeline, but have potential to disrupt emotional bonds; reliance on special services may preclude later use of ordinary facilities.

Adopting a consistent, practical approach to managing toddlers, including developing healthy sleep patterns, regular meal times, and toilet routines, is no less important for preschool children with ID than their peers, although it may be challenged by communication difficulties and family distress. If it is accepted that all preschool children have similar basic needs (e.g. for affection, security, nourishment, play), then inclusion into ordinary nurseries and other children's provision, with extra support where required, could be easiest at a time where differences are less pronounced.

Further reading

Contact a Family: for families with disabled children ⬚ www.cafamily.org.uk

Down's Syndrome Association ⬚ www.downs-syndrome.org.uk

School-aged children

The statutory right to education is now well established for every child, including children with the most profound ID who were previously excluded. In some areas, for example Finland and various American States, the school entry age is 7yrs, while in England the current legal requirement is for children to be educated between 5yrs and 16yrs of age, with initiatives promoting continuance to 18yrs and beyond. In reality many children enter full-time Reception classes shortly after their 4th birthday (i.e. in the school year during which they will be 5yrs), or attend preschool facilities half-time from 3yrs. Even prior to this, day nurseries and child minders are inspected against educational standards, e.g. by the Office for Standards in Education, Children's Services and Skills (Ofsted).

Starting school is recognized in our culture as a rite of passage. Children with diagnosed or suspected ID may have been protected from direct comparisons with peers, but at this point difficulties may be brought sharply into focus. In other cases ID will be recognized for the first time.

Society is increasingly competitive, valuing ability and appearance, and exclusion for the child[1] can occur as a result of failure to conform to expectations. This can affect parents, particularly where their self-esteem is intertwined with their child's achievements. Practitioners should develop their expertise in understanding and supporting this potential emotional impact.

Although the detail of procedures may vary, in Western countries identification of special educational needs (SEN) normally follows a systematic, staged process:

- Possible SEN brought to the attention of the coordinator within provision
- Action
  - Collaboration between parents, teacher, and coordinator; changes made to teaching, extra support or equipment offered
- Action plus
  - As action but with involvement of external specialists, e.g. speech and language therapy service
- Statutory assessment
  - Collects views of child, parents, school, educational psychologist, doctor, social services (if child is known), anyone else the local authority thinks it should get advice from to get a clear picture of child's needs
  - Parents access support and advice from local parent partnership service, voluntary organization, and other parent support groups
- Issuing of statement
  - Sets out child's needs and the help they should have. Reviewed annually to ensure that any extra support given continues to meet child's needs.

Transition planning

At the first annual review following a child's 14th birthday, a transition plan should be made, with the aim of easing the path into adulthood by identifying aspirations for continuing education, occupation, leisure etc, and planning for their availability. Despite increasing efforts to combine this with person-centred planning, it remains a time fraught with potential difficulty for young people and their families. Some services have attempted to address this by appointing dedicated transition teams or workers.

In relation to children with ID, perhaps the greatest, and still hotly debated, issue is the provision of integrated or segregated education in ordinary or special schools. This is often presented as a polarized argument, without recognition that children are individuals. Proponents of social inclusion highlight the rights of all children to be educated together, suggesting that to do so sets a standard for a more inclusive adult life. For example, attending the local school rather than being taken by bus to an area special school may promote children with disabilities building supportive friendships, leisure, and sporting networks in their local communities. This is perhaps seen more in the 5–11yrs group, but less as children progress to larger, faster paced, attainment focused educational provision, where more complex social relationships develop. The potential widening of the gap between teenagers with ID and their peers, and the attendant difficulties, provides for some the impetus to revert back to a more protected, but less integrated (possibly segregated), educational position. Increased use of personal assistance may offer a social counterpoint in such circumstances, promoting maintenance of relationships and activities outside of school.

1 Mencap (2007). *Don't Stick It, Stop It!* Mencap: London.

Adolescents

This turbulent period marks the transition from childhood to adulthood, when physical, psychological, and cognitive changes occur. The development of independence and autonomy is the ultimate aim for all adolescents, including those with ID. For young people it can be overwhelming to come to terms with their personal identity and it may be the first time they begin to perceive themselves as different from their peers. Simultaneously this period of development becomes anxiety provoking for parents, who often express concern regarding their adolescent's rebelliousness, mood swings, and time wasting activities; hence conflict is often the result.

Self-identity

As pubescent changes occur and young people's bodies begin to alter, adolescents begin to question themselves. Coupled with this are the concurrent major changes that adolescents experience, going through puberty, changing school, and the possibility of losing established peer relationships, all impact on young people's ability to cope with everyday pressures.

Family relationships

- Parent–child relationship; are challenged as the adolescent continues to dispute boundaries and family rules
- Relationships with siblings may change as brothers' and sisters' perception of adolescent with ID alters
- Conflicts may arise concerning peers and peer relationships
- Anxieties may occur as parents become concerned for their adolescent's physical safety as risk-taking behaviours increase
- As adolescents strive to become more independent, parents concerns grow regarding their vulnerability to emotional, sexual, and financial abuse.

Health issues relating to adolescence

- Young person may appear clumsy due to accelerated growth rate.
- Nutrition intake becomes important, because if insufficient, intellectual and biological development may be affected
- Energy needs may vary according to gender, age, and puberty
- Eating styles may change (skipping meals) and may need to be encouraged to eat a healthy balanced diet
- Emotional well-being becomes important, as greater incidence of depression is reported, and this is especially so for young people with ID; this is possibly related to hormonal changes[1]
- Adolescents require more sleep because they release a growth hormone during sleep that is essential for their growth spurt.

Considerations for practitioners

- Allow young people the time and opportunity to discuss their fears and anxieties e.g in a group or one-to-one situation
- Provide a rationale and support to families to assist them to comprehend changes in behaviour e.g. where possible, normalize behaviours and put them into context of the young person's development
- Encourage a healthy lifestyle e.g. promote exercise and a balanced diet

- Promote independence across all areas of daily living e.g. assist the young person to develop self-care skills
- Assess risk and promote positive risk taking where appropriate e.g. encourage independent travel.

1 Nehring WM, Faux SA (2005). School-age and adolescence. In: Nehring WM. *Core Curriculum for Specializing in Intellectual Disabilities*. Jones and Bartlett: London.

Puberty

Definitions

The word puberty derives from the Latin *pubertas*, which means the age of manhood. However, the word puberty is now associated with the complex process that involves changes to both male and female bodies. These occur as a result of alterations in hormonal activity. It is particularly important for all young people, including those with ID, to be prepared for the physical, emotional, and psychological changes that occur, so that they know what to expect and therefore have less anxiety.

Onset

Puberty can occur in males as early as 9yrs or as late as 15yrs, and in females from 7yrs up to 14yrs. It is characterized at the age of onset by menstruation in females and testicular enlargement in males. For most young people with ID, physical changes will occur at the same time as their peers. However, for some people with ID, the emotional changes may be delayed by several years.

Physical changes

During puberty numerous physical changes occur in both male and female:

Male
- Testicles and scrotum become larger
- Pubic hair develops
- Penis increases in length and circumference
- Growth and weight spurt occurs
- Spermarche occurs (first ejaculation)
- Body and facial hair develops
- Shoulders become wider and muscle develops
- Body odour and acne can become noticeable
- Larynx becomes bigger and voice becomes deeper.

Female
- Breast buds develop under one or both nipples
- Growth and weight spurt occurs
- Pubic and body hair develops
- ~2yrs after breast development commences, menarche (first menstruation) is experienced
- Body shape alters—the waist appears to become smaller as body fat becomes stored on the hips, buttocks and legs
- Body odour and acne become noticeable
- Menstruation becomes regular as ovaries mature and begin to produce eggs regularly.

Considerations for intellectual disability nursing

- Be prepared to provide advice on hygiene as skin changes occur
- Nutrition and exercise become important issues in maintaining a healthy BMI, the statistical measure of the weight of a person according to height

- Increased aggressive behaviour and mood swings may be reported as some adolescents could test boundaries and others might feel unsure of how to deal with the emotional changes that are occurring
- Provide appropriate material and support parents in educating their children on body changes and sexual development
- The physical changes often occur at a similar chronological age; for some people with ID the emotional changes may be delayed by several years. This may result in physically developed 'adults', who may still lack the accompanying maturity, which may leave them significantly at risk of exploitation or abuse.

Further reading

Coleman JC, Hendry LB (1999). *The Nature of Adolescence*. 3rd edn. Routledge: London.

Adulthood

Definition

Becoming an adult is generally associated with gaining independence and creating your own life. In most countries people are viewed as adults when they reach 18yrs. However, this is not always applied to people with ID. For example, people with ID are often described by the media in relation to their mental age, an approach that places them, in the eyes of society, as perpetual children.

Aspirations

More people with ID, particularly those with profound and multiple disabilities, are surviving into adulthood. At this time people aspire to:

• become more independent
• manage their own finances
• develop close relationships with other adults, including sexual relationships, possibly leading to the birth of children (see 📖 Parents with intellectual disability, p.128)
• engage in meaningful occupation
• choose how, and with whom, to spend free time.

Many people with ID will share these aspirations, but to fulfill these desires will pose a greater challenge for them and their supporters. Hence all efforts should be made to ensure that a person-centred approach is adopted (see 📖 Person-centred planning, p.250).

Transition to adulthood

To aid smooth transition from adolescence to adulthood, the following considerations must be made:

The individual with intellectual disability may find the prospect of adulthood daunting. Alternatively, they may be perceived as having unrealistic expectations, leading others, perhaps unintentionally, to seek to protect them from disappointment. The practitioner's role should be to assist the individual to develop knowledge and skills related to independence, and to respond appropriately to the fears and anxieties associated with positive risk taking (see 📖 Risk management, p.444).

Parents and family may be more protective, citing vulnerability and risk of abuse, perhaps favouring substitute family care (e.g. staffed group homes) over more individualized options. It may distress parents when their son or daughter appears to reject their advice or lifestyle by desiring an alternative. Acknowledging that people with ID are vulnerable to bullying, deliberate harm, and exploitation, can be a first step to building resilience.

Practitioners can experience tension when someone they are supporting, who has capacity, makes decisions that they feel are 'unwise'. The practitioner should collaborate with colleagues and seek supervision to ensure that the approach they take is consistently person-centred.

Proactive interventions

Adults with ID have rights, accompanied by responsibilities; therefore when working with adults, practitioners should:

- provide accessible information (see ⬚ Developing accessible information, p.68)
- assess risk, promoting positive risk taking (see ⬚ Risk assessment, p.100)
- minimize potential for harm.

Specific health issues associated with adulthood

Although evidence suggests that people with ID are likely to have increased health needs (see ⬚ Chapter 6, pp.139–212), there are some health issues that potentially affect all adults, so the nurse should encourage:

- access to primary health surveillance and health promotion services (see ⬚ Primary care, p.220), and support access to secondary provision where required
- regular vision, hearing, and dental checks, to monitor and treat age-related changes
- use of ordinary facilities (e.g. gyms and weight reducing clubs) to facilitate general fitness and weight control
- self-help groups to address issues associated with managing stress and promoting emotional well-being (see ⬚ Promoting emotional well-being, p.216).

Personal relationships

People with ID need to have meaningful and respectful relationships in order to maintain their mental health and well-being; this is the same for every person living within our society. Certainly, with the development of person-centred planning, people's needs are better understood and respected more. The person-centred plan provided the opportunity for people to make choices, develop personal relationships, and be involved within their local community, which for many people had never occurred before, because services sought to protect people from the harshness of life.

It is time spent with friends and family, laughing, enjoying local amenities, and being involved within the community, that are the very things which make life rich for us all. A life without personal relationships can be very limiting and these aspects of a person's life with ID may at times not be fully understood, or ignored. A recent study by Emerson found that many people continued to lack friendships in their lives—2 out of 3 people had contact with friends at least once a year, and 1 in 3 people had no contact with friends.[1] This was also apparent for contact with family members—while 1 in 3 people saw a family member every year, 1 in 5 people never saw their family, and 1 in 20 people had no friends and did not see anyone from their family.

What are the barriers to developing or maintaining relationships?

- A person's family may have problems with travelling or live too far away. This should always be taken into consideration when people move away from home or move into residential/assessment or treatment services
- Not enough time—people working and/or have other family commitments
- Lack of money—the costs of travelling and social functions can be prohibitive
- Not enough support—a person with high support needs may need extra support to be able to go out, as they need help with toileting or need more than one person to support them
- People cannot get out or are too ill to be able to leave the home
- People are afraid to get out or leave the home.

What could you do differently?

- Always seek to support and maintain friendships and relationships with family members; ensure that this is part of the person-centred plan
- Always think about what would be in the person's best interests when a care home move is being considered
- Support the person to maintain contact with family and friends; this might be by supporting writing letters, sending photographs, video clips, text messages or emails.

---

1 Emerson E, Malam S, Davies I, Spencer K (2005). *Adults with Learning Disabilities in England 2003/4*. National Statistics: London.

Marriage and family life

People with ID have the same rights in law to marry as others. A person who is at least 18yrs can legally marry without parental consent, providing the registrar or minister is satisfied that they understand what marriage means (the capacity to consent). If a person is 16–17yrs, permission needs to be sought from the person's parents/legal guardian (see 📖 pp.260–271).

Can anyone refuse to marry a person with an intellectual disability?

The registrar or clergy can refuse to marry someone, but only if they believe that either of the intending spouses does not have the capacity to understand the consequences of their actions.

What could the intellectual disability nurse do?

- Offer support and guidance to the person(s)
- Discuss the implications and consequences with the person(s) concerned
- Assess the help and support the person(s) may need
- Only involve the parents with the person's consent (parents' support in any marriage is helpful, starting married life without this support would be difficult for many).

Remember

- Having an ID does not mean that the person is unable to have a happy or successful marriage.
- While every person believes that their marriage will last for ever, there are no guarantees and this is the same for people with ID.
- Marriage should be entered into only with the free and full consent of the intending spouses.[1]

There are occasions, however, when people with ID have been forced into marriage by harassment, trickery, assault, kidnapping, and blackmail. Having an ID can cause difficulties for the person in reporting abuse, or for the person to remove themselves from a difficult or abusive relationship, because they may be dependant on others for the care they need. A person may be subject to unwanted sexual acts and become pregnant as part of an abusive relationship.

What are the warning signs?

- The person is accompanied to appointments by people who restrict their opportunities to talk freely and in confidence to a health professional
- Withdrawal of the person from social networks
- Unreasonable financial control
- Inability to attend outside activities.

What to do?

Take any concerns raised seriously and speak to your supervisor/manager as soon as is practicable, contact the child or adult protection services (depending on the age of the person).

Further reading

Foreign and Commonwealth Office (2007). *Dealing with Cases of Forced Marriage; Practice Guidelines for Health Professionals.* Foreign and Commonwealth Office: London.

Parents with intellectual disability

People with ID are now mostly living the same lives as their peers, and this includes becoming a parent. If a person has an ID, however, it is more likely that their child will be placed on an 'At Risk Register' or taken 'into care', and it is more likely that they will have to prove their ability to parent before they can keep their child. Recent studies have highlighted that nearly 50% of parents with ID had their children removed because of concerns of a lack of support.

Possible barriers to successful parenting for people with intellectual disability

- Lack of knowledge, skills or capacity in the person with ID
- Lack of opportunities to develop new knowledge and skills required
- People's attitudes
- Assumptions that if a person has an ID they will not be able to parent
- Being watched at all times by different people and agencies
- A real lack of understanding of how to work with people with ID who become parents
- Conflicting advice from professionals and agencies
- Too many people being involved
- Having to be the perfect parent at all times.

What can help?

- Early identification of pregnancy
- Support during the pregnancy
- Building trusting relationships with the person, their partner and family members
- Early identification of the person's needs
- Skills training, for example helping mum and dad prepare feeds and prepare for bedtime routines
- Help in the home
- Parenting groups
- Agencies and staff working together
- Involving family members in support
- Keep information clear and straight forward; provide easy to read and accessible information to the person on all aspects of parenting. This is especially important at child protection proceedings or involvement with the courts
- Training for staff, e.g. how to communicate effectively with people with ID; not giving too many instructions at once
- Review attitudes and values of staff members (not all people think that a person with an ID should become a parent).

Who can help?

There are a number of people from a variety of agencies that can help a person to parent (see 📖 Chapter 10, pp.333–398). This includes midwives, health visitors, community ID nurses, psychologists, speech and language therapists, occupational therapists, social workers and care officers, and advocacy and voluntary services. These services range from assessing a person's ability to parent, to providing day-to-day hands-on support.

It needs to be recognized that these services will be needed long term, supporting the mother (parents) through the pregnancy, in the early days/months and thereafter as the child grows, and particularly during the normal childhood difficulties i.e. 'terrible 2s', going to school, at puberty etc.

Further reading

Change. *You and Your Baby 0-1*. CD-ROM available from 🖳 www.changepeople.co.uk

Kent A (1999). *Helping Parents to Parent*. Report from a Florence Nightingale Study tour.

Morris J, Wates M (2006). *Supporting Disabled Parents and Parents with Additional Support Needs*. SCIE: Bristol.

Tarleton B, Ward L, Howarth J (2006). *Finding the Right Support*. Norah Fry Research Centre: Bristol.

Women and menopause

Definitions
- Menopause refers to the last menstrual bleed of women, and can be defined as the permanent cessation of menstruation resulting from the loss of ovarian follicular activity.
- Perimenopause is the period immediately before the menopause. Endocrinological, biological and clinical features of approaching menopause become evident and continue until at least the first year after menopause.
- Postmenopause cannot be determined until 12mths of spontaneous amenorrhoea have been observed.

Onset
The onset of menopause usually occurs late 40s to early 50s, although it can occur as early as 45 or as late as 56. For women who have Down syndrome, onset may occur in their mid-40s.

Symptoms
Early recognition of menopausal indicators can assist women with an ID to be empowered rather than disempowered by acknowledging symptoms that may previously have been ignored or misrepresented. 75% of women experience acute symptoms, including;
- Vasomotor instability
  - Hot flushes
  - Night sweats
- Urogenital tissue atrophy
  - Vaginal dryness
  - Dry skin
  - Stress incontinence
- Emotional and psychological
  - Insomnia
  - Depression
  - Irritability
  - Lethargy
  - Poor memory.

Treatments
HRT is an option for women with perimenopausal symptoms, and can be administered:
- orally
- transdermally
- vaginally
- implants
- nasal spray.

HRT usually comprises two hormones—oestrogen and progestogen. Women who have had a hysterectomy can safely take oestrogen on its own.

Women prescribed psychotropic medication may require lower doses, because of diminishing levels of oestrogen.

The role of the intellectual disability nurse

- Enable women to live healthily and promote access to primary health care
- Prepare women for changes that may occur using pictures and visual resources where appropriate
- Encourage women to live active and meaningful lives to maintain and develop their self-esteem
- Be a resource to other health professionals to ensure symptoms of menopause are not misrepresented or misdiagnosed in women with ID

Further reading

Abernethy K (2002). *The Menopause and HRT*. 2nd edn. Baillière Tindall: London.

McCarthy M (2003). Discussing the menopause with women with learning disabilities. *British Journal of Learning Disabilities* **31**, 9–17.

Robinson GE (2002). Women and psychopharmacology. *Medscape General Medicine* **4**(1).

Older people with intellectual disabilities

There have been marked changes in the life expectancy of people with ID, but their life expectancy still remains less than that of the general population. Data from the Republic of Ireland show a steady increase in the number of people with ID >35yrs.[1] In 1974, 28.5% of registered persons were >35yrs; in 1996, 38%, and in 2007 the figure was 48%. Additionally, 48% of people with a moderate, severe, or profound ID were 35yrs or over.

Health status of older people with intellectual disabilities

Individuals with ID have a greater variety of healthcare needs than those of the same age and gender in the general population, and are reported to have 2.5 times the health problems of other persons.[2] Common concerns include—hypertension, obesity, congenital heart disease, abdominal pain, respiratory disease, cancer, gastrointestinal disorders, diabetes, chronic urinary tract infections, oral diseases, musculoskeletal conditions, osteoporosis, thyroid disease, hypothermia, pneumonia, vision impairment, and hearing impairment. Poor nutrition and polypharmacy, social disadvantage, syndrome-specific disorders, and improved survival rates for those with profound and severe disabilities increase such risks.

Psychological health

In a review of available studies, Parry reported that depending on the instruments and definitions of old age used, 20–40% of older persons with ID have a mental health problem.[3] Social, cultural, environmental, and developmental factors and stressors appear to have significant impact on the expression of both psychiatric and behavioural disorders in older people with ID. Gender issues have been poorly investigated, and polypharmacy and inadequate medication reviews increase the risk for drug interactions, leading in old age to sedation, increased confusion, constipation, postural instability, falls, incontinence, weight gain, endocrinological or metabolic effects, impairments of epilepsy management, and movement disorders.[4]

The health service needs of older people with intellectual disabilities

People with ID are more likely to lead unhealthy lifestyles, which contribute to the development of physical ailments in later life. Health problems are often not recognized, and people with ID do not access health promotion and health screening services to the same extent as non-disabled peers. There are additional access barriers because many people with ID are reliant on health management by proxy. People with ID often experience discrimination, inequality and barriers (e.g. attitudinal and physical) when using healthcare. For people with ID who are terminally ill, concerns have been raised about a lack of specialist knowledge and training among front-line ID nurses, as well as lack of experience among specialist palliative care staff who work with this population (see 📖 End of life, p.136).[5]

Living situations

Better health has been reported for those in community settings compared to those living in nursing homes, and quality of life increases when people move from homes with institutional features to community settings.[6] Living with family may also have the benefit of a community based lifestyle, natural social networks, continuity and consistency in care, familiarity of environment, greater acceptance by family members, and greater respect for the needs of the older person and the contribution of the person with ID to activities of daily living.[7] Yet, similar to USA data,[8] the National Intellectual Disability Database noted a greater likelihood for living in out-of-home settings, including institutions, with increasing age—3.6% of all 0–19-yr-olds are in receipt of full-time residential services, compared with 27.1% of 20–34-yr-olds, 55.0% of 35–54-yr-olds, and 74.6% of 55yrs or over.[1]

1 Kelly F, Kelly C, Craig S (2007). *Annual Report of the National Intellectual Disability Database Committee*. Health Research Board: Dublin.

2 van Schrojenstein Lantman-De Valk HM, Metsemakers JF, Haveman MJ, Crebolder HF. Health problems in people with intellectual disability in general practice: a comparative study. *Family Practice* **17**, 405–407.

3 Parry JR, Ed. (2002). *Overview of Mental Health Problems in Elderly Persons with Developmental disabilities*. NADD: New York.

4 Thorpe L, Davidson P, Janicki MP (2000). *Healthy Ageing—Adults with Intellectual Disabilities: Biobehavioural Issues*. World Health Organization: Geneva.

5 McCarron M, Fahey-McCarthy E, Connaire K, McCallion P (2008). *Supporting Persons with Intellectual Disability and Advanced Dementia: Fusing the Horizons of Intellectual Disability, Dementia and Palliative Care*. School of Nursing and Midwifery, Trinity College: Dublin.

6 Heller T, Miller AB, Factor A (1998). Environmental characteristics of nursing homes and community-based settings and the well-being of adults with intellectual disability. *Journal of Intellectual Disability Research* **42**, 418–428.

7 McCallion P, Janicki MP (1997). Area agencies on aging: Meeting the needs of persons with developmental disabilities and their aging families. *Journal of Applied Gerontology* **16**, 270–284.

8 Fujiura GT (1998). Demography of family households. *American Journal of Mental Retardation* **103**, 225–235.

Older people with Down syndrome

Life expectancy for people with Down syndrome has improved dramatically from reports of death at 9yrs and 12yrs through the 1940s, to 30yrs by the early 1970s, to late 50s by the 1990s, and anecdotal reports today of some people living to their 9th decade.[1]

The active treatment of two issues in persons with Down syndrome, still of concern in older years, are believed to have influenced this growing longevity—upper respiratory tract infection and heart anomalies.[1] There is also some suggestion that perimenopausal women with Down syndrome are more prone to heart problems, given pre-existing heart anomalies. At the very least ID nurses must be observant for the complications associated with these heart and respiratory condition, and make prompt referrals to appropriate primary or secondary healthcare services.

It is also likely that living in the community, greater quality of life, and opportunities for self-determination have made important contributions to longevity. People with Down's syndrome will therefore be more likely to maintain good health and quality of life if ID nurses work to ensure continued living in the community.

A popular myth that adults with Down syndrome will not exercise is not true. Systematic programmes offering exercise and health education improve attitudes to exercise, and offer better exercise outcomes, improved life satisfaction, and lower depression.[2] Attention to exercise by ID nurses therefore offers an opportunity for people with Down syndrome to be active partners in the pursuit of their own good health.

Old age will not always be without health complications. Comorbid health conditions are of particular concern in older adults with Down syndrome. Many of these health issues, even those associated with ageing in the general population, appear to begin in earlier years. There are also high levels of obesity, low levels of exercise, and poor nutritional intake.[2] By 50yrs:

- 40% of people with Down syndrome have developed a thyroid disorder
- there are sensory losses in 40–80%
- 28% have hip disease
- 50% have adult onset epilepsy
- diabetes, osteporosis and depression are more prevalent
- dementia occurs at higher rates than in the general population.[3]

Dementia is reported to be present in 15–45% of people with Down syndrome >40yrs,[4] increasing with age, and there is also evidence that people with Down syndrome experience an early and more abrupt decline in memory, behaviour, and day-to-day functioning and work skills. There is also a danger that all health concerns and symptoms in persons with Down syndrome will be attributed to dementia. This robs people with Down syndrome of the potential to have these symptoms treated, when they are more appropriately attributed to other treatable conditions. This approach also fails to recognize that people with Down syndrome and dementia are also prone to other conditions. Among people

with Down syndrome and dementia, epilepsy is reported to be as high as 80%, and compared with those without dementia there are:
• higher levels of depression
• higher levels of arthritis, gastric problems, and immobility
• higher levels of balance problems, falls, gastrointestinal disorders, night-time incontinence, diarrhoea, malnutrition, and musculoskeletal disorders.[5]

Failure to recognize that other conditions are present means that those conditions will be not be treated effectively, decreasing quality of life for older people with Down syndrome and increasing the likelihood of premature death. Therefore screening for dementia among people with Down syndrome and other people with ID is important and more likely to be accurate when using assessment specifically designed for use with these populations rather than generic screening tools.

Important roles for ID nurses are:
• monitoring for likely health concerns
• screening for dementia symptoms
• advocating for community maintenance and self-determination
• treating health concerns
• supporting care as dementia progresses, should it be ascertained.

Above all, the risk that health concerns and dementia may lead to long-term residential care must be recognized, and ID nurses must work with interdisciplinary teams to address treatable health concerns, and to modify expectations programmes and living situations to ensure successful ageing in their community residence for as long as possible.

1 Bittles AH, Glasson EJ (2004). Clinical, social and ethical implications of changing life expectancy in Down syndrome. *Developmental Medicine & Childhood Neurology*, **46**, 282–286.

2 Heller T, Hsieh K, Rimmer JH (2004). Attitudinal and Psychosocial Outcomes of a Fitness and Health Education Program on Adults with Down Syndrome. *American Journal of Mental Retardation* **109**,175–185.

3 Janicki MP, Henderson CM, Davidson PW *et al.* (2002). Health characteristics and health services utilization in older adults with intellectual disabilities living in community residences. *Journal of Intellectual Disability Research* **46**, 287–298.

4 Prasher VP, Krishnan VHR (1993). Age of onset and duration of dementia in people with Down's syndrome. *International Journal of Geriatric Psychiatry.* **8**, 923–927.

5 McCarron M, Gill M, McCallion P, Begley C (2005). Health Comorbidities in Ageing Persons with Down syndrome and Alzheimer's dementia. *Journal of Intellectual Disability Research* **49**, 560–566.

End of life

Death—a normal part of life

Death is an important part of life, and caring for dying people is an important facet of healthcare. However, many ID services are more concerned with the process of supporting people to live well, rather than supporting people to die well. Death remains an indicative part of life, and for many may be one of the most important times of that life. As people approach the end of life, navigating new services and systems of health and social care become vital to the patient, the families, and the nurses involved. All nurses have a responsibility to ensure that this process is managed appropriately, involving the patient and their family wherever possible, and that death is as pain free and easeful as is feasible and indeed possible. Everyone becomes potentially vulnerable at the end of life, as the body becomes weaker and health needs increase, but for people who have additional needs (such as ID) that vulnerability becomes compounded, for a variety of reasons. (see 📖 Responding to bereavement, p.246).

Dying with an intellectual disability

Many people with ID die without fully understanding the nature and severity of their illness, and often experience disenfranchised death.[1] This is where the death is not openly acknowledged with the dying person; where the dying person is socially excluded from the dying process and deliberately excluded from any decision-making surrounding their impending death (Fig. 5.1).

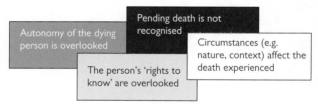

Pending death is not recognised

Autonomy of the dying person is overlooked

Circumstances (e.g. nature, context) affect the death experienced

The person's 'rights to know' are overlooked

Fig. 5.1 Features of disenfranchised death.

Communication challenges, and the ability of the person to understand the concept of death and the meaning of illness may cumulatively compound to make dealing with their death more difficult. Individuals with an ID may have difficulties at the end of life with:
- not knowing that death is imminent
- cognition, understanding difficult concepts (such as treatments, importance of treatment regimens, palliative care, consent)
- sharing feelings and talking about the illness with others
- being treated differently because they have a disability
- understanding the reality of the situation and how to cope with it
- letting people know when symptoms worsen or when they are frightened
- loss of control/autonomy/choice throughout the dying process
- preparing for death (making a will, identifying funeral preferences).

Nursing the patient with an intellectual disability

Numerous reports have identified the difficulties that people with ID have in accessing healthcare, and this includes end of life care too. General nurses may have little experience in caring for this client population, and rely on familiar carers to work alongside them at this time. Hence collaborative working is the key to effective palliative care and support. Nurses may have difficulties supporting the person with an ID at the end of life because of:

- reciprocal communication difficulties
- recognition of health deterioration
- pain and symptom assessment and management
- diagnostic overshadowing
- communicating and explaining about complex issues such as diagnosis, prognosis, death; collusion (between families and professionals); and concordance (with medication and treatments)
- ethical considerations and consent.[2]

Effective support at the end of life

Professionals need to remember that people with ID have more similarities to the rest of the population than differences from them; particularly as end of life approaches. Their need for comfort, support, to die in a place of their own choosing, among friends, family or familiar people, to be pain free, to have symptoms relieved (acknowledging spiritual, physical, psychosocial and emotional needs), and to be treated with dignity and respect are important to anyone at this time. Providing effective care at the end of life involves a collaborative, skilled approach (see 📖 End of life care, preferred place of care, p.206).

Further reading

Blackman N, Todd S (2005). *Caring for People with Learning Disabilities who are Dying.* Worth Publications: London.

Brown H, Burns S, Flynn M (2005). *Dying Matters: A Workbook on Caring for People with Learning Disabilities Who are Dying.* The Mental Health Foundation: London.

---

1 Read S (2006). Communication in the dying process. In: Read S, Ed. *Palliative Care for People with Learning Disabilities.* Quay Books: London.

2 Department of Constitutional Affairs (2005). *Mental Capacity Act.* HMSO: London.

Physical health and well being

Introduction

Physical ill health and challenges to well-being are common in people with ID. Consequently it is important that they have early access to assessment, treatments, and interventions, thereby reducing complications, maintaining physical health and well-being, and leading to an improved quality of life.

As a population, children, adults and older people with severe ID all have higher health needs compared with the general population. They also have a different pattern of physical health needs, many of which go unrecognized and remain untreated. However, in the absence of a specific syndrome, the health profile of people with mild ID is the same as the general population once socioeconomic factors are taken into account, although they may experience more difficulty in accessing health promotion and primary and secondary care services. Such difficulties may contribute to increased health problems for some individuals.

As a result of a range of factors, which include unmet health needs, many die unnecessarily at a premature age. This section provides comprehensive coverage of the very many factors that can compromise the health and well-being of this group of people, along with a range of strategies that ID nurses can adopt to support them.

Further reading

Mencap (2007). *Death by Indifference*. Mencap: London.

Michael J (2008). *Healthcare for All: Report of the independent inquiry into access to healthcare for people with learning disabilities*. Department of Health: London. ▣ www.iahpld.org.uk/

Health inequalities

Definition

Health inequalities may be described as the gap in access to healthcare, or in the health status, between different and discrete populations. These populations may include people from different ethnic communities and social groups, as well as people with ID or people living in defined geographical localities. Many people with ID are known to experience persistent and multiple factors that can result in health inequalities and social exclusion. These factors may include:

• Living in poverty and greater physical and mental health needs
• Difficulties in accessing primary and secondary healthcare
• Lower nutritional status and poorer quality of healthcare provision
• Limited access to good health information and health education
• A higher likelihood of living in poor quality housing and reduced access to reliable transportation
• Less employment opportunities
• Increased experiences of hate crime and organizational/individual discrimination.

Tackling health inequalities

The need to tackle health inequalities is identified in numerous documents, which are directed across various agencies and departments, as being central to key government policy. These documents include all 4 UK learning disability policies: in Wales, *Fulfilling the Promises*,[1] in Scotland, *The Same as You*,[2] in Northern Ireland, *Equal Lives*,[3] and in England, *Valuing People*.[4] The focus of delivery of programmes developed to tackle health inequalities is directed towards local action. Leadership for these is expected through local authorities, education departments and health services, including PCTs. Within England, LSPs have a key role in tackling health inequalities.

What are Local Strategic Partnerships (LSPs)?

An LSP is a single body that brings together people from the public, private, voluntary, and business sectors, to provide an integrated approach to tackling health issues, at a local level. Each local government area in England has an LSP. Their role is to identify shared priorities and write joint targets as a means of tackling local health inequalities.

Tackling health inequalities in people with intellectual disabilities

Everyone working with people with ID, whether in health, social care, leisure or housing, has a role in reducing health inequalities. The following four principles underpin how health inequalities are tackled in practice. These are presented along with examples of actions that have been taken when applying them to reducing health inequalities for people with ID.

Working through general services making all services more accessible to the needs of disadvantaged groups

Ensuring that accessible health information on chronic health conditions and health treatments are available at GP surgeries and hospital outpatient clinics. Providing training on the health and communication needs of people with ID to all primary care and hospital care staff

Preventing inequalities from getting worse by addressing underlying causes of ill health

Introducing annual health checks and the opportunity for health action plans to all people with ID. Running regular health information groups for people with ID, to help them gain greater knowledge and personal control. Supporting people with chronic health conditions access the Expert Patient Programme.

Finding new ways of meeting needs, particularly in areas that are resistant to change and targeting interventions at these

Working with acute hospitals to develop acute liaison nurse posts, and support the development of resources to improve the care of people with ID in hospitals. Working with local police departments, to help them understand the needs of people with ID, in relation to the management of local hate crime.

Developing policies and supporting coordinated action on these from a central point

National guidance on the NHS Cancer Screening Programme on breast and cervical screening for women with ID, highlights the importance of the issue, informed consent and sets national standards for practice.

Further reading

Department of Health (2003). *Tackling Inequalities: A Programme for Action.* Department of Health: London.

Department of Health (2004). *Choosing Health: Making Healthy choices Easier.* Public Health White Paper. Department of Health: London.

Mencap (2007). *Death by Indifference.* Mencap: London.

Michael J (2008) *Healthcare for All: Report of the independent inquiry into access to healthcare for people with learning disabilities.* Department of Health: London.

1 Welsh Office (2001) *Fulfilling the Promises.* Welsh Assembly: Cardiff.

2 Scottish Executive (2000). *The Same as You? A Review of the Services for People with Learning Disabilities.* Scottish Executive: Edinburgh.

3 Department of Health, Social Services and Public Safety (2005). *Equal Lives.* Department of Health, Social Services and Public Safety: Belfast.

4 Department of Health (2001). *Valuing People. A New Strategy for Learning Disability for 21st Century.* Department of Health: London.

Principles of health promotion

Health promotion comprises a broad span of activities that work towards achieving the positive health and well-being of individuals, groups, and communities.

The focus of health promotion work includes health education, lifestyle and preventative approaches, alongside environmental, legal, and fiscal measures.

Key health promotion principles

- Equity
- Participation
- Collaboration
- Empowerment
- Sustainability.

> ### What health promotion barriers do people with intellectual disability experience?
>
> - Limited skills of primary and secondary care staff in accessible communication and in the knowledge of the population's health needs
> - A lack of policy promoting health to the ID population
> - Reduced access to health screening and health education
> - A lack of accessible health promotion resources
> - Low priority given to the health of the population
> - Reduced health ownership and control, with less opportunity for decision making and informed choice.

Everyone who works with people with ID has a role to play in tackling health inequalities through health promotion activities. Health promotion comprises a complex and wide ranging area of activities, which at times may require radical thinking. It facilitates opportunities to focus on developing choice, promoting independence and rights, and enabling inclusion. Health promotion activities may take place with individuals or collectively within small or large groups. It may be necessary, in order to meet the needs of people with ID to the same level as that of the general population, to adopt different kinds of solutions.

The following list identifies 5 key principles of health promotion that may be used in work relating to people with ID.

Equity

- Promoting the need for and supporting GPs and their staff in developing and introducing annual health checks
- Highlighting and working with public/private/voluntary sector employers in raising the need for developing an accessible application process to help people with ID to apply for and get jobs
- Keeping up to date with new projects at a local level. Working with staff in education, housing, health and leisure projects to help make projects accessible to people with ID.

Participation
- Informing people with ID on the role of links and other local consultation groups. Supporting them to participate in these groups
- Employing people with ID as co-trainers in the delivery of training to health and other staff
- Involving people with ID in the recruitment of staff
- Ensuring meetings and their minutes are accessible.

Collaboration
- Working in partnership with people in local advocacy groups in developing local strategies and policies
- Working across service boundaries to ensure the needs of people with ID are incorporated into local services e.g. older people's services, sexual health, drug and alcohol, mental health
- Working with health visitors in the delivery of training to staff on the needs of parents with ID.

Empowerment
- Promoting and using person-centered approaches to care
- Organizing and delivering health education related activities, either individually or in groups
- Consulting with user-led groups, e.g. black and minority ethnic groups, on their needs in local service development
- Involving people with ID in the commissioning strategy
- Sharing responsibility.

Sustainability
- Developing and using accessible health education resources to help people understand and take greater control of their health
- Undertaking inclusive research activities (see 📖 Working with people with intellectual disabilities in the research process, p.514)
- Supporting self-advocacy groups to run health information related activities
- Being innovative in the collection of evidence to promote the need for new service developments
- Ensuring that the needs of people with ID are included in disability equality schemes.

Promoting public health

Definition

The Faculty of Public Health has described public health as, 'The science and art of preventing disease, prolonging life and promoting health through the organized efforts of society'.

Overview

The role of public health is strongly driven towards the reduction of health inequalities. Public health may be referred to, and considered from, four different approaches. These are:

- A multidisciplinary profession, whose wide range of skills are focussed on, predominantly, proactive work, directed towards improving the health of the population
- A set of diverse skills, including specific skills in working with populations, as well as collecting, interpreting, and using evidence to direct, and develop programmes of service delivery, to meet identified need
- A range of desired outcomes originating from both individuals and populations, relating to the aim of achieving lasting improvements across mainstream health service delivery
- Factors that contribute to health and illness, focused on tackling the root causes of ill health. These include addressing personal lifestyle issues such as diet, exercise, and smoking, as well as wider determinants, which may include housing, or the quality of healthcare.

Public health delivery

The assessment and delivery of public health initiatives are increasingly being delivered in working partnerships. At a local level an increasing number of directors of public health are joint posts, which cover both the NHS and local authorities that share geographical boundaries. This joint approach is reflected in some shared delivery of health promotion and public health practice. Coordinated approaches to public health are set out in LAAs.

What are Local Area Agreements (LAAs)?

An LAA is a 3yr agreement. It sets out the priorities and objectives for a local area, represented by a local strategic partnership of representatives of all key organizations, and central government. LAAs are designed to:

- improve central and local government relationships
- improve efficiency in public services
- strengthen partnership and enhance leadership of local authorities on a range of public service outcomes.

Public health in practice
People working in public health consider their role, and its application in practice, in 3 domains:
- Health protection and prevention
- Improving health and social care
- Health improvement.

People with ID experience extreme and multiple health inequalities; however, their needs are often neglected in the work of public health departments. This has been recognized and there is currently a strong national push to rectify this.[1] Initiatives include public health departments employing a staff member to take a lead in ID, or ID staff working with multiagency services to include the needs of people with ID in local audits, strategies and projects. However, public health departments cannot be considered the only agency responsible for meeting the health inequalities of people with ID. The promotion of public health needs to be considered as central to everyone working with this population. The above domains can be used as a framework to list examples of work that may be required.

> ### How do the three public health domains translate into examples of work related to intellectual disability?
> *Health protection and prevention*
> - Facilitating accessible sex education to children and adults
> - Educating and supporting women with ID to access breast and cervical screening
> - Providing education on home/road safety.
> - Promoting and supporting annual health checks
> - Working with police in addressing management of hate crime.
>
> *Improving health and social care*
> - Developing and auditing quality standards in primary/acute hospitals
> - Conducting local needs assessments to inform local service delivery
> - Facilitating groups to enable people with ID to understand local service provision and contribute to local consultation
> - Undertaking local/national research and reporting on findings.
>
> *Health improvement*
> - Ensuring availability of accessible health promotion resources
> - Developing and facilitating health, housing, employment projects
> - Influencing/working with public health specialists to ensure ID is included in local strategies e.g. older people, exercise, diet, and obesity.

Further reading
Care Services Improvement Partnership (CSIP) (2007). *The Role of Public Health in Supporting the Development of Integrated Services*. National Institute for Mental Health in England: Leeds.

1 Michael J (2008). *Healthcare for All: Report of the independent inquiry into access to healthcare for people with learning disabilities*. Department of Health: London.

Promoting physical well-being of individuals

Good health is the foundation on which a good quality of life can be built. Good physical well-being, that includes a sense of personal ownership and a personal locus of control, is strongly linked with positive mental well-being. People with ID experience many barriers in the achievement of optimum physical health. Multiple sources of evidence from the UK, and wider, have found that people with ID experience worse physical health, due to many different causative factors. In addition they receive worse treatment from health services, with both primary and acute hospital system failures. It is also widely acknowledged that insufficient priority is given within health services in addressing the specific health needs of this population.

What do we know about the health of people with intellectual disabilities?

- They have an increased risk of an early death, and have a different picture of health needs, than the general population
- Some syndromes associated with ID (e.g. Down syndrome, Prader–Willi syndrome) are accompanied by an increased range of specific health conditions
- They have high levels of unmet physical and mental health needs and higher rates of some chronic or long-term health conditions, e.g. epilepsy
- They have higher rates of vision and hearing difficulties and are less likely to have received regular physical health, dental, vision, and hearing checks
- Women with ID are much less likely to access breast mammography or cervical screening
- They are more likely to experience mental health problems
- They are less likely to have access to health education or to live healthy lives, and they have reduced ownership and control of their personal health needs.

The aim of developing local approaches in meeting the health needs of people with ID in England was identified in *Valuing People* that stated the aim to be:[1]

'To enable people with a learning disability to access a health service designed around their individual needs, with fast and convenient care, delivered to a consistently high standard, with additional support, where necessary'

Practical steps to consider when promoting physical well-being

Individual

- Be pro-active in considering and promoting health needs within all working roles and care environments; facilitate a healthy living environment, ensuring availability to accessible information; facilitate each individual making informed decisions on health treatments, health screening, and lifestyle choices.
- Enable each individual to select someone they know and trust to be their health facilitator (HF), to support them in thinking about their health, building knowledge, health ownership, and responsibility.
- If not initiated by the local GP practice, the HF should support each individual to arrange and attend a health screening check. This should help each person to identify individual health needs, and consider how these will impact on their wider lifestyle aspirations and future plans
- Working with the individual, record the needs identified by the health check. Consider how these needs will be met, by whom, and in what timescale. Support the person to put these into a plan, where possible, in a style and format accessible to the individual. This may be known as a health action plan (HAP).
- Plan and prepare for any health or hospital visits, where possible, in advance. Write any special requirements down in a patient passport, to share and leave with medical staff.

Organizational

- Raise the health profile of people with ID across commissioning, health, social, and voluntary agencies at local levels. Also offer support and initiate partnership working with local primary care teams, acute hospitals, and dental and other heath agencies.
- Ensure health strategy planning group has multi-agency membership. Also offer and deliver staff training to a wide range of health staff and health students. Employ people with ID to share this role.
- Develop a resource base that contains a wide range of accessible resources on physical health conditions, health screening, and medical procedures. Make these resources or the links to them easily available to all. Also build a local resource of examples of HAPs, to support training, and work in partnership with self-advocacy groups in building health knowledge in people with ID.
- Link with national networks to share and learn from national best practice.
- Develop surveys, research, audit or other approaches that record evidence of local health needs.

Further reading

Disability Rights Commission (2007). *Equal Treatment: Closing the Gap—One Year On*. Equality and Human Rights Commission

Michael J (2008). *Healthcare for All: Report of the independent inquiry into access to healthcare for people with learning disabilities*. Department of Health: London.

---

1 Department of Health (2001). *Valuing People. A New Strategy for Learning Disability for 21st Century*. Department of Health: London.

Physical health assessment of people with intellectual disability

People with ID experience a wide range of inequalities in relation to their physical health. These include an increased prevalence of a number of specific health conditions along with poor health outcomes. Other evidence suggests that they are less likely than the general population to access regular health checks or health screening. This inequality leads to increased likelihood of suffering from a range of specific conditions, and poor health outcomes. There is a sound rationale for introducing systematic physical health assessments for this population. An additional legal rationale, the Disability Discrimination Act, Disability Equality Duty, requires all public bodies to address meeting these inequalities within local disability equality schemes; failure to do this could make them liable to prosecution.

What is physical health assessment?

Physical health assessment is the process of gaining a fuller understanding of the health needs of an individual, in order to detect, treat, and manage any health conditions.

National recommendations are that physical health assessment may be best managed in people with ID, by the provision of individual health checks. It is recommended that these are offered annually. Health checks should be offered by GP practices to all adults with ID registered with the practice. Annual health checks should include the key areas of health risks known in the ID population.

To ensure an integrated approach between each person's health check and well-being, the outcomes of the health check, with any actions, by whom and the timescale to be achieved, should be recorded within the HAP.

Preparing people with intellectual disability for a health check

People with ID may need support in preparing to have a health check so that they can give informed consent for it. Prior to the appointment, work should be undertaken with the person to help them understand what investigations may be required during the health check. It may be helpful to obtain accessible information leaflets.

Accessible information may be available from:
- The GP surgery
- The local NHS health information resource centre
- The local community learning disability service
- Health information websites e.g. ⌨ www.easyhealth.org.uk

What areas of physical health warrant assessment in a health check?

- Family history and risk factors
- Immunization record
- Drug and alcohol use
- Vision and hearing
- Review of chronic illness including epilepsy
- Physical examination including skin condition, mobility and posture
- Syndrome specific check
- Medication review
- Oral health
- Sexual health
- Continence
- Review of mental health and emotional needs
- Behavioural disturbance, sleep issues
- Carer details and constraints
- Referrals made and any follow up
- Identified areas of risk and actions to be taken.

Supporting physical health assessment in practice

The implementation of annual health checks for people with ID across the UK is extremely patchy. The Welsh Assembly introduced regular health checks into their GP contracts from 2006/2007. In other parts of the country, different areas have introduced them using Local Enhanced Services payments to GPs.

Resources

A number of resources have been developed to promote and support the introduction of health checks. These include:
- Primary care service commissioning framework July 2007
- The management of healthcare for people with ID in primary care

⌨ www.primarycarecontracting.nhs.uk/204.php

This is an extensive package of practical resources to support the development and implementation of health checks. It includes:
- Health checks—a summary of steps and support
- Templates for GP IT systems
- Job description of a HF
- GP practice step-by-step guide at a glance
- Health checks—role of the CLDT
- Health checks—role of the PCT

Blood pressure, temperature, pulse

Blood pressure

Blood pressure is a measure of the levels of force exerted on the walls of blood vessels, due to the flow of blood from the heart. Blood pressure is dynamic, and varies from minute to minute. It is measured by an instrument called a sphygmomanometer, a gauge that measures the pumping (systolic) and resting (diastolic) stages of the heart. Readings of blood pressure are usually performed by trained health professionals.

Blood pressure is influenced by a large number of factors. These include temperature, respiration, environmental noise, pain, fear, anxiety, exercise, smoking, eating, and drinking. Body position can also affect blood pressure readings.

High blood pressure is known as hypertension, and low blood pressure is hypotension. Consistent readings of 140/90 mmHg and above are likely to be associated with hypertension. Hypertension is an increasing medical concern, being commonly associated with obesity, diabetes, and high levels of fat in the blood. If left untreated, a combination of the above can lead to cardiovascular (heart) disease, stroke, kidney failure, dementia, and early death. Treatment is usually based on lifestyle changes and drug interventions.

People with ID are known to have higher rates of obesity than the general population, and receive fewer health checks. In meeting the health needs of people with ID, carers have a key role in the prevention, detection, and management of hypertension. It can be difficult to detect without measuring blood pressure, therefore blood pressure measurement is required in any regular health check. In preparing a person for the procedure, people need to be aware of the discomfort of a tightening cuff on the upper arm—distraction interventions may help. There are a number of less uncomfortable wrist readers, but these are less accurate.

Preventative lifestyle measures include healthy eating, eating a well balanced, low-salt diet, maintaining a healthy weight, regular exercise, low alcohol intake, reduced caffeine intake, stopping smoking, stress reduction, and learning free relaxation techniques.

Temperature

Body temperature varies from person to person—the normal range is 36–37.5°C. It is always useful to have a record of each individual's normal temperature, as what may be a normal temperature for one person, may be high or low for another. Normal body temperature is slightly lower in the morning than in the evenings.

A wide range of factors influence body temperature. These include age, exercise, circadian rhythms, hormonal actions, stress, and environmental factors. Hypothermia, or low body temperature, develops when the body temperature becomes too cold, and when the usual body mechanism of heat production cannot maintain a thermal balance. This is most often seen in older people, or people overly exposed to very low temperatures for a long time. A high temperature, known as pyrexia, or hyperthermia, is symptomatic of infection, neurological injury, extreme drug reaction, or heat exhaustion.

Body temperature is recorded using a thermometer. There are different types of thermometer, including glass thermometers, tympanic (ear) battery operated devices, fever brow (chemical disposable strips), and electronic readers.

The most commonly used thermometer, in the home, is the glass thermometer. Under the tongue, in the mouth, is the most commonly used site for recording temperature. The mouth, however, should never be used for infants, small children, people with poorly controlled tonic clonic epilepsy, or people with ID who are confused or have poor cognitive understanding. In these situations the thermometer should be placed, and held, in the axilla (arm pit), or another type of thermometer should be used. On rare occasions, body temperature may be taken using a special rectal thermometer.

Pulse

The measurement of pulse rate is another aspect of a person's health assessment, closely associated with temperature, respiration, and blood pressure. Taking a pulse reading is one common technique used to assess how well the heart is working, and therefore, to assess the general health of the patient. A pulse reading measures the force of blood pumped from the ventricle, in the left side of the heart, into the aorta, the main artery that then sends blood around the body. Pulse points are places in the body where an artery can easily be felt when pressed against a bone. There are 10 common pulse points, the most common being the wrist (radial pulse), the neck (carotid pulse), and the inner arm of the elbow (brachial pulse). Placing a finger or a stethoscope over a pulse point is referred to as 'taking a pulse'. This gives information on the number of times the heart beats in a min, the rhythm and regularity of the pulse, and its strength. If taken over several pulse points, it can also measure consistency of blood flow throughout the body.

A normal adult pulse rate is 60–100 beats/min. Depending on the age, a child's pulse rate is significantly faster. Exercise, temperature, anxiety, pain, body posture, and drugs or medication can all influence pulse rate.

Respiration and oxygen saturation levels

Respiration

When a body is at rest, and the person is in good general health, respiration, or breathing, should be regular, require minimal effort, and be quiet. By discreetly observing a patient's respiration, much can be indicated relating to general health. The measurement of respiration involves counting the rate, depth, and pattern of chest wall movement. Breathing rates are extremely variable, being influenced by age, emotion, and pain. The normal adult respiratory rate is 12–18 breaths/min.

> ### What is respiration?
>
> Respiration is another word for breathing. It involves a process of gaseous exchange in the lungs. This involves air constantly moving in and out of the lungs, bringing oxygen into the body and removing carbon dioxide.

The observation of respiration is something that can be done by anyone working with people with ID, and may be the first observation to identify physical ill health. Changes in respiration may include coughing, either dry or productive; that may be different at different times of the day, or in different postural positions. This could indicate the presence of infection, asthma, or allergy. Coughing during eating or drinking may suggest that the person is aspirating (breathing) food or liquid into their lungs, and should be referred to the GP as a matter of urgency. In observing seizures in epilepsy, particular attention needs to be given to ensure that the airway to the lungs does not become blocked. Halitosis, bad smelling breath, may indicate poor oral hygiene, infection, or severe constipation. Sweet smelling breath may indicate diabetes.

Oxygen saturation levels

The body cannot function well without high levels of oxygen in the blood. Oxygen is carried in the haemoglobin of the red blood cells, which take oxygen to all parts of the body. Levels of blood gases may be monitored using a noninvasive method of pulse oximetry, in which a probe is placed on the end of a finger, covering the fingernail. If more detailed information is required, a blood test known as ABG (arterial blood gases) is undertaken to measure oxygen, carbon dioxide, and acidity levels of blood. These levels relate to how well body organs, predominantly the lungs, are working.

An ABG test is carried out on blood taken from an artery. It is likely to be requested to:
- check for breathing problems in lung disease, such as asthma, cystic fibrosis or chronic obstructive airways disease
- check how well lung treatments are working
- check whether more oxygen is needed if the person is on oxygen treatment
- measure the acid levels in the blood of people with heart failure, uncontrolled diabetes, severe infections, or drug overdoses.

Epilepsy

Epilepsy is a condition where a person has a continuing tendency to have seizures resulting from an abnormal electrical discharge from a group of brain cells, caused by a disruption to the electrical and chemical balance of neurons. The type of seizure the person experiences depends on which part of the brain the discharge originates, and how far and quickly it spreads.

Diagnosis of epilepsy

Diagnosis of epilepsy involves identification of seizure type, and relies on a description of the episode provided by the individual, where possible, and/or an eyewitness. Detailed information, *before* (what the person was doing, environment, time of day, how did they feel/appear, warning or partial onset, any potential 'trigger'), *during* (sudden onset, fall, body movements, eyes open/closed, incontinence, gum/tongue bite, level of consciousness, behaviour, duration), and *after* (recovery time, confusion, behaviour, injury) is essential. Video recording is increasingly being used to assist with diagnosis. Tests including EEG, MRI, and blood screening may be performed to support a diagnosis of epilepsy and/or assist in differential diagnosis. If possible, epilepsy syndrome should be identified, the disorder defined by the type(s) of seizures seen, EEG findings, age of onset, family history, response to treatment, and prognosis (e.g. Lennox Gastaut Syndrome).

Main seizure types

Focal or partial seizures affect only part of the brain.

Simple partial seizures—consciousness is not impaired, and duration is less than a minute. Can present with:
- localized motor signs e.g. twitching of mouth (may spread to other areas), head turning, lip smacking, rhythmic jerking of one part of body
- special sensory symptoms e.g. taste, smell, tingling, light flashes, sound
- autonomic symptoms e.g. epigastric sensation, pallor, sweating, flushing
- psychic symptoms e.g. déjà vu, distortion of time, fear, anger, dreamy.

Complex partial seizures—consciousness is impaired, duration approximately 1–3mins, difficult to tell exactly start and finish of seizure, some confusion after, and no memory of event. Can present with complex automatic behaviour e.g. dress and undress repetitively, sucking, chewing or swallowing movements, inappropriate urination, frantic running, and uncontrollable laughing. May develop from simple partial seizures, and may evolve to secondary generalized seizures.

Generalized seizures affect more or less all the brain.

Absence seizures—brief impairment of consciousness, will stare normally for less than 10s, may be some mild motor movements e.g. eye blinks, mouth movements, rubbing the fingers together.

Atypical absence—similar to above but last longer, may be somewhat responsive, and motor movements are more pronounced.

Myoclonic seizures—very quick muscle jerks usually of arms, legs or trunk, may be one sided or both sides, frequently happens soon after waking.

Clonic seizures—rhythmic jerking movements of the arms and legs, sometimes on both sides of the body, rare seizure type.

Tonic seizures—sudden stiffening of limbs, body, and facial muscle, will fall if standing, lasts seconds, can cause injury, fairly quick recovery.

Atonic seizures—sudden loss of muscle tone, person drops to the floor, lasts a few seconds, can cause injury, quick recovery.

Tonic–clonic seizures—may be preceded by partial seizure activity, may experience a 'prodrome' (feeling unwell for some days before). Sudden contraction of muscles (tonic stage), will fall if standing, may cry as air is expelled from lungs, may bite gum or side of tongue. Intermittent relaxation and contraction of muscles follows (clonic stage); results in rhythmical jerking of body. Person may become blue, usually around the lips, exaggerated by dilation of blood vessels in the face caused by pressure from the contraction of the chest. May be excess saliva, snorting noises may be heard, and the person may be incontinent. Periods of relaxation become more prolonged, eventually contractions stop, usually within 1–2mins. Full consciousness may not return for 10–60mins, confusion and tiredness may persist for hours or days.

Unclassified seizures—seizures may present which are unclassifiable.

Treatment of epilepsy

The effective treatment of epilepsy is important in order to provide opportunities for an enhanced quality of life for the person, and reduce the risk of sudden unexplained death in people with ID (see ⬚ Supporting people with epilepsy, p.158). AEDs are the mainstay of treatment for epilepsy; the aim of their use is to maintain a normal lifestyle by complete seizure control without drug-related side effects. Some 70–80% of newly diagnosed cases of epilepsy have a good outcome with AEDs; however, complete control may not always be achievable. Choice of AED depends on seizure type and individual circumstances. One prescribed AED at a time is preferable; however, more than one may be required. Published guidelines provide recommendations for AED treatment.[1]

Non-pharmacological approaches to the treatment of epilepsy include psychological and alternative therapies, and avoidance of obvious 'triggers', and these may help seizure control for some individuals. Generally a healthy lifestyle approach is recommended to help seizure control; consideration should be given to diet, exercise, and compliance with medication, along with a regular sleep pattern, and controlled alcohol intake. Vagal nerve stimulation or neurosurgery, under certain circumstances, may be considered if satisfactory control cannot be obtained with AEDs.

1 Stokes T, Shaw EJ, Juarez-Garcia A, Camosso-Stefinovic J, Baker R (2004). *Clinical Guidelines and Evidence Review for the Epilepsies: Diagnosis and Management in Adults and Children in Primary and Secondary Care.* Royal College of General Practitioners: London.

Supporting people with epilepsy

Up to 25% of people with ID have epilepsy, compared with 0.7% of the general population. The more severe the ID the higher the prevalence of epilepsy will be. The aim of epilepsy management is to maintain or improve seizure control without drug-related side effects, or if seizures are unavoidable then to reduce physical and psychological injury as much as possible.

Epilepsy management plan (EMP)

Know the individual's seizures—having an individual EMP will assist carers in recognizing and managing the person's epilepsy on a day-to-day basis. The EMP should include the following.

Description of seizure—what happens before, during and after the seizure, and recovery details (see ⬚ Diagnosis of epilepsy, p.156). It may take time to observe and record seizure activity in various settings.

Usual duration of seizure—care should be taken to detail the time of actual seizure activity and recovery period separately.

Management of seizure—detail the first aid required for particular seizure types (see ⬚ First aid for seizures, p.159) and consider individual needs.

Emergency management—this should detail after how many minutes or the number of seizures when emergency services should be contacted. Alternatively when emergency medication should be administered, if the individual is prescribed them, and staff are trained to administer—this will require an individual emergency management plan.

Other relevant information—e.g. how often do seizures occur, what time of day, are they in a particular environment, are there any triggers and how can these be avoided.

Epilepsy and risk

When specific concerns are raised, individual risk assessments should be carried out. This is because a balance is required to minimize risk while simultaneously achieving optimum quality of life for the individual. There may be a tendency to over protect, so individual choice, capacity, and consent are issues must be considered.

Supporting individuals to maintain or improve seizure control

Correct diagnosis—diagnosis should be reviewed by a specialist if seizure control does not improve. Observation and detailed description of seizures is essential for correct diagnosis; involve individual, family, and consider video recording to assist with this. Note that challenging behaviour, repetitive stereotyped behaviour, and behaviour relating to mental ill heath can make diagnosis difficult. A structured approach to differentiation is needed and may require behavioural analysis. Communication difficulties further complicate the diagnosis and treatment of epilepsy.

Regular review—individuals should have a yearly review, or more frequently if seizure control does not improve, deteriorates, or AED side effects occur.

Medication compliance—make sure education is provided and memory problems are identified. Records should be inspected for missed medication;

consider use of alarms, pill dispensers, timing, and slow-release preparations to increase compliance.

Identifying triggers—isolate factors unique to the individual if apparent e.g. physical stress—pain, pyrexia, constipation, lack of sleep, emotional stress, missed meds, alcohol, drugs (prescribed and illegal), and hormonal impact on women.

Comorbidity—be aware of drug interactions and their effect on seizure control or other treatments, particularly drugs used for mental ill health.

Complementary therapies—some find these helpful although no evidence suggests they are successful in controlling or curing epilepsy.

Lifestyle choices—a healthy lifestyle approach is recommended to help seizure control, including diet, exercise, regular sleep pattern, structured routine, avoidance of drugs, and controlled alcohol intake.

Education for individuals with epilepsy, their family and support staff, including information on voluntary organizations e.g. Epilepsy Action, National Society for Epilepsy.

First aid for seizures

Simple partial seizures—simply stay with person and offer reassurance.

Complex partial seizures—stay with the person, speak calmly and reassure, do not restrict movements (as it may be misinterpreted as aggression and they may respond aggressively), guide the person away from danger if necessary. Even if confused for a short period most people recover quite quickly and can continue with their work/activity. If complex partial seizures persist (non-convulsive status epilepticus), the person will require medical assistance and possible hospitalization.

Absence seizures—usually no help is needed; if walking they may require guidance and reassurance.

Myoclonic seizures—usually so short lived little can be done other than reassure when over; may be unbalanced, help to steady them, if they fall check for injuries.

Clonic—stay with person, prevent injury from jerks, reassure.

Tonic and atonic seizures—these are over very quickly therefore little can be done during the seizure; check for injuries, which may need medical attention, stay with the person and reassure. *Tonic–clonic seizures*—try to stay calm, time seizure, assess danger to self and client, and only move if in danger. Protect the person's head, loosen tight clothing, and remove glasses. Move objects away if you can or try to protect all from injury. When seizure has ceased, if the person does not regain consciousness place them in the recovery position. Monitor breathing, and skin colour, maintain airway. Wipe away excess saliva, do all you can to minimize embarrassment, quietly reassure, keep others from gathering around. Assess for injury. Allow to rest if they indicate need. Observe as they may be confused. Inform carer where appropriate.

See Emergency management of a person in a seizure, p.542.

Cardiorespiratory disorders

This section outlines some of the health challenges that some people with ID face because of cardiac and or respiratory problems. Cardiac disorders experienced by some people with ID may result from the underlying cause of their disability. For example people with Down syndrome experience a range of cardiac disorders that require effective management. People with Down syndrome have a high prevalence of cardiac septal defects, Tetralogy of Fallot, ductus arteriosus, mitral valve disorder, and aortic insufficiency. Some may go on to experience pulmonary hypertension as a consequence of their cardiac disorder, with associated further complications such as heart failure. It is important, therefore, that cardiorespiratory disorders are assessed effectively and managed across their lifespan.

Respiratory disease is the most common cause of death for people with moderate or severe ID.[1] This point is significant and is a major factor in the premature death of some people with ID, and nurses who practice in all care settings should recognize this. For example, gastric aspiration is associated with swallowing, specific nutrition, and feeding problems—and this is experienced by some in this population. Gastro-oesophageal reflux disorder (GORD) is common and is experienced by some 70% of people with ID.[2,3,4] As can be seen in 🕮 Gastrointestinal disorders, p.180 this may lead to them regurgitating the acidic gastric contents back up the oesophagus, resulting in inflammation of the respiratory tract that in turn leads to infection. Another example is illustrated in a recent study that identified respiratory disorders as common reasons for hospital admission for people with Prader–Willi syndrome.[5]

Cardiovascular disease is the second most common cause of death of people with moderate or severe ID.[6] This contrasts with the general population, where it is the most common cause. Congenital heart disease is common in people with ID, and as this population is now living longer, it is anticipated that more will experience the complications of cardiovascular disease associated with the ageing process. As a consequence, some people with ID will experience conditions such as hypertension, vascular dementia, myocardial infarction, and cerebral vascular accident. Therefore it is important for nurses working in primary care, general hospital, and specialist assessment and treatment services, to be aware of the increased likelihood of these physical disorders being present.

As a consequence of these physical disorders, children, adults and older people with ID will be regular users of primary care and general hospital services.[7,8] Nurses working in these care environments must familiarize themselves with the distinct needs of people with ID in their care to ensure that their needs are appropriately addressed.[1]

Some people with ID who have cardiorespiratory disorders will also require assessment and treatment from specialist ID health services, because of the nature of their complex health needs. Nurses practising in such services need to be familiar with the physical health problems that can be experienced by people with ID in their care. They have an important contribution to make in supporting them during the assessment and treatment of their physical healthcare, and have a responsibility to liaise and communicate effectively with colleagues in primary and general hospital care settings, to ensure that issues relating to communication, behaviours, mental illness, and ASD are reflected within nursing care plans.

1 Hollins S, Attard MT, von Fraunhofer N, McGuigan S, Sedgwick P (1998). Mortality in people with learning disability: risks, causes, and death certification findings in London. *Developmental Medicine & Child Neurology* **40**, 50–56.

2 Galli-Carminati G, Chauvet I, Deriaz N (2006). Prevalence of gastrointestinal disorders in adult clients with pervasive developmental disorders. *Journal of Intellectual Disability Research* **50**(10), 711–718.

3 Böhmer C, Klinkenberg-Knol E, Niezen-de Boer R, Meuwissen S (1997). The prevalence of gastro-oesophageal reflux disease based on non-specific symptoms in institutionalized, intellectually disabled individuals. *European Journal of Gastroenterology & Hepatology* **9**, 187–190.

4 Böhmer C, Niezen-de Boer M, Klinkenberg-Knol E, Deville W, Nadorp J, Meuwissen S (1999). The prevalence of gastroesophageal reflux disease in institutionalized intellectually disabled individuals. *American Journal of Gastroenterology* **94**, 804–810.

5 Thomson A, Glasson A, Bittles A (2006.) A long-term population-based clinical and morbidity review of Prader–Willi syndrome in Western Australia. *Journal of Intellectual Disability Research* **50**(1), 69–78.

6 NHS Health Scotland (2004). *People with learning disabilities in Scotland: The health needs assessment report*. NHS Health Scotland: Glasgow.

7 Morgan C, Ahmed Z, Kerr M (2000). Healthcare provision for people with a learning disability: record-linkage study of epidemiology and factors contributing to hospital care uptake. *British Journal of Psychiatry* **176**, 37–4.

8 Melville C, Cooper S-A, Morrison J et al. (2006). The outcomes of an intervention study to reduce the barriers experienced by people with intellectual disability accessing primary healthcare services. *Journal of Intellectual Disability Research* **50,** 11–17.

Obesity

Obesity is a growing issue in developed countries. The level of obesity is higher in people with ID than in the general population.[1] There are a range of factors that contribute to this situation, which include limited physical activity, poor nutritional practices, and the lack of nutritional knowledge, that collectively results in a population that is overweight.[2] Obesity is a significant risk factor among people with ID for the development of coronary heart disease, cardiovascular disease, cerebrovascular accident, and type II diabetes.[3] Obesity is linked to genetic conditions such as Prader–Willi syndrome and women with Down syndrome. Men with Down syndrome have been found to be obese, but less so than in people with ID without Down syndrome. Obesity results in a decrease in life expectancy and an increase in health needs.[4] In recognition of the increasing life expectancy of people with ID, obesity is a significant health issue that needs to be addressed.

Inactivity plays an important part in contributing to obesity in this population. People with ID lead more sedentary lifestyles when compared with the general population, and have limited opportunities to exercise. Many people with ID are dependent on a carer, be it family or paid, to provide living support. Studies have found that people who receive care in care homes and from family carers are more likely to be obese.[5] Evidence further suggests that increasing the amount of vigorous exercise, reducing carbohydrates, and improving the daily diet can bring about benefits.[6]

Following assessment that includes identifying dietary habits and other risk factors, it is necessary to monitor and record weight regularly, and to set weight parameters appropriate to the individual. There is an opportunity to work collaboratively with people with ID and their carers to effect longer term change. Treatment needs to include a focus on providing education for carers and others involved in the care.

Primary care has an important role in assessing for diabetes, hypertension and cardiovascular disease. Preventative strategies are important, and effectiveness is increased when delivered in partnership with ID specialists such as nurses, physiotherapists, and dieticians. Nurses have an important role in working in partnership with dietitians to provide support, advice, and regular monitoring, thereby enabling reduction or maintenance of weight. Medications used to treat mental illness need to be reviewed, as they can contribute to obesity.[7] Structured approaches need to be in place, including the development of weight management services that can provide a focus for supporting weight maintenance, and where possible weight reduction.

1 Bhaumik S, Watson J, Thorp C, Tyrer F, McGrother C (2008). Body mass index in adults with intellectual disability: distribution, associations and service implications: a population-based prevalence study. *Journal of Intellectual Disability Research* **52**(4), 287–298.

2 Hamilton S, Hankey C, Miller S, Boyle S, Melville C (2007). A review of weight loss interventions for adults with intellectual disability. *Obesity Reviews* **8**, 339–345.

3 van Schrojenstein Lantman-de Valk H, van den Akker M, Masskant M *et al.* (1997). Prevalence and incidence of health problems in people with intellectual disability. *Journal of Intellectual Disability Research* **41**(1), 42–51.

4 Melville C, Cooper S-A, McGrother C, Thorp C, Collacott R (2005). Obesity in adults with Down syndrome: a case-control study. *Journal of Intellectual Disability Research* **49**(2), 125–133.

5 Robertson J, Emerson E, Gregory N *et al.* (2000). Lifestyle related risk factors for poor health in residential settings for people with intellectual disability. *Research in Developmental Disability* **21**(6), 469–86.

6 Rimmer J, Braddock D, Marks B (1995). Health characteristics and behaviours of adults with mental retardation residing in three living arrangements. *Research in Developmental Disabilities* **16**(6), 489–499.

7 Virk S, Schwartz S, Jindal N, Jones N (2004). Psychiatric medication induced obesity: an aetiological review. *Obesity Reviews* **5**, 167–170.

Nutrition

Nutrition plays an important part in everyone's life. Food has a central role in relation to socialization, and is generally an enjoyable experience. It is recognized that nutrition plays an important part in the lives of people with ID, and there are high rates of obesity when compared with the general population.[1] Obesity contributes to a range of important risk factors, such as the development of coronary heart disease, reduced mobility, musculoskeletal problems, and diabetes.[2] This emphasizes the need to develop opportunities for people with ID to participate fully in community activities, and experience regular physical activity and exercise.[3] Ensuring health promotion information is fully accessible is vital in supporting people with ID and their carers to make informed food choices.

The nutrition issues impacting on the lives of people with ID have important public health significance as the population ages and more people live into old age.

Whereas there is clear evidence of the prevalence of obesity within the ID population, for others, particularly those with profound and multiple impairments, there is the risk of being underweight or malnourished.[4] The prevalence of being underweight increases with the severity of the ID, and is common in conditions such as cerebral palsy. People with profound and multiple ID are at increased risk of swallowing and feeding problems such as choking, regurgitation, vomiting, and gastric aspiration.[5,6] As a consequence, comprehensive assessment is required of the gastro-oesophageal tract and swallowing mechanism, and of nutritional needs to maintain weight and appropriate hydration.

Nurses have a role to play in providing additional support during hospitalization when investigations are necessary. The issue of consent to treatment is important, particularly in those with profound intellectual impairment, and where capacity may be lacking. Effective individual nutrition plans are required to minimize the possibility of dehydration, gastric aspiration and pneumonia. The prevention of aspiration pneumonia is important as it is the highest cause of death in this population, and with appropriate assessment and management can be prevented. Nurses have an important role in working collaboratively with people with ID, their families, and carers, to promote healthy lifestyles that includes a focus on improving nutrition and physical activity wherever possible.

1 Robertson J, Emerson E, Gregory N et al. (2000). Lifestyle related risk factors for poor health in residential settings for people with intellectual disability. *Research in Developmental Disability* **21**(6) 469–86.

2 van Schrojenstein Lantman-de Valk H, van den Akker M, Masskant M et al. (1997). Prevalence and incidence of health problems in people with intellectual disability. *Journal of Intellectual Disability Research* **41**(1), 42–51.

3 Bryan F, Allan T, Russell L (2000). The move from a long-stay learning disabilities hospital to community homes: a comparison of clients' nutritional status. *Journal of Human Nutrition & Dietetics* **13**, 265–270.

4 Bhaumik S, Watson J, Thorp C, Tyrer F, McGrother C (2008). Body mass index in adults with intellectual disability: distribution, associations and service implications: a population-based prevalence study. *Journal of Intellectual Research* **52**(4), 287–298.

5 Galli-Carminati G, Chauvet I, Deriaz N (2006). Prevalence of gastrointestinal disorders in adult clients with pervasive developmental disorders. *Journal of Intellectual Disability Research* **50**(10), 711–718.

6 National Patient Safety Agency (2004). *Understanding the patient safety issues for people with learning disabilities*. National Patient Safety Agency: London.

Mobility

There are high rates of mobility problems experienced by people with ID. Some mobility problems will be evident, such as those experienced by people with cerebral palsy and more severe forms of ID. Mobility may be reduced as a consequence of falls and injuries that result in deformity and pain which impacts on the ability and confidence to mobilize. Some anti-psychotic and anti-epileptic medication can impair mobility, thereby contributing to falls and injuries.[1,2] People with ID participate in lower levels of physical activity, well below those recommended to protect and improve health. As a result for the population there is an increased prevalence of obesity. Exercise, as part of the structured preventative approach, has the potential to increase life expectancy and improve health and well-being.[3]

In people with severe physical disabilities and those in older age, the role of postural management is relevant, and plays an important role in minimizing and preventing deformities and breathing difficulties in order to maximize mobility potential.[4] Providing appropriate access to assessment and management by specialists such as ID nurses, physiotherapists, occupational therapy, and specialist services contributes to promoting and maintaining mobility.[5] Ensuring regular attendance at podiatry services is important because of the higher prevalence of foot and toenail problems in this population. Access to specialist footwear may also be required. Addressing these issues helps to reduce pain, falls, and accidents, and offers people with ID increased mobility, which in turn creates the opportunity to participate in community activities.[1,6]

Some people with ID experience visual and hearing disorders that can be treated easily, which helps to improve mobility and self-confidence.[7] Nurses have a role to play in facilitating access to audiology and ophthalmology services, orthotics and wheelchair clinics, and the necessary aid to promote mobility. Regular review of medication used to treat mental illness and epilepsy is important in this population to minimize possible side effects.

1 Hsieh K, Heller T, Miller A (2001). Risk factors for injuries and falls among adults with developmental disabilities. *Journal of Intellectual Disability Research* **45**(1), 76–82.

2 McGrowther C, Bhaumik S, Thorp C, Hauck A, Branford D, Watson J (2006). Epilepsy in adults with intellectual disability: Prevalence, associations and service implications. *Seizure* **15**, 376–386.

3 Hamilton S, Hankey C, Miller S, Boyle S, Melville C (2007). A review of weight loss interventions for adults with intellectual disability. *Obesity Reviews* **8**, 339–345.

4 Janicki M, Davidson P, Henderson C et al. (2002). Health characteristics and health services utilization in older adults with intellectual disability living in community residences. *Journal of Intellectual Disability Research* **46**(4), 287–98.

5 NHS Health Scotland (2004). *People with Learning Disabilities in Scotland: The Health Needs Assessment Report.* NHS Health Scotland: Glasgow.

6 Evenhuis H, Henderson C, Beange H, Lennox N, Chicoine B (2001). Healthy ageing – adults with intellectual disability: Physical Health Issues. *Journal of Applied Research in Intellectual Disability Research* **14**(3), 175–194.

7 Evenhuis H, van Splunder J, Vink M, Weerdenburg C, van Zanten B, Stilma J (2004). Obstacles in large-scale epidemiological assessment of sensory impairments in a Dutch population with intellectual disability. *Journal of Intellectual Disability Research* **48**(8), 708–718.

Exercise

Regular exercise is important for everyone and brings about positive benefits to both physical and mental well-being. Undertaking regular exercise increases community visibility and presence, and offers opportunities to establish and develop new relationships and friendships.

Ensuring that people with ID of all ages have access to and participate in regular exercise has become an issue of increasing importance and concern.[1] As a population, people with ID are unhealthy, overweight, and undertake limited exercise.[2] It is recognized that physical activity among people with ID offers an effective way to improve health and well-being.[3] Inactivity is common within this population and there is lack of light, moderate, and vigorous exercise.[3]

Many of the health conditions and restrictions resulting from living environments impacts significantly on the ability of people with ID to exercise regularly.[1,4] Many people with ID live in supported living or with families, and continue to attend congregated day activities with limited opportunities for physical activity.[3,5] As the population ages and increases there is an opportunity to develop and incorporate physical activity within the supports and services offered to people with ID. This is important, because few people with ID achieve the recommended daily level of physical activity.[4,6]

Nurses and others working with people with ID have an important part to play in supporting the development of healthy lifestyle choices. It is important to ensure that regular exercise appropriate to the individual is incorporated within their daily activities. Identifying opportunities to participate in local leisure and exercise activities offers the potential to bring about the benefits of regular exercise, which in the longer term impacts on physical and mental well-being. By developing collaborations with people with ID, their carers, and creating opportunities whereby people with ID can be supported and enabled to undertake regular daily physical activity is vital in promoting and improving their overall health and well-being.

1 Messent P, Cookes C, Long J (1998). Daily physical activity in adults with mild and moderate learning disabilities: is there enough? *Disability and Rehabilitation* **20** (11), 424–427.

2 Evenhuis H, Henderson C, Beange H, Lennox N, Chicoine B (2001). Healthy ageing – adults with intellectual disability: Physical Health Issues. *Journal of Applied Research in Intellectual disability Research* **14**(3), 175–194.

3 Robertson J, Emerson E, Gregory N *et al.* (2000). Lifestyle related risk factors for poor health in residential settings for people with intellectual disability. *Research in Developmental Disability* **21**(6), 469–86.

4 Hamilton S, Hankey C, Miller S, Boyle S, Melville C (2007). A review of weight loss interventions for adults with intellectual disability. *Obesity Reviews* **8**, 339–345.

5 Rimmer J, Braddock D, Marks B (1995). Health characteristics and behaviours of adults with mental retardation residing in three living arrangements. *Research in Developmental Disabilities* **16**(6), 489–499.

6 Temple V, Anderson C, Walkley J (2000). Physical activity levels of individuals living in a group home. *Journal of Intellectual and Developmental Disability* **25**(4), 327–341.

Diabetes

Glucose is necessary for normal body functioning, and circulates in the blood, where it is used by the cells and muscles as energy. Insulin is a hormone produced by the Islets of Langerhan's in the pancreas and is necessary for the uptake of glucose by cells, to enable their normal functioning. Diabetes is an endocrine disorder affecting glucose metabolism. In diabetes, the pancreas produces little or no insulin or, for reasons that are poorly understood, the body cannot effectively use the insulin that is produced. As a result there is a build up of glucose in the bloodstream, which is disposed of by the body in the urine.

There are two main forms of diabetes, type I and type II. People with type I diabetes have difficulty manufacturing insulin; it is more common at a younger age. Insulin is required for treatment. In type II diabetes there is an inadequate amount of insulin produced to enable glucose metabolism. This form of diabetes is more common in adults, particularly those who are overweight. The clinical features of diabetes can include fatigue, an increase in micturition, glycosuria, and an increase in thirst and hunger.

There are a range of risk factors associated with the development of diabetes, including obesity, coronary heart disease, and poor diet.[1] The link with obesity and the development of type II diabetes is clear, and this is an important issue for people with ID.[2] Within the ID population, where diagnostic overshadowing is possible,[3] the existence of diabetes may be overlooked, and therefore go untreated. It is important, therefore, to recognize the possibility of diabetes within the ID population, and support the opportunity to access health screening, appropriate management and, if required, treatment.

The ID population is increasing and ageing, and evidence further points to many of the population being overweight, which results in a reduction of their life expectancy and increases the risk of associated health complications, including diabetes.[2] The effective prevention and management of obesity is therefore an important issue for many people with ID, and requires a range of coordinated interventions to improve health outcomes and quality of life.[4]

Interventions include the need to ensure that there are effective and systematic health screening programmes that support a treatment element, including weight reduction, behavioural interventions, and physical activity, and health promotion interventions.[5] There is an important role for carers in the management of diabetes, and specific education and support needs to be available for them. Nurses have an important role in supporting people with ID and carers to manage their weight effectively as a means to reduce possible consequences of diabetes, coronary vascular disease, and obesity. Where diabetes is identified it is necessary to ensure that the treatment regimens in place are adhered to, and this could include compliance with hypoglycaemic medication and insulin. There is also a need to ensure effective monitoring and recording of weight, urinalysis, and blood results where appropriate. Effective management of diabetes can therefore require a coordinated approach to care, including the person with ID, their carers, primary care services, specialist diabetes services, and specialists for ID health services.

1 van Schrojenstein Lantman-de Valk H, van den Akker M, Masskant M et al. (1997). Prevalence and incidence of health problems in people with intellectual disability. *Journal of Intellectual Disability Research* **41**(1), 42–51.

2 Melville C, Cooper S-A, McGrother C, Thorp C, Collacott R (2005). Obesity in adults with Down syndrome: a case-control study. *Journal of Intellectual Disability Research* **49**(2), 125–133.

3 Reiss S, Syzszko J (1983.) Diagnostic overshadowing and professional experience with mentally retarded persons. *American Journal of Mental Deficiency* **87**, 396–402.

4 Evenhuis H, Henderson C, Beange H, Lennox N, Chicoine B (2001). Healthy ageing – Adults with intellectual disability: Physical Health Issues. *Journal of Applied Research in Intellectual Disability Research* **14**(3), 175–194.

5 Hamilton S, Hankey C, Miller S, Boyle S, Melville C (2007). A review of weight loss interventions for adults with intellectual disability. *Obesity Reviews* **8**, 339–345.

Thyroid

The thyroid gland is an endocrine organ responsible for making thyroid hormone, which is responsible for regulating some of the physiological functions of the body. The gland itself is situated behind the thyroid cartilage below the larynx in the neck. It comprises a right and a left lobe, joined in the middle by an isthmus. The thyroid gland produces the hormones thyroxin (T4) and triiodothyronine (T3), which are responsible for the regulation of metabolism and growth. T3 and T4 hormones are regulated by thyroid-stimulating hormone (TSH), which is released by the pituitary gland in the brain.

Thyroid disorders commonly take the form of hypothyroidism (myxoedema), where there is under production of the thyroid hormone, or hyperthyroidism (thyrotoxicosis), where there is over production of the thyroid hormone. Hyperthyroid disease can result in conditions such as Grave's Disease, characterized by goitre (a swelling in the neck), tachycardia, arrhythmias, exophthalmus, over activity, sweating, and non-pitting oedema of the lower limbs.

Hypothyroidism is more common to people with Down syndrome, and the incidence of this condition increases with age.[1,2,3,4] The clinical features associated with an under-active thyroid gland include;

- Tiredness
- Lethargy
- Dry skin
- Weight gain
- Depression
- Reduced concentration
- Memory impairment
- Constipation.

Diagnosis of thyroid disorders is made by measuring TSH T3 and T4 levels in the blood, and in some cases by biopsy.

In people with ID, hypothyroidism may not be detected until the later stage of the disease, and recognition is important to supporting health and well-being.[5,6] Treatment is with levothyroxine tablets, and annual screening is recommended in people with Down syndrome.[4]

Nurses have an important role to play in the possible detection of hypothyroidism. A detailed history obtained from families and carers familiar with the person with ID can provide useful insight and background information regarding their usual behaviours and presentation, and changes that have occurred over a period of time. Regular recording of weight can indicate an increase, which, when coupled with other symptoms, may indicate the need for screening by primary care services. Health checks should include blood tests to check for thyroid disorders, and ongoing monitoring and review is required by those with active hypothyroidism and for older people with Down syndrome, where the condition is more common.[4]

1 Pueschel S, Jackson I, Giesswein P, Dean M, Pezzullo J (1991). Thyroid function in Down syndrome. *Research in Developmental Disabilities* **12**, 287–96.

2 Prasher V (1999). Down syndrome and thyroid disorders: a review. *Down's Syndrome Research and Practice* **6**, 42.

3 van Schrojenstein Lantman-de Valk HM (2005). Health in people with intellectual disability: current knowledge and gaps in knowledge. *Journal of Applied Research in Intellectual Disability* **18** (4), 325–333.

4 Prasher V, Gomez G (2007). Natural history of thyroid function in adults with Down syndrome: 10-year follow-up study. *Journal of Intellectual Disability Research* **51**, 312–317.

5 Evenhuis H, Henderson C, Beange H, Lennox N, Chicoine B (2001). Healthy ageing – Adults with intellectual disability: Physical Health Issues. *Journal of Applied Research in Intellectual Disability Research* **14**(3), 175–194.

6 McCarron M, Gill M, McCallion P, Begley C (2005). Health co-morbidities in ageing persons with Down syndrome and Alzheimer's dementia. *Journal of Intellectual Disability Research* **49**(7), 560–566.

Cancer

Cancer comprises a large number of diseases where abnormal cells divide uncontrollably and infiltrate normal body tissue. Cancer can spread throughout the body from the primary source, and is a disease that is found across age groups and genders. It is recognized that there are risk factors associated with the development of cancers, such as smoking, harmful chemicals such as asbestos, a family history, and conditions such as ulcerative colitis. Tumours may be benign or malignant. Malignant tumours can involve the invasion of tissues throughout the body, resulting in metastatic spread. Leukaemia is a cancer that involves blood, bone marrow, the lymphatic system, and the spleen, and does not form into a tumour.

People with moderate or severe ID experience a different cancer pattern compared with the general population that contributes to their mortality.[1,2] In the general population respiratory cancer is the leading cancer for men and women, with breast cancer being prevalent in women and prostate cancer in men. People with ID experience lower levels of prostate cancer, respiratory cancer and urinary tract cancer, with evidence suggesting an increased risk of stomach, oesophageal, and gallbladder cancer.[3] Cancers of the stomach and oesophagus may be related to the high prevalence of gastrointestinal disorders, and in particular GORD and *Helicobacter pylori*.[2]

Leukaemia is a cancer of the white blood cells, and there are two main types: lymphocytic leukaemia and myeloid leukaemia.

Lymphocytic leukaemia affects the lymphocytes, and myeloid leukaemia arises from an immaturity of the myeloid stem cell. White blood cells have an important role to play in protecting the body from infection. People with Down syndrome are at risk of leukaemia, with rates being significantly higher than the general population.[4] People with Prader–Willi syndrome are at increased risk of myeloid leukaemia.[5]

Cancers are diagnosed by examining a biopsy of a tumour, blood analysis, by CT scan, or mammography. A range and combination of treatments may be used, including surgery, bone marrow transplants, chemotherapy, and radiotherapy.

Preventing cancer is important. Ensuring that women with ID are supported to access national cervical and breast screening services is important, as uptake is poor. Nurses have an important role in ensuring adjustments to care are made to help obtain consent and to ensure cooperation. Men with ID may need support and advice to assist with testicular self-examination. Screening for *Helicobacter pylori* should be undertaken, and treatment initiated. Some patients may require admission to hospital for further investigations, such as endoscopy. GORD should be treated with proton-pump inhibitors.

For those diagnosed with a cancer, additional support and information is required during investigations, diagnosis, and treatment.[6] The issue of capacity to consent to treatment needs to be considered, and communication needs identified and addressed. With the population of people with ID there is a need to consider and identify their information and support needs, as some will require care from palliative care services as a consequence of cancer or other life-limiting conditions.[7]

1 Hollins S, Attard MT, von Fraunhofer N, McGuigan S, Sedgwick P (1998). Mortality in people with learning disability: risks, causes, and death certification findings in London. *Developmental Medicine & Child Neurology* **40**, 50–56.

2 Patja K, Molsa P, Livanainen M (2001). Cause-specific mortality of people with intellectual disability in a population-based, 35-year follow-up study. *Journal of Intellectual Disability Research* **45**, 30–40.

3 NHS Health Scotland (2004). *People with Learning Disabilities in Scotland: The Health Needs Assessment Report.* NHS Health Scotland: Glasgow.

4 Hasle H, Clemmensen I, Mikkelsen M (2000). Risks of leukaemia and solid tumours in individuals with Down's syndrome. *Lancet* **355**, 165–169.

5 Davies H, Leusink G, McConnell A *et al.* (2003). Myeloid leukemia in Prader–Willi syndrome. *Journal of Pediatrics* **142**, 174–178.

6 Tuffrey Wijne I, Bernal J, Jones A, Butler G, Hollins S (2006). People with intellectual disability and their need for cancer information. *European Journal of Oncology Nursing* **10**, 106–116.

7 Tuffrey-Wijne I, Hogg J, Curfs L (2006). End-of-life and palliative care for people with intellectual disability who have cancer or other life-limiting illness: A Review of the literature and available resources. *Journal of Applied Research in Intellectual Disability* **20**, 331–344.

Stopping smoking

People with moderate or severe ID tend to have a lower incidence of smoking when compared with the general population.[1,2] This may in part be attributed to social and occupational factors, which could account for the lower rates.

Even though the overall level of cigarette smoking is lower, some people with ID are cigarette smokers and they require access to information, education, and support to assist them to stop.

Information available for the general population about the risks of cigarette smoking may be inaccessible to people with ID who may have difficulty reading. Therefore accessing health promotion information at an appropriate level and in an accessible format is necessary.

Alternative methods of providing health information are being developed by way of symbolized and pictorial health improvement material.[3,4,5]

Smoking cessation clinics and self-help groups have been developed for the general population. People with ID who smoke should have the opportunity to attend and participate in these.

It is important to recognize, however, that some people with ID may need additional support to enable them to access clinics and groups that support smokers to quit. Modified counselling may be necessary as part of a treatment programme tailored to individual needs.

CBT approaches have been developed to assist smokers to quit, and include preparation to quit, coping with the challenges after quitting, and becoming a long-term non-smoker.

Health screening programmes targeted at people with ID need to include a specific focus on smoking, and the possibility of associated respiratory problems. Primary care and specialist ID health services, as a result of the health screening, have the opportunity to identify people with ID who require education and support to enable them to stop smoking.[6] Assisting people with ID to stop smoking will bring about wider improvements in their health.

Consideration and recognition needs to be given to the possibility of weight gain in a population that face challenges with their weight. It is appropriate, therefore, to consider support for stopping smoking, in the wider context of a plan aimed at supporting healthy lifestyles and choices for people with ID.[7]

Medication options to help people with ID to stop smoking need to be considered carefully, to ensure that they are appropriate to the individual, and that any additional support needs are identified, and clearly set out and agreed by them and their carers in the patient's care plan. Ongoing review and monitoring is necessary.

1 Tracy J, Hosken R (1997). The importance of smoking education and preventative health strategies for people with intellectual disability. *Journal of Intellectual Disability Research* **41**, 416–421.

2 Robertson J, Emerson E, Gregory N *et al.* (2000). Lifestyle related risk factors for poor health in residential settings for people with intellectual disability. *Research in Developmental Disabilities* **21**, 469–486.

3 Bradshaw J (2000). A total communication approach towards meeting the communication needs of people with learning disabilities. *Learning Disability Review* **5**, 27–30.

4 Bradshaw J (2001). Complexity of staff communication and reported level of understanding skills in adults with intellectual disability. *Journal of Intellectual Disability Research* **45**, 233–243.

5 Karreman J, van der Geest T, Buursink E (2007). Accessible website content guidelines for users with intellectual disability. *Journal of Applied Research in Intellectual Disability* **20**(6), 510–518.

6 Cooper S-A, Morrison J, Melville C *et al.* (2006). Improving the health of people with learning disabilities: outcomes of a health screening programme after 1 year. *Journal of Intellectual Disability Research* **50**, 667–677.

7 van Schrojenstein Lantman-de Valk HM (2005). Health in people with ID: Current knowledge and gaps in knowledge. *Journal of Applied Research in Intellectual Disability* **18**, 325–333.

Accidents

People with ID frequently experience accidents, falls, fractures, and trauma.[1,2,3] Accidents and falls are associated with epilepsy, the side effects of medication, such as anticonvulsants, visual impairments, impulsivity, and epilepsy, and are multifactorial. People with profound and multiple ID are at significant risk from fractures.[4]

Epilepsy is common in people with ID and can be related to specific syndromes and conditions such as Angelman syndrome, Tuberose sclerosis, Fragile X, Rett syndrome, and Down syndrome. Epilepsy has been implicated in contributing to injuries and sudden unexplained death in people with ID.[5,6] Seizures can cause fractures, subluxation, joint dislocation, and soft tissue injury. Fractures to the skull may result from trauma to the head following a seizure.

It is now recognized that people with ID are more at risk of developing osteoporosis due to vitamin D deficiency and lower bone density than the general population.[7,8,9] Osteoporosis can go unrecognized and may contribute to bone fractures that result from falls, nutritional issues, and the menopause.[8,9,10] There is also the possibility that fractures can occur even with very minor injury, and this needs to be borne in mind if people with ID stumble, trip, or fall. Women with ID are at risk of fractures, and should be recommended to have bone density tests and medication to improve the bone's density.[10]

Nurses working in unscheduled care services, such as accident and emergency departments, need to be aware of the possibility of fractures. The detection and treatment of fractures is important as it eliminates pain and suffering, as well as the possibility of deformity and reduction in functioning. Exercise, good nutritional supplements, and medication for the treatment of osteoporosis can reduce the progress of this disorder.

People with ID can experience mobility problems due to associated conditions such as cerebral palsy and severe intellectual disabilities.[4] Mobility problems may also be associated with disorders of the foot, which if not treated can contribute to falls, and associated trauma and injury in this population.

Some people with ID are prone to become overweight, and ensuring the issue is addressed is important in terms of accident prevention and improving health. Poorly managed respiratory disease can impact on the ability of people with ID to mobilize, and conditions such as asthma may reduce the ability and confidence of people with ID to participate in community activities. As this population ages, many will experience cardiovascular disease such as diabetes, high blood pressure, and cerebral vascular accidents, and these conditions can impact on the mobility of people with ID, thereby increasing their disadvantage.[11] Nurses have an important contribution to make in collaborating with dietitians, physiotherapists, primary care colleagues, carers, and people with ID to minimize the impact of health conditions and associated complications, thereby helping to reduce the possibility of accidents that in some circumstances result in further disability and can contribute to premature death.

Further reading

Kelly K, Stephen L, Sills G, Martin B (2002). Topiramate in patients with learning disability and refractory epilepsy. *Epilepsia* **43**(4), 399–402.

Kerr M (2001). Clinical guidelines for the management of epilepsy in adults with an intellectual disability. *Seizure* **10**, 401–409.

McGrowther C, Bhaumik S, Thorp C, Hauck A, Branford D, Watson J (2006). Epilepsy in adults with intellectual disability: Prevalence, associations and service implications. *Seizure* **15**, 376–386.

1 Grant H, Pickett W, Lam M, O'Connor M, Ouellette-Kuntz H (2001). Falls among persons who have developmental disabilities in institutional and group home settings. *Journal on Developmental Disabilities* **8**(1), 57–73.

2 Hsieh K, Heller T, Miller A (2001). Risk factors for injuries and falls among adults with developmental disabilities. *Journal of Intellectual Disability Research* **45**(1), 76–82.

3 Wagemans A, Cluitmans J (2006). Falls and fractures: a major health risk for adults with intellectual disability in residential settings. *Journal of Policy and Practice in Intellectual Disability* **3**(2), 136–138.

4 Glick N, Fischer M, Heisey D, Leverson G, Mann D (2005). Epidemiology of fractures in people with severe and profound developmental disabilities. *Osteoporosis International* **16**(4), 389–396.

5 van Schrojenstein Lantman-de Valk HM, Metsemakers J, Haveman M, Crebolder H (2000). Health problems in people with intellectual disability in general practice: a comparative study. *Family Practice* **17**, 405–407.

6 Espie C, Watkins J, Duncan R, Sterrich M, McDonagh E, Espie A, McGarvie C (2003). Perspectives on epilepsy in people with intellectual disability. Comparison of family carer, staff carer and clinician score profiles on the Glasgow Epilepsy Outcome Scale. *Seizure* **12**, 195–202.

7 Center J, Beange H, McElduff A (1998). People with mental retardation have an increased prevalence of osteoporosis: A population study. *American Journal on Mental Retardation* **103**, 19–28.

8 Jaffe J, Timell A, Elolia R, Thatcher S (2005). Risk factors for low bone mineral density in individuals residing in a facility for the people with intellectual disability. *Journal of Intellectual Disability Research* **49**(6), 457–462.

9 Vanlint S, Nugent M (2006). Vitamin D and fractures in people with intellectual disability. *Journal of Intellectual Disability Research* **50**(10), 761–767.

10 Schrager S, Kloss C, Ju AW (2007). Prevalence of fractures in women with intellectual disability: A chart review. *Journal of Intellectual Disability Research* **51**(4), 253–259.

11 NHS Health Scotland (2004). *People with learning disabilities in Scotland: The health needs assessment report.* NHS Health Scotland: Glasgow.

Sexual health and personal relationships

People with ID are unique individuals who have their own relationships and friendship needs.[1,2] They are sexual beings and have the right to express their sexuality in line with their peers and all other members of society, but their sexuality and sexual health needs have historically been ignored and their rights not recognized. They need to access information relating to their rights and responsibilities regarding relationships as well as their sexuality and sexual health.

Young people and their parents

There is a need to include young people with ID in sex education programmes within schools, and materials have been developed to assist in this regard. Regardless of age they have to have accessible sexual health information that enables and supports them to make choices within their relationships. Nurses have an important role in supporting and facilitating them to form relationships and express their sexuality. By working with small groups nurses can support and develop understanding of puberty, menstruation, masturbation, and contraception. It is important to recognize the needs of parents, and differences in views and opinions that may be expressed by them regarding relationships and friendships that their adult son or daughter may form. Parents may have anxieties regarding the ability of their son or daughter to enter into sexual relationships, and may be concerned about abuse and exploitation.

Women with intellectual disability

Women with ID have sexual and reproductive health needs. Additional support and education may be required by some young women at the onset of menstruation to enable them to understand and meet their personal care needs. Contraception and the additional information that may be required to enable choices to be made by these women offers opportunities for nurses in sexual health services, primary care teams, and specialist ID teams to support these women. Sexually active women should attend regular cervical screening; women with ID are sometimes not included because it can be distressing and embarrassing, so nurses working in specialist services should work collaboratively with colleagues in primary care and sexual health services to overcome this. Women should attend for breast screening, and as this group is now living longer, breast screening is indicated, because there is the possibility of an increase in cervical and breast cancer.[3] Nurses should ensure that health screening programmes take account of their sexual health, and contraception needs, and that they are included in national screening programmes.[4,5] As women age they will also experience the menopause. Literature highlights a delay or absence of puberty in some women with ID, whereas others, as a result of syndrome-based conditions, may fail to produce sex hormones.

Men with intellectual disability

Men with ID have their own distinct sexual health needs, and yet many are not included in well-men activities, and this is an issue that needs to be addressed. Testicular cancer can occur in young men and it is important to ensure that men with ID have the necessary knowledge and support to examine their testicles and seek help if indicated. As men age there is a need to recognize the possibility of prostate disease and prostate cancer; all social and healthcare workers must ensure that their care needs are addressed within screening and well-men programmes, and they are given information, advice, and support about relationships, sexuality, their sexual health, and options available to them to make informed choices.

Sexual health and abuse in intellectual disability

People with ID who are sexually active may be at risk of developing STIs, such as gonorrhoea, syphilis and *Chlamydia*, and the possibility of HIV and hepatitis. It is important to recognize that they may enter into same-sex relationships, and this may bring with it an increased risk of STI.[6,7,8] People with ID have been victims of a range of abuses, and this includes sexual abuse.[9,10] As a result of their cognitive impairment and communication difficulties, perpetrators may target such people and all social and healthcare workers need to be mindful of this.

1 Scottish Executive (2000). *The Same as You? A Review of Services for People with Learning Disabilities.* The Stationary Office: Edinburgh.

2 Department of Health (2001). *Valuing People: A New Strategy for Learning Disability for the 21st Century.* HMSO: London.

3 Durvasula S, Beange H, Baker W (2002). Mortality of people with intellectual disability in northern Sydney. *Journal of Intellectual and Developmental Disability* **27**, 255–264.

4 Cowie M, Fletcher J (1998). Breast awareness project for women with learning disabilities. *British Journal of Nursing* **7**(13), 774–778.

5 Parrish A, Marwick A (1998). Equity and access to healthcare for women with learning disabilities. *British Journal of Nursing* **7**(2), 92–96.

6 Cambridge P (1997). How far is gay? The politics of HIV in learning disability. *Disability and Society* **12**(3), 427–453.

7 Brown E, Jemmott L (2002). HIV prevention among people with developmental disability. *Journal of Psychosocial Nursing & Mental Health Services* **40**(11), 14–21.

8 Rurangirwa J, Van Naarden Braun K, Schendel D, Yeargin-Allsopp M (2006). Healthy behaviors and lifestyles in young adults with a history of developmental disabilities. *Research in Developmental Disabilities* **27**, 381–399.

9 Joyce T (2003). An audit of investigations into allegations of abuse involving adults with intellectual disability. *Journal of Intellectual Disability Research* **47**(8), 606–616.

10 Brown H (2004). A rights based approach to abuse in women with learning disabilities. *Tizard Learning Disability Review* **9**(4), 41–44.

Gastrointestinal disorders

Gastrointestinal disorders are common in people with ID and increase with the severity of their disability.[1]

GORD is experienced by ~70% of people with ID.[1,2] Gastric aspiration and pneumonia are associated with the swallowing, nutritional, and feeding problems experienced by this population. As a consequence of GORD, people with ID, particularly those with cerebral palsy, scoliosis, and severe and profound ID, may regurgitate the acidic gastric contents up the oesophagus, which is then inhaled into the lungs. Material inhaled results in inflammation of the respiratory tract, which in turn results in pneumonia, which if not promptly and effectively treated and managed, results in death. Trial treatments with proton-pump inhibitors such as omeprazole and lansoprazole are indicated, and should be instigated without an endoscopy.[3]

It is important to identify and treat gastric disorders in people with ID, because they cause pain and distress, and have been linked to cancers.[4] Nurses have an important role in working with carers, dietitians, physiotherapists, speech and language therapists, and colleagues in gastroenterology units in general hospital services, to ensure that risk assessments are undertaken, and plans of care developed and implemented, thereby ensuring that nutritional and care needs are met.

Some people with ID may require nasogastric nutrition or a PEG tube (see 🕮 PEG and PEJ feeding, p.190). This requires the surgical insertion of a tube into the stomach where it remains *in situ* and is used to provide nutrition. Nurses need to be familiar with the care needs of people with ID who have additional nutritional needs, and the safe management of the equipment they require. They also have a key role in providing education and support for carers and family members, and in reassessing care needs.[5]

Helicobacter pylori is a Gram-negative bacterial infection of the stomach lining and small intestine, that if untreated results in gastritis and ulceration of the mucosal lining. It is more common in people with ID than the general population, and many do not present with symptoms.[6,7] Diagnosis is made by breath, blood tests or endoscopy, and biopsy and obtaining specimens can be challenging.[8] Treatment is with antibiotics; it can recur and further treatment may be required. Side effects are common.[7,9] Evidence suggests a link with the increased risk of stomach cancer, oesophageal cancer, and gallbladder cancer within this population.[3] Nurses need to be aware of the possibility of *Helicobacter pylori* within the ID population, and of the presence of symptoms such as vomiting, weight loss, haematemesis, and melaena, which may indicate infection. Good infection control measures are required, such as scrupulous attention to hand hygiene, and particular attention is required when dealing with faeces and salivary secretions to minimize the spread of infection.

1 Galli-Carminati G, Chauvet I, Deriaz N (2006). Prevalence of gastrointestinal disorders in adult clients with pervasive developmental disorders. *Journal of Intellectual Disability Research* **50**(10), 711–718.

2 Böhmer C, Niezen-de Boer M, Klinkenberg-Knol E, Deville W, NadorpJ, Meuwissen S (1999). The prevalence of gastroesophageal reflux disease in institutionalized intellectually disabled individuals. *American Journal of Gastroenterology* **94**, 804–810.

3 NHS Health Scotland (2004). *People with Learning Disabilities in Scotland: The Health Needs Assessment Report.* NHS Health Scotland: Glasgow.

4 Cooke L (1997). Cancer and learning disabilities. *Journal of Intellectual Disability Research* **41**(4), 312–316.

5 Liley A, Manthorpe J (2003). The impact of home enteral tube feeding in everyday life: a qualitative study. *Health and Social Care in the Community* **11**(5), 415–422.

6 Wallace R, Webb P, Schluter P (2002). Environmental, medical, behavioural and disability factors associated with Helicobacter pylori infection in adults with intellectual disability. *Journal of Intellectual Disability Research* **46**(1), 51–60.

7 Wallace R, Schluter P, Webb P (2004). Effects of Helicobacter pylori eradication among adults with intellectual disability. *Journal of Intellectual Disability Research* **48**(7), 646–654.

8 Wallace R, Philip J, Schluter P, Forgan-Smith R, Wood R, Webb P (2003). Diagnosis of Helicobacter pylori infection in adults with intellectual disability. *Journal of Clinical Microbiology* **41**(10), 4700–4704.

9 Wallace R, Schluter P, Webb P (2004). Recurrence of Helicobacter pylori infection in adults with intellectual disability. *Internal Medicine Journal* **34**, 131–133.

Constipation

Constipation is difficulty in passing faeces or a change in the person's usual pattern. Having a bowel movement is a routine activity of daily living, although having a bowel movement does not necessarily happen every day, and what is normal varies from individual to individual. People with ID are more likely to be constipated than those in the general population.

What are the causes of constipation?
- Not drinking enough fluids
- Not having enough fibre in the diet
- Not being active enough
- Side effects of medications
- Being stressed

Why are people with intellectual disability at a greater risk?
- They may be at risk of not eating a balanced diet.
- They may not drink enough fluids and/or have limited food choices, particularly if they are dependant on others.
- They may engage in less physical exercise than is recommended, the prevalence is greater if they are less mobile.
- They may be taking medications that have side effects, including constipation.
- They may be over reliant on laxatives and or PRN (as necessary) medications.
- They may be unable to communicate the urge to defecate or of being hungry/thirsty.
- They may be unable to sit on the toilet in the right position or to use toilet safely.
- They may have problems with eating and drinking (dysphagia).
- Their carers may lack understanding of the effects of food and fluid on the bowel.

Bristol Stool Chart
This is a recognized general measure of consistency and form that is understood by many. This tool classifies faeces into seven types, according to their appearance. Type 1 has spent the longest in the colon, type 7 the least time, with type 4 being the easiest to pass with little discomfort (see Fig. 6.1).

Think about?
Fluid intake—a person needs on average 2L/day of fluid, depending on the person's age and weight. On average a person needs 30ml/kg every 24hrs. For further details seek advice from a dietitian.

Food intake—a person should eat regular balanced meals that contain both soluble fibre (porridge oats, fruit, beans, lentils, baked beans) and insoluble fibre (wholemeal bread/flour, pasta, wholegrain breakfast cereals, brown rice). Consider keeping a food diary over a 7 day period. Any increase in dietary fibre should be done gradually to prevent any abdominal discomfort. This could mean starting ¼ wholemeal products with refined white products and gradually increasing to ½ and then ¾. Further advice should be sought from a dietitian.

Position on the toilet—a person should be able to sit on the toilet comfortably, with their hips at a right angle to the floor, with both feet on the floor or firm base. See a physiotherapist or occupational therapist for further advice.

Increasing exercise—if a person has limited mobility, abdominal massage could be included as part of a total bowel management programme. This is performed to promote peristaltic action within the bowel. Seek further advice from a qualified physiotherapist or community nurse

Use of laxatives—these can be prescribed while dietary or other measures begin to take effect, or for drug-induced constipation, or when other measures fail. Laxatives can be divided into 4 main groups; bulk forming, stimulant, faecal softeners, and osmotic laxatives. Discuss further with either a non-medical prescriber or the person's GP. It is important that these are reviewed once the food and fluids, and/or exercise have begun to take effect on the bowel.

Privacy and dignity—think how you would feel if were trying to defecate while someone was caring for you. Think about how you communicate with the person at this time.

The gastro-colic reflex—this occurs 20–30mins following a hot drink or food hitting the gut; having a bowel movement is more likely at these times and should be encouraged. While straining should not be encouraged, blowing into a balloon can be helpful and fun for children at this time, as this uses the muscles needed to bear down and defecate.

THE BRISTOL STOOL FORM SCALE		
Type 1	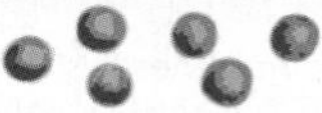	Separate hard lumps, like nuts (hard to pass)
Type 2	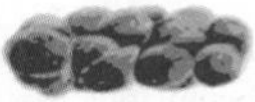	Sausage-shaped but lumpy
Type 3	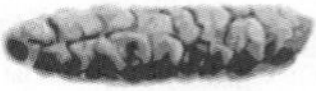	Like a sausage but with cracks on its surface
Type 4	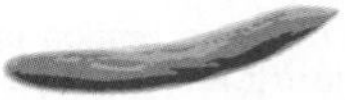	Like sausage or snake, smooth and soft
Type 5	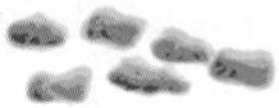	Soft blobs with clear-cut edges (passed easily)
Type 6	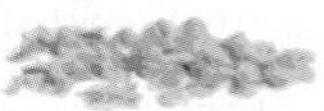	Fluffy pieces with ragged edges, a mushy stool
Type 7	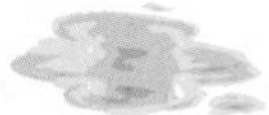	Watery, no solid pieces ENTIRELY LIQUID

Fig. 6.1 Bristol Stool Chart. Reproduced by kind permission of Dr KW Heaton, Reader In Medicine at the University of Bristol. © 2000 Norgine Pharmaceuticals Ltd.

Spirituality

Spirituality is defined as *'the essence of our being, and it gives meaning and purpose to our existence'.*[1] Our spirituality gives us a sense of personhood and individuality. It is the guiding force that gives us our uniqueness, and acts as an inner source of power and energy, which enables us to 'tick over' as a person. Spirituality drives some of us to search for meaning and purpose, and establish positive and trusting relationships with others. Some people may use religion as a medium to express their spirituality and as a way of relating to the transcendent.[2] Spirituality is a journey and religion may become the transport to help people through their journey in life.

Spiritual needs

Spiritual needs may be attained through meaning and purpose, loving and harmonious relationships, forgiveness, hope and strength, trust and personal beliefs and values, spiritual practices, concept of God/Deity, beliefs and practices, and creativity.[3]

Spiritual care

Nurses should use a problem-based approach to plan care to meet the spiritual needs of their patients. Concentrating on helping patients in their growth can improve patients' overall well-being. The following steps of the nursing process may be used for spiritual care.

Assessment

Valuable information central to spiritual needs should be obtained from patients (for Spiritual Assessment Guide, see Narayanasamy 2001, 85–86).[4]

Planning

The information from a spiritual assessment may contribute to the formulation of spiritual care plans. When formulating the care plan, careful consideration should be given to the patient's individuality, the willingness of the nurse to get involved in the spirituality of the patient, the use of the therapeutic self, and the nurturing of the inner person (the spirit).

Implementation (giving spiritual care)

Implementation is about spiritual care intervention based on an action plan that reflects caring for individual. It is necessary to develop a caring relationship, which signifies to the person that he or she is significant. It requires an approach that combines support and assistance in growing spiritually.

Evaluation

As part of evaluation, the following questions may be helpful:
- Is the patient's belief system stronger?
- Do the patient's professed beliefs support and direct actions and words?
- Does the patient gain peace and strength from spiritual resources (such as prayer and minister's visits) to face the rigours of treatment, rehabilitation, or peaceful death?
- Does the patient seem more in control and have a clearer self-concept?
- Is the patient at ease in being alone? In having life plans changed?

- Is the patient's behaviour appropriate to the occasion?
- Has reconciliation of any differences taken place between the patient and others?
- Are mutual respect and love obvious in the patient's relationships with others?
- Are there any signs of physical improvement?
- Is there an improved rapport with other patients?

Further reading

Koenig HG (2001). *Spirituality in Patient Care: Why, How, When and What?* Templeton Foundation Press: Radnor, Pennsylvania.

O'Brien ME (2003). *Spirituality in Nursing: Standing on Holy Ground.* Jones and Bartlett: Boston.

Swinton J (2001). *Spirituality and Mental Healthcare.* Jessica Kingsley: London.

1 Narayanasamy A (2004). The puzzle of spirituality for nursing; a guide to practice assessment. *British Journal of Nursing* **13**(19), 1140–1144.

2 MacKinlay E (2001). *The Spiritual Dimensions of Ageing.* Jessica Kingsley: London.

3 Narayanasamy A (2006). *Spiritual and Transcultural Healthcare Research.* Quay: London.

4 Narayanasamy A (2001). *Spiritual Care: A Practical Guide for Nurses and Healthcare Practitioners,* 2nd Edn. Quay: Wiltshire.

Profound and multiple learning disabilities

Definition

In the UK, the most widely cited definition of profound and multiple learning disabilities (PMLD) was provided by Lacey,[1] who suggested that the term is applied to a group of people who can be described as having; *profound intellectual impairment, and additional disabilities which may include sensory disabilities, physical disabilities, autism, or mental illness.* The WHO state that profound intellectual impairment refers to people who score <20 on an IQ test.[2] They need high levels of support and supervision in all aspects of their lives. They will have significant difficulties with communication and be reliant on others to anticipate their needs and interpret their non-verbal communication.

Problems with labeling

A number of labels have been used to refer to this group of people including; 'profound disabilities and complex needs', 'profound learning disabilities' and 'the most severely disabled'.[3] This can lead to confusion, not least for parents and carers, and also to difficulties with accessing appropriate services. Although definitions and labels are arguably necessary for the planning and delivery of care, people with PMLD are all different and should be treated as individuals.

Prevalence

According to Mencap,[4] PMLD was the fastest growing part of the population of people with ID, and this is thought to be due to developments in medical technology, better control of epilepsy, and an increase in the use of tube feeding. Between 1985 and 2001, the number of children and adults with profound and multiple ID living in England and Wales rose from 25,000 to 40,000.[4]

Assessment of needs

Assessment should be holistic and include physical, psychological, emotional, and spiritual needs. Some areas that may need to be addressed are:

- Mobility—many people with PMLD have difficulties with movement and control of posture. Specialized equipment may be required to aid mobility, support posture, and protect and restore body shape
- Sensory disabilities—specialist assessment of hearing and visual impairment may be necessary
- Respiratory difficulties, epilepsy and mental health
- Eating and drinking—some people with PMLD are unable to take food by mouth and require gastrostomy feeding; others may experience severe swallowing difficulties, which must be assessed by a speech and language therapist
- Continence
- The nature and complexity of the needs of people with PMLD, and/or lack of appropriate support may affect behaviour.

Learning

Despite the severity of the disabilities, people with PMLD can continue to learn throughout their life if they are given the right opportunities. Learning takes place slowly, and constant repetition may be needed to develop the most basic skills.

Services and multidisciplinary support

Assessment and care should involve a multidisciplinary team, which may include:
- family and carers
- school/education professionals and day services
- respite care
- GP, community nurse, physiotherapist, occupational therapist, speech and language therapist, psychologist, and psychiatrist.

When planning care, consideration should be given to issues of informed consent. Many people with PMLD will be unable to give informed consent, both for day-to-day decisions and major health and welfare decisions. Decisions should therefore be made in accordance with relevant legislation (Mental Capacity Act 2005; Human Rights Act 1998).

Attitudes and social exclusion

People with PMLD are one of the most marginalized groups in Western society. Clark and Gates have argued that there remains considerable ignorance both in the general public, and health and social care professions about this group of people.[5] However, the PMLD Network have argued vehemently that people with profound ID and complex needs have a fundamental right to life,[3] and the Human Rights Act 1998 has enshrined their right to life in law. Lacey[1] and the PMLD Network[3] have pointed out the positive contributions that such people make to the lives of people around them.

1 Lacey P (1998). Meeting complex needs through collaborative multidisciplinary teamwork. In: Lacey P and Ouvry C, Eds. *People with Profound and Multiple Intellectual Disability: A collaborative approach to meeting complex needs.* David Foulton: London.

2 World Health Organisation (1992. *The ICD-10 Classification of Mental and Behavioural Disorders: Clinical descriptions and diagnostic guidelines.* WHO: Geneva.

3 PMLD Network (2002). *Valuing People with Profound and Multiple Intellectual Disability (PMLD).* Mencap: London.

4 Mencap (2001). *No Ordinary Life: The support needs of families caring for children and adults with profound and multiple intellectual disability.* Mencap: London.

5 Clark J, Gates B (2006). Care planning and delivery for people with profound intellectual disability and complex needs. In: Gates B, Ed. *Care Planning and Delivery in Intellectual Disability Nursing.* Blackwell Publishing: Oxford, 277–301.

Dysphagia

Dysphagia is a disorder of swallowing that may involve problems with any of the phases of a swallow—the reception and oral preparation of a bolus, the initiation of the reflexive swallow, and the pharyngeal or the oesophageal phase.[1] Dysphagia can cause increased risk of mortality, dehydration, malnutrition, respiratory tract infections, and aspiration.

The normal swallowing process

Oral—food in the mouth is chewed, sucked, and mixed with saliva to create a bolus to allow food to be swallowed.

Pharyngeal—the swallowing reflex is triggered, allowing the bolus to be moved into the oesophagus. The epiglottis lowers to protect the airway and prevent aspiration of food.

Oesophageal—the bolus is moved along the oesophagus towards the stomach by peristalsis.

Signs and symptoms of dysphagia[2]

- Difficulty chewing—food spills from lips, excessive mastication, tongue, jaw or lip weakness
- Difficulty in swallowing—mouth dryness, lip/tongue weakness
- Drooling—lip/tongue weakness, infrequent swallows
- Swallow delay—food is held in the oral cavity for excessively long periods of time
- Food sticking—food residue in mouth, pharynx or oesophagus after swallowing
- Coughing/choking—because of food entering the airway instead of the oesophagus
- Coughing when not eating—aspiration of saliva or lung abnormality
- Regurgitation—undigested food in the mouth; food returning from the oesophagus to the pharynx, acid reflux
- Weight loss—unexplained weight loss/weight below ideal standard.

Management of dysphagia[3]

- Any concerns regarding the capacity of an individual to swallow effectively, should be referred to a speech and language therapist for a full assessment.
- Dysphagia management procedures developed by speech and language therapists should be strictly adhered to. A multidisciplinary approach is required. Ensure that all members of the multidisciplinary team are aware of the risk factors and management procedures in place for those who present with dysphagia.
- Correct positioning of the individual, in a chair with their head and trunk slightly forward will aid the passage of food through the pharynx and oesophagus.
- Desensitizing the oral cavity prior to feeding may be beneficial for some individuals, by massaging the cheeks or tooth brushing to reduce hypersensitivity. Liaise with speech and language therapists to identify best approach.

- Tilting the chin down, turning/tilting the head to the left/right may be beneficial for some people. However, a speech and language therapist should determine which position is best for each individual.
- Ensure the individual is comfortable and free from distractions.
- Use adapted equipment, spoons, and feeding cups to maximize food intake, as required.
- Ensure food is presented in an appetizing manner, at an appropriate temperature. This may require preparation of small amounts of food at a time, particularly if the feeding process is protracted.
- Allow enough time to feed the individual involved, pace the intake of food to meet the person's needs, and give appropriate amounts of food at a time.
- Determine the portion of food the person will eat.
- Ensure the consistency of the food is right (pureed versus soft, thin versus thickened). If using commercial thickeners, follow manufacturer's directions. Observe for changes in food bolus consistency; some foods become thicker/thinner as they heat up/cool down.
- Use verbal/non-verbal cues to direct the person's attention to eating.
- Observe the individual closely during and following feeding. The person should remain upright for 30mins following feeding. Clear any remaining food from the person's mouth when finished feeding.
- Record dietary intake on appropriate recording charts, and monitor the person's weight regularly.
- Carefully observe the person's preference for different foods, and reassess regularly as people's tastes change over time.
- Continuous assessment is required through direct observation and a diet history to monitor the condition.
- Any deterioration in the condition, such as increase of incidences of aspiration, respiratory tract infections, weight loss, may be an indication of the need for enteral feeding.
- It is essential to remember that not all individuals present with visible signs of aspiration. Silent aspiration is difficult to detect; individuals present with recurrent respiratory tract infections or pneumonia, which may be fatal. Video fluoroscopic[†] swallow evaluation is required to identify silent aspiration.
- Care of the oral mucosa is essential for people with dysphagia; food must be removed carefully after feeding.

1 Rubin L, Crocker A (2006). *Medical Care for Children & Adults with Developmental Disabilities.* Paul H Brookes Publishing Company: Canada.

2 Crary MA, Groher ME (2003). *Adult Swallowing Disorders.* Butterworth Heinemann: London.

3 Mager D, Pencharz P (2007). Nutritional considerations in children with intellectual and developmental disabilities. In: Brown I, Percy M. *A Comprehensive Guide to Intellectual and Developmental Disabilities.* Paul H Brookes Publishing Company: Canada.

PEG and PEJ feeding

PEG and PEJ feeding are forms of enteral feeding. PEG feeding requires the insertion of a tube through a surgically created opening, known as a fistula, in the abdominal wall (see Fig. 6.2). This creates an artificial tract into the stomach through which feeding can occur. A peg is a flexible silicone transabdominal tube, which following insertion is held in place by an internal retainer disc and external skin bumper disc. 6 months following insertion, a balloon tube or low profile button tube may be inserted. Some individuals who are at risk of severe GORD may need PEJ feeding, where the tube is placed in the jejunum, bypassing the stomach, thus reducing the risk of GORD. This is usually undertaken in association with gastroscopy, with jejunal extension (PEG-J) or direct percutaneous jejunostomy. Issues and care of PEG/PEJ tubes and feeding regimens are similar.

Indicators for use of PEG/PEJ feeding[1]

- Aspiration and or anorexia, respiratory difficulties, dysphagia, limited gag reflex, poor appetite, cerebral palsy, cleft lip and palate, individual unable to meet nutritional requirements.

Advantages of PEG/PEJ feeding

- An effective means of long-term nutritional support. Ensures a person is adequately hydrated, enables an individual to take in orally what they can while ensuring adequate nutritional intake is achieved, reduces the risk of aspiration, can be used in the presence of significant medical illness, and are concealed by clothing therefore are more cosmetically acceptable than nasogastric tubes.

Disadvantages of PEG/PEJ feeding

Gastrointestinal problems

- Diarrhoea, constipation, nausea, vomiting, gastroesophageal reflux (associated more with PEG feeding).

Tube related

- Invasive procedure, requires general anaesthetic, wound infection, blockage, kinking or dislodgement of tube, can be difficult to relocate (associated more with PEJ feeding).

Quality of life

- Unnatural method of feeding, social element of mealtimes may be lost, loss of enjoyment, pleasurable experience of food, rapid or excessive weight gain, continuous feeding (12–20hrs/d) may limit mobility and level of activity, care of oral mucosa may be overlooked.

Feeding

With PEG tubes methods of feeding may include:

- Bolus—given via syringe 3–6 times/d (feed is instilled by force of gravity)
- Intermittent—via feeding pump (large volume 3–4 times/d)
- Continuous—via feeding pump (12–20hrs/d).

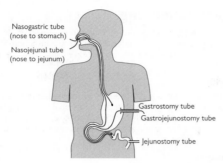

Nasogastric tube
(nose to stomach)

Nasojejunal tube
(nose to jejunum)

Gastrostomy tube

Gastrojejunostomy tube

Jejunostomy tube

Fig. 6.2 Routes for enteral feeding. Reproduced with kind permission.
©Burdett Institute 2008.

With PEJ, feeding is continuous; PEJ feed needs to be given more slowly, and any water put into the PEJ needs to be sterile or boiled. Always confirm correct positioning of the tube using pH indicator strips; a pH of 5.5 or less indicates correct positioning of the tube. Before starting feeding, gain consent and reassure the individual. Never lay the person flat during a feed—elevate the head and upper body at least 30°. Maintain this position during and post feeding for 1hr. The feeding regimen developed for the individual should be adhered to, and manufacturer's guidelines for storage and use followed. The tube should be flushed out after each feed using cool boiled water or sterile water, to prevent blockage. Carefully document feeds in appropriate recording charts.

Caring for PEG/PEJ tubes[2]

Use of standard infection control procedures is necessary. Observe for:
- leakage of stomach contents, blockage of the tube (clear by flushing the tube with cool boiled water or pineapple juice), granulation of tissue at the site, which may indicate friction, bleeding around the tube, which may indicate tissue erosion from pressure or granulation tissue, bleeding through the tube, which may indicate gastritis/ulcer or tissue erosion caused by the tube, erythema around the tube caused by cellulitis or yeast infection, treatable with topical or oral antibiotics as required.

1 Gates B (2007). *Learning Disabilities. Towards Inclusion.* Churchill Livingstone: Edinburgh.

2 Rubin L, Crocker A (2006). *Medical Care for Children & Adults with Developmental Disabilities.* Paul H Brookes Publishing Company: Canada.

Nasogastric feeding

NG feeding is used to supplement feeding of individuals of all ages who have swallowing or feeding difficulties. It requires the insertion of a disposable plastic feeding tube into the nose, extending into the stomach[1] (see Fig. 6.2).

Advantages

- Ensures adequate nutritional intake, allows individuals to take in orally what they can while ensuring adequate nutritional intake is achieved, ensures a person is adequately hydrated, reduces the risk of aspiration, less invasive procedure than gastrostomy, and can also be used as a trial prior to gastrostomy.

Disadvantages

Gastrointestinal problems
- Diarrhoea or constipation, nausea and vomiting

Tube related
- Erosion of nasal and oral mucosa, sinusitis and/or nasal ulcers, skin irritation, from fixing the tube to the individual's cheek, blockage, kinking or dislodgement of tube

Respiratory
- Pulmonary aspiration, incorrect insertion of tube

Quality of life
- More 'visible' than gastrostomy, can cause distress when inserted, unnatural method of feeding, social element of meal times may be lost, long-term use can impact on swallowing and oral feeding.

Nasogastric care and feeding

Types of nasogastric tubes
NG tubes come in varying sizes for children and adults. There are 2 main types of NG tubes:
- Silicone tubes can be used for up to 1wk and are less expensive than silk tubes.
- Silk tubes can be used for up to 6wks.

It is important to adhere to local health service providers and manufacturer's guidelines for timescale for use and disposal of NG tubes.

Insertion of nasogastric tubes
- Wash your hands prior to gathering required equipment, put on gloves, select the tube required, and take time to explain the procedure to the person. Gain consent, and offer reassurance, ensuring the person is in an upright position.
- Identify the length of tube required by using the tube itself to measure from the person's nose to their ear and down to the epigastric area. Make sure to lubricate the tip of the tube and gently insert the tube into the nostril in an upward and backward motion, and encourage the person to swallow or offer a drink if possible while passing the tube.

- Continue to swiftly and steadily pass the tube through the nose and down into the stomach, until the desired length of tubing has been inserted. Then temporarily secure the tube to the person's cheek and behind the ear prior to checking that the tube is positioned correctly in the stomach.

Confirming correct positioning of tube

It is essential to check the position of the tube before every feed. So using a syringe, aspirate fluid from the tube (~0.2–1ml of aspirate will suffice). Place a few drops of the aspirate on a pH indicator strip, and allow 10–15s for any colour change to occur. Match the pH indicator strip with the colour code chart on the strip box. A pH of 5.5 or below indicates that the tube is correctly positioned, and feeding can start. A pH of 6 or over suggests that the tube may be incorrectly positioned. Consider rechecking or re-passing the tube. Seek advice if the situation remains unchanged. Having confirmed correct positioning of the tube, it must be attached securely with tape to either the left or right cheek. Observe the person for any adverse reaction to the insertion of the tube.

Feeding

Feeding via an NG tube can take the form of a bolus feed, where the prepared feed is administered via a syringe barrel, held above the height of the person, and the feed is instilled by gravity. Feeding may also be continuous, where the feed is administered via a pump. On completion of each feed flush out the tube to ensure it is clean and to avoid blockages, and document input and output in appropriate recording charts.

Important points to remember

If the person can take fluids and food orally, then feeding via NG tube should only be used to supplement their oral intake as required. Particular attention should be given to oral hygiene, particularly to alleviate mouth dryness. Care of the nasal mucosa is also important.

1 Batshaw ML, Pellegrino L, Roizen NJ (2007). *Children with Disabilities*. Paul H Brookes Publishing: Canada.

2 Sense Scotland and Women and Children's Directorate, NHS Greater Glasgow. *Meeting the Healthcare Needs of People with Multiple Disabilities. Training and development packs for support staff*. Pavilion Publishing: Brighton.

Hearing

In developing and maintaining communication skills, information from all five senses is important. However, the main channels for communication are the distance senses of hearing and sight. Many people with ID have additional difficulties in communication because of sensory impairment. Clarke-Kehoe estimate that as many as 45% of people with ID may have some level of visual or hearing impairment.[1] Hearing is vital for the development of spoken language. Those with a pre-lingual profound hearing loss will not have access to speech sounds and therefore will not develop verbal communication.

Behaviours that may indicate hearing loss

- Pulling/poking the ears
- Watching the speaker's face and lips constantly
- Tilting the head to one side towards the source of sound
- Speaking loudly—this is typical of a sensorineural hearing loss, where people raise their voice so that it is audible to themselves
- Speaking softly—this is typical of conductive hearing loss, where people match their own voices to the level at which they hear others voices
- Appearing startled when someone approaches
- Visible signs of discharge from the ears, or excessive wax
- Dislike of loud sounds—this may be due to recruitment, where people have a reduced range between the point where they can just hear sounds and the point where sound is perceived as unbearably loud.[2]

Causes of hearing impairment

- Conductive hearing loss—sounds have difficulty passing through the outer or middle ear; hearing loss is usually mild/moderate
- Sensorineural hearing loss—the cause of the hearing loss is in the cochlea or auditory nerve; hearing loss is usually severe or profound.

Some people may have the same type and degree of hearing loss in each ear, or it may be different in each ear. A hearing test will identify the type of hearing loss the person presents with and the appropriate intervention that is required.

Levels of hearing loss

- Mild hearing loss—falls within the range 25–40db. The sounds heard may be compared to listening to sounds when you have a heavy cold.
- Moderate hearing loss—falls within the range 40–70db. This may be compared to listening to someone talking in the next room with the door closed.
- Severe hearing loss—falls within the range 70–90db. Many sounds cannot be heard at this level. A person with a severe hearing loss would experience gaps in what they hear.
- Profound hearing loss—exceeds 90db. The person will not hear normal speech, but would be able to detect rhythms in loud music and feel the vibration of sound.

Hearing aids

Hearing aids may be recommended post assessment. Nurses and carers will have a vital role in assisting the individual to maintain and use them effectively.

Communication

When communicating with a person presenting with hearing loss, it is necessary to follow certain measures:

- Ensure you have the person's attention and that they are looking at you. This promotes lip-reading and the use of facial expression to aid communication
- Slow your speech
- Do not shout
- Cut out background noise where possible
- Get reasonably close to the person. If a hearing aid is worn, the optimum distance apart is ~1m—beyond this point background noise will sound as loud as speech
- Be aware in group settings; changing speakers may be confusing for the listener
- Ensure that the person has had a recent ophthalmological assessment; when someone has a hearing impairment, it is particularly important to know the person's visual acuity
- Use pictures, symbols, facial expression, gesture and Makaton signs to augment speech
- Thorough communication assessment of the individual will allow for accurate intervention, using the most appropriate communication tool.

1 Clarke-Kehoe A, Harris P (1992). It's the way that you say it. *Community Care* **9**, 15–20.

2 Gates B (2007). *Learning Disabilities. Towards Inclusion*. Churchill Livingstone: Edinburgh.

Integration of sensory experiences

There is an increased prevalence of sensory impairments within the population of people with ID when compared with the general population.[1,2,3] Hearing and visual impairments are common, and may be apparent from birth. Others may be acquired in later life and may be associated with genetic conditions related to the cause of the ID, such as Down syndrome, where visual and hearing problems are common.[3,4] Some people with ID can experience congenital cataracts, retinal abnormalities, optic atrophy, or abnormalities of the eye structure that result in visual impairment.[5] Access to assessment and remedial prosthesis, and other treatments such as cataract surgery, can be beneficial, and therefore early detection, treatment, and regular review is important and will contribute to reducing the possibility of accidents and injury resulting from visual impairments. Attention should also be paid to the sense of smell and touch, and there have been developments in the provision of therapies such as reflexology and aromatherapy provided for people with ID and cerebral palsy. As people with ID are ageing and living longer they will also experience visual changes and hearing loss associated with the ageing process.[1,6] Their possible changing needs must be recognized, and routine health screening programmes provide an ideal opportunity for nurses to incorporate visual and hearing screening at the same time. Effective screening and management can have positive benefits to the quality of life of the person with ID; barriers can exist, however, when undertaking assessment of vision and hearing.[7] Nurses should play an important role in enabling access to visual and hearing assessments, and in ensuring there is support to adapt to their prosthesis, such as glasses and hearing aids, and in educating carers of their importance.[3]

1 Janicki M, Dalton A (1998). Sensory impairments among older adults with intellectual disability. *Journal of Intellectual & Developmental Disability* **23**(1), 13–11.

2 Carvill S (2001). Sensory impairments, intellectual disability and psychiatry. *Journal of Intellectual Disability Research* **45**(6), 467–483.

3 Meuwese-Jongejeugd A, Vink M, van Zanten B *et al.* (2006). Prevalence of hearing loss in 1598 adults with an intellectual disability: Cross-sectional population based study. *International Journal of Audiology* **45**(11), 660–669.

4 Evenhuis HM, Mul M, Lemaire E, de Wijs J (1997). Diagnosis of sensory impairment in people with intellectual disability in general practice. *Journal of Intellectual Disability Research* **41**(5), 422–429.

5 Evenhuis HM, Theunissen M, Denkers I, Verschuure H, Kemme H (2001). Prevalence of visual and hearing impairment in a Dutch institutionalized population with intellectual disability. *Journal of Intellectual Disability Research* **45**(5), 457–464.

6 Evenhuis H, Henderson C, Beange H, Lennox N, Chicoine B (2001). Healthy ageing – adults with intellectual disability. Physical Health Issues. *Journal of Applied Research in Intellectual Disability Research* **14**(3), 175–194.

7 Evenhuis H, van Splunder J, Vink M, Weerdenburg C, van Zanten B, Stilma J (2004). Obstacles in large-scale epidemiological assessment of sensory impairments in a Dutch population with intellectual disability. *Journal of Intellectual Disability Research* **48**(8), 708–718.

Oral health

Oral health *'is a standard of health of the oral and related tissues which enables an individual to eat, speak and socialize without active disease, discomfort and embarrassment and which contributes to general well-being'.*[1] People with ID experience poorer general and oral health than the general population. In the past oral disease has not been given as much priority as other complex medical problems experienced by people with ID, despite the severity of the impact of oral disease on this population.[2]

Impact of oral disease

- Dental caries, coronal caries (of the crown part of the tooth)
- Root caries (of the root part of the tooth)
- Periodontal disease (of the gum and supporting bone)
- Lower number of natural teeth
- Higher level of tooth extraction and lower levels of restorations
- Significant pain
- Inability to consume nutritious food
- Poor quality of life (destruction of self-image, lack of confidence).

Oral disease has been linked to other systemic diseases such as:

- Cardiovascular disease
- Cerebrovascular disease
- Diabetes
- Respiratory infection
- Periodontal bone loss
- Osteoporosis.

Specific factors such as bruxism (involuntary grinding of the teeth), altered salivary flow resulting in xerostomia (dry mouth), and hypertrophy or overgrowth of the gingival tissues, due to long-term use of certain medications need to be addressed.[3]

Effective oral care.

Oral assessment—simple oral assessment can initially be carried out by carers; healthy gums are firm in texture and do not bleed when brushed. Inflamed gums are swollen and often bleed. Observe for any changes in teeth, such as cavities, signs of trauma, or loose teeth. Observe the lips, gums, tongue, palate, and soft tissue of the oral cavity for damage and mouth ulcers. A full assessment by a dentist needs to be undertaken to identify signs and symptoms of oral disease. An annual review with a dentist should be standard for each individual with and without teeth. People with ID may require an advocate or health facilitator to arrange dental visits and to ensure an effective oral care plan is developed.

An oral care plan should:

- Ensure a person's teeth are brushed effectively, using an ordered approach to brushing to ensure no part of the mouth is missed. If an individual has difficulty tolerating this, brush different parts of the mouth throughout the day. Record oral care appropriately, including any abnormalities noted. If an individual can brush their teeth with assistance, this should be encouraged, to promote independence.

Skills training programmes can also be developed to teach individuals to brush their teeth.

- When brushing teeth, always explain to the individual what is to happen, and gain consent if possible. Brushing someone's teeth is an invasive procedure and can be frightening for the individual involved. Be aware of how long a person can tolerate having their teeth brushed, brush more frequently and for shorter lengths of time if required. Encourage the individual to cooperate as much as he/she can.

- Stand behind and to one side of an individual and gently draw back the lips with thumb and forefinger on one side of the mouth to gain access to the teeth. Commence with the upper teeth, brush teeth with short motions paying particular attention to the gum margins. Brush the inner and biting surfaces of all teeth as far as possible. If possible, gently brush the tongue. Assist the person to rinse their mouth, or clean around the mouth with a damp swab if required.

- Proper nutrition is required to ensure good oral health; sugary snacks and drinks should be kept to a minimum. Self-cleansing foods such as apples and celery should be given as snacks between meals, for those who can tolerate them. No drinks (other than water) should be given after tooth brushing at night. It is important to remember that people who are fed via enteral feeding devices also require effective oral healthcare.

- Medication can impact on oral health; more than 400 medications cause xerostomia (dry mouth), and anticonvulsant therapy has been linked to gingival overgrowth. Medications can often have a high sugar content, 'sugar free' options should be used where available.

- Denture care is important, and individuals with dentures should be assessed regularly to ensure that their dentures fit properly. When cleaning dentures, follow manufacturer's instructions when using cleaning agents. Do not use very hot water as this may warp dentures. They should be stored in a container of cool water, as they can become dry and warp. They can break easily if dropped onto a hard surface, so care must be taken when cleaning.

1 Waldman B, Perlman S (2007). Oral health, nurses and patients with developmental disabilities. *International Journal of Nursing in Intellectual and Developmental Disabilities* **3**(1):4. See ▣ http://journal.hsmc.org/ijnidd

2 Department of Health, Social Services and Public Safety (2005). *Survey of Dental Services to People with Learning Disabilities in Northern Ireland.* See ▣ http://www.dhsspsni.gov.uk

3 Doyle S, Dalton C (2008). Developing clinical guidelines on promoting oral health: an action research approach. *Learning Disability Practice,* **11**(2).

Healthy skin

The skin is the largest organ of the body, covering 1.5–2.0m². It is made up of a number of layers and contains nerve endings, sweat glands, and blood capillaries.[1]

Functions of the skin

- Protects the body against noxious agents and infectious organisms
- Helps to regulate body temperature
- Assists with the body's fluid and chemical balance
- Sensitivity to pain, temperature, pressure, and touch
- Production of vitamin D with exposure to sunlight
- By being visible to the outside world, the skin is also integral to an individual's personal identification.

People with ID are at greater risk of suffering from skin complaints than the general population.[2] For example, dryness and eczema is common in people with Down syndrome, and a variety of skin lesions and abnormalities are associated with phenylketonuria and tuberose sclerosis. Good assessment and care is therefore essential for this group.

Assessment

Skin care is integral to person-centred health action planning. Assessment should be individualized and holistic, and take account of personal preferences and cultural factors. Carers should be mindful of the impact of skin colour on the presentation of skin conditions. For example, lesions that appear red or brown in white skin may appear black or purple in pigmented skin, and mild degrees of redness (erythema) may be masked completely in black skin. Personal and intimate care can provide an opportunity for carers to assess the skin. People with ID who are able to carry out their intimate care independently should be educated to examine their skin and to report any worrying changes they notice to a carer or their GP. Assessment of the skin should include consideration of:

- Family history of skin disease
- Medication and its side effects
- Seasonal effects
- Allergies and changes in the use of cleansing agents, washing liquid and cosmetics.

Use of skin care products and cleansing agents

A balanced diet and drinking plenty of water is thought to be important for the health of the skin. Good personal and intimate care is also essential for maintaining the health of the skin, and the use of appropriate skin care products can promote healthy skin. Products should be chosen according to an individuals' particular skin type, and based on individual assessment and preference. Soap and perfumed products should be used with caution because they can cause dryness and irritation, and soap substitutes, known as emollients, are more suitable for many people. Dry skin can be itchy, sore, and unsightly. This can be reduced and prevented with the use of appropriate emollients and moisturizers. Excessive washing, the use of detergents (such as soap), failing to remove soap from the skin, extensive soaking, and very hot bath water, can cause dryness and lead to dermatitis.

Common skin conditions and their symptoms

- Eczema—dry, red, scaly skin that can be intensely itchy
- Psoriasis—the most common forms appear as patches of silvery scales on top of areas of red skin
- Leg ulcers—swelling, brown discolouration of white skin, presence of eczema
- Pressure sores—initially appear as an area of red skin and feel warm and spongy or firm to the touch. In people with darker skin, the mark may appear to have a blue or purple cast, or look flaky or ashen. If pressure is not relieved, an open sore may develop that looks like a blister, and in advanced stages can appear as a deep crater-like wound.
- Herpes simplex—ulcers or sores, found particularly on the face, hands and genitals
- Dandruff—white, oily-looking flakes of dead skin appearing on the hair and shoulders, and an itchy, scaling scalp
- Cellulitis—a bacterial infection resulting in redness, swelling, warmth, pain and tenderness.

A GP should be consulted for advice on specific skin complaints.

Care of the skin in the sun

The risk of skin cancer as a result of over-exposure to the sun has been well documented and established. The risk can be greatly reduced by taking the following precautions:

- Stay out of the sun during the hottest part of the day. In the UK, this is usually 11–3pm in the summer months. Particular caution should be taken for people who are on psychotropics, or any medication, that can cause skin sensitivity to sunlight
- Wear clothing made of cotton or natural fibres that are closely woven and offer good protection against the sun
- Protect the face and neck by wearing a wide-brimmed hat
- Use a high-factor sunscreen (SPF 30 or above) whenever you are exposed to the sun. Follow the instructions on the bottle and reapply as recommended, particularly after swimming
- Never allow the skin to burn
- Report mole changes or unusual skin growths to the GP promptly.

1 Holland K, Jenkins J, Solomon J, Whittma S (2003). *Applying the Roper Logan Tierney Model in Practice*. Churchill Livingstone: London.

2 Sines D, Appleby F, Frost M (2005). *Community Healthcare Nursing*. Blackwell Publishing: London.

Personal and intimate care

Personal and intimate care includes: bathing and showering, dressing, changing continence pads, helping someone use the toilet, changing sanitary towels or tampons, shaving, skin care, hair care, and brushing teeth.

Good personal and intimate care is essential for health, hygiene, psychological well-being, and self-esteem. Many people with ID are dependent on others for their personal and intimate care. This might be as a result of deficits in cognition, sensory disabilities, or physical disabilities, which restrict movement and the ability to carry out fine and gross motor skills that are required for self-care. Personal and intimate care is carried out for hygiene, comfort, pleasure, and personal appearance.

Good hygiene

Skin cleanliness reduces the number of microorganisms on the skin that can cause infections. The genital and anal areas are particularly prone to bacteria and bodily secretions. Thorough hygiene is necessary to prevent infections and unpleasant odours in these areas.

Male hygiene

Perineal-genital care for an uncircumcised male involves retracting the foreskin to expose the glans or head of the penis, washing and drying the glans, and then replacing the foreskin. Inadequate hygiene and over washing with soap is associated with an increased risk of balanitis (inflammation and itchiness (of the head of the penis)), and viral infections.

Female hygiene

The vulva and perineal area should be washed daily, although the use of strong solutions of any kind in this area should be avoided because these can damage the mucus membrane. The use of deodorants, or clinging or synthetic clothes in this area can also lead to irritation and potentially vulvitis. Females should always be washed from cunnus to anus (i.e. front to back) in order to avoid transferring germs. Skin creases, such as beneath the breasts of women, are areas that are particularly prone to skin problems, and it is important that these areas are washed and dried gently but thoroughly, and with care.

Assessment and planning

Planning should be based on assessment of the individual's physical and cognitive abilities, as well as their personal preferences. Other issues that need to be considered when assessing and planning care are:
- Informed consent and capacity to consent
- Maintaining and promoting independence
- Particular needs around continence care
- Choice of products (men and women with black and dark skin should use oils or moisturizers after bathing to keep the skin supple and smooth).

Cultural and religious considerations

In Hindu, Muslim, and Sikh religions, physical cleanliness is extremely important. Many people who belong to these religions have a preference for washing under running water; for these people showering is more appropriate than bathing. Modesty is important, particularly for women; legs and upper arms may need to be covered. The necessity for washing rituals prior to prayer time may need to be considered. In the Muslim faith genitals are washed with the left hand, because the right hand is used for eating. In Sikhism, hair and beards may need to be kept uncut; men and women fix their hair on their head with a plastic comb known as a 'kangha'. Hair should not be cut without permission of the person or family.

Risk assessment, policies, and training

Areas that need to be addressed in risk assessments, policies and training include:

- Prevention of abuse, and cross-gender care
- Epilepsy and environmental safety (e.g. water temperature, need for slip mats)
- Moving and handling
- Infection control (consider use of gloves, aprons and good hand hygiene).

Good practice tips

- Be discrete when talking about incontinence to others and in front of others; prepare the environment and ensure all items are close to hand.
- Respect dignity at all times, e.g. do not undress the person until the last min when they need to be undressed, and use appropriate communication strategies, which may include short simple sentences and objects of reference. Allow the person time alone in private to masturbate, if they indicate by touching themselves that they would like to, and if it is safe for them to do so.
- Intimate and personal care can be used as an opportunity for one-to-one communication and intensive interaction.
- Clothing and appearance are important for self-expression.

Further reading

Cambridge P, Carnaby S (2000). *Making it Personal: Providing Intimate and Personal Care for People with Intellectual Disability*. Pavilion Publishing: Brighton.

Clark J (2006). Intimate care: theory, research and practice. *Learning Disability Practice* **9**(10), 12–17.

Continence

Definition

Continence is the voluntary control over urinary and faecal discharge. Failure to achieve continence is referred to as 'incontinence' and is the involuntary loss of urine or faeces. Incontinence ranges from occasional leakage to an inability to control voiding.

Prevalence

Prevalence of incontinence is difficult to determine because a variety of definitions have been used, and also because of the stigma associated with it. Incontinence can happen to anyone and occurs across all age groups. It is, however, more common in older age. In people with ID, continence is more likely to be delayed later into childhood and some people remain incontinent throughout adulthood. Incontinence is more common in people with ID than the general population, and presents a greater problem to those with more severe disabilities.

Causation

Continence is dependent on hormonal, muscular, and neurological control. Incontinence is therefore associated with a variety of conditions, and the primary cause for people with ID is likely to be related to the nature of their learning and/or physical disability. Neurological and physical disabilities can be the root causes of incontinence and urinary tract infections, and renal abnormalities can exacerbate the problem. Many people with ID may have problems achieving continence if they are unable to understand the biological signals for urination and defecation. There may also be psychological and behavioural reasons for failing to urinate and defecate appropriately.

Assessment

Assessment should:
- Be individualized, holistic and lead to person-centred treatment package
- Be made by a multidisciplinary team, which might involve a GP, community nurse, continence advisor, physiotherapist, carers and social workers
- Identify underlying problems and the type of incontinence
- Include consideration of mobility, physical and mental health
- Involve the measurement of fluid and dietary intake and output
- Determine bladder and bowel habits and patterns.

Consider also the following factors, which may contribute to incontinence:
- Medication
- Constipation/diarrhoea
- Lack of access to toilet facilities and lack of privacy
- Difficulties with psychomotor skills needed for undressing and using the toilet independently.

Treatment

Incontinence is often viewed as an inevitable consequence of having ID, and therefore treatment is not always prioritized or even considered. However, with assessment, planning, and appropriate support, many people with ID have a significant chance of becoming continent.

A training programme for incontinence might include:
- Positive reinforcement for appropriate voids
- Teaching skills required for dressing and undressing
- Regulating fluid and dietary intake
- Making toilet facilities accessible
- Training in pelvic floor exercises to increase muscle control for continence.

Management of incontinence

Good, person-centred personal and intimate care is essential when caring for someone who suffers from incontinence. This involves prompt skin care after defecation to reduce odour and skin problems. Brisk scrubbing should be avoided to prevent damaging the skin, and moisturizing cream or ointment can be applied to protect the skin from future exposure to urine and stool. Appropriate use of continence aids, such as the correct size of pads is important. Catheterization can be considered, and may be successful for people with neurological conditions.

The impact of incontinence

Incontinence can have serious effects on physical, psychological, and emotional well-being, both for the person and their carers. Some of the potential impacts are:
- Increased risk of skin infections and perineal dermatitis and discomfort
- Reduced independence and problems with access to social opportunities, school and work, and difficulties with accessing the community for extended periods of time due to limited changing facilities
- The effects of stigma from a society that tends to undervalue people who have not mastered continence
- Shame, embarrassment, depression and anxiety, lowered self-esteem, and negative body image
- Barriers to sustaining relationships and leading a sexually fulfilling life
- Physical, emotional and financial burden to carers and family; dealing with incontinence can be unpleasant and is a factor that leads to request for residential care.

Further reading

Stenson A, Danaher T (2005). Continence issues for people with learning disabilities. *Learning Disability Practice* **8**(9) 10–14. ▣ www.continence-foundation.org.uk

End of life care, preferred place of care

Planning for the future

As people approach the end of life, it is important to consider preferences regarding where they wish to be cared for and ultimately where they would prefer to die. While it is recognized that most people would prefer to die at home, many do not manage to do so and are often admitted to hospital in the last few days or hours of life.[1] Reasons for this in the general population are complex, but are compounded for marginalized groups (such as people with ID or elderly people) who may lack the vocal ability to understand, make informed choices, and make their personal needs and wants known at this difficult time.

End of Life Care Programme

In recognition of the needs that all patients who are suffering and dying should have equivalent access to palliative care and opportunities for a good death, in the place of their choosing, the Department of Health launched their End of Life Care Programme. This initiative recognizes the importance of service user involvement in healthcare and aims to reduce the number of emergency admissions to acute care for those wishing to die at home, and it supports nationally recognized tools for end of life care. These include the Liverpool Care Pathway and the Preferred Place of Care (PPC). The PPC originated in Lancashire and South Cumbria Cancer Network, as part of a District Nurse education programme. From 2008, the PPC document will be known as the Preferred Priorities of Care (PPC), reflecting the importance of discussing priorities, preferences, and wishes with the patient and their family.

Preferred Priorities of Care

The PPC is a patient-held tool to record patient and carer preferences and priorities in relation to care and ultimate place of death, following the patient into different care settings as required. It recognizes that views are likely to change over time, and encourages discussions among the patient, the family, and other professionals associated with care delivery and support. Indicative to this process is the knowledge and ability of the care staff involved to facilitate the process in a meaningful fashion, that the individuals involved have the ability to communicate in a fairly sophisticated manner (both at staff and patient levels), and patients being supported to make informed, sometimes difficult, choices about sensitive and important issues. Such tools have been developed for the general population, and as such may not be easy to translate across to those within ID services.

Issues for people with intellectual disability

Marginalized groups such as people with ID have an increased risk of disenfranchised death resulting from a lack of autonomy, choice, and social exclusion, particularly at the end of their life. Challenges to reciprocal communication, an inability to comprehend complex information, and limited writing skills, are all factors that compound to make end of life choices around PPC difficult for both the staff facilitating the process and the patient who has an ID who is at the centre of that care. The Government's White Paper, *Valuing People*,[2] has advocated a person-centred approach to planning care for people with ID, which is a useful framework as end of life approaches.

Person-centred approaches to end of life care

Discussions regarding end of life preferences with people with ID should not be left until death is imminent, but as early as is possible and feasible after a prognosis is known. Person-centred approaches to care planning promote inclusion, civil rights, and independence for people with ID. Planning should start with the individual, not with services, taking into account their wishes and preferences. To this end, person-centred planning and palliative care share similar philosophies with regards to taking a holistic approach, incorporating active listening to the patient and those who know them best. Health action plans or essential lifestyle plan are well suited to facilitating holistic, palliative/end of life care.[3]

Supporting the individual who has an ID to make complex choices at the end of life may not be easy for those nurses involved. Shared value bases across different professional groups will promote collaborative working to support this initiative and help individuals to die in places of their own choosing. Research around this topic will provide a sound evidence base for future development and support.

Further reading

National End of Life Care Programme ◪ www.endoflifecare.nhs.uk

1 Higginson IJ (2003). *Priorities and preferences for end of life care in England, Wales and Scotland.* National Council for Palliative Care.

2 Department of Health (2001). *Valuing People: A New Strategy for Learning Disability for the 21st Century.* London: Department of Health: London.

3 Read S, Elliott D (2006). Care planning in palliative care. In: Gates B, Ed. *Care Planning and Delivery in Intellectual Disability Nursing.* Blackwell Publishing: Oxford.

Medicines management

For a range of reasons, people with ID are sometimes prescribed a lot of medicines. This may partly be because of their poor physical health, e.g. high prevalence rates of mental health problems and challenging behaviour, and comorbidity, e.g. epilepsy, which often require long-term use of medication. New standards for medicines management, recently published by the Nursing and Midwifery Council,[1] outline 26 standards that nurse registrants need to consider and apply in whatever setting they work. However, it is also important to recognize and understand that these standards will not cover every eventuality that nurses will face with respect to medicines management, and that they will continue to be required to apply professional judgement and expertise in decision making. The use of medicines for people with ID presents a number of significant challenges/problem areas. These include polypharmacy (the use of two or more drugs), the detection of adverse/side effects of drugs, consent, choice and compliance, the high use of PRN medication, inadequate regular and/or routine monitoring and review, and the provision of information to service users and carers. Nursing staff can improve medicines management by reflecting on their competencies in the following 6 key areas.

1. Knowledge of drugs

People with an ID will be prescribed the same range of drugs as the general population, e.g. antipsychotics, analgesics, hypnotics, corticosteroids, laxatives, antidepressants, and anticonvulsants. Such medicines may be prescribed to be administered via a range of routes, e.g. topical, oral, and parenteral. If a nurse is involved in the administration of any medication to anyone with ID, then they must ensure that they have adequate knowledge, and have access to information about indications for use, normal dose parameters, expected effects, contraindications, precautions, side effects, and interactions with other prescribed medicines.

2. Delegation of care

Most medicines are administered by unqualified carers. Nursing staff will be expected to develop, enhance, maintain, and assess competence in the unqualified workforce, and should ensure that they have access to robust systems, guidelines, and policies to do so.

3. Consent

Individuals with an ID have the right to accept or refuse their medication. Significant difficulties can occur in the administration of medicines to this population due to refusal, or inability to express consent. For consent to be legal and valid the individual in question must:

• have adequate competence to make the decision
• be given adequate information
• not be placed under any form of duress or coercion.

In obtaining consent, all three of these components may present significant challenges to everyone involved in caring for people with ID. It is vital, therefore, that nurses have adequate understanding of consent and capacity principles, and relevant law in this area.

4. Information to service users and carers

Nurses must be responsive to the information needs of service users and carers. By doing so, efficacy of medicines will be enhanced, and adverse effects reduced. Information about medicines should be provided in a format that can be understood. The Elfrida society (🖳 www.elfrida.com) provides a series of easy to read information leaflets about a range of medications that could be used for this purpose.

5. Regular review and monitoring

Due to the potential for polypharmacy for people with ID, nurses should ensure that adequate reviews of medication take place on a regular basis and are undertaken by the appropriate physician. This should occur at least yearly, and twice yearly for individuals taking 4 or more medicines. Nurses must also equip themselves to use side effect rating scales for neuroleptic medication, and 2 examples are provided below:

Dyskinesia Identification System: Condensed User Scale (DISCUS) is a well-established measure for the assessment of tardive dyskinesia among individuals with an ID.[2]

Liverpool University Neuroleptic Side Effect Rating Scale (LUNSERS) provides information relating to a range of side effects of neuroleptic medication.[3]

6. Adherence to fundamental standards

Nursing staff should be guided by a range of policy guidance documents in this area, and should ensure that they are aware of, and comply with, key standards in respect of e.g. transporting medicines, use of controlled drugs, PRN prescriptions, self-administration, documentation, and the management of adverse events and errors.

1 Nursing and Midwifery Council (2008). *Standards for Medicines Management*. Nursing Midwifery Council: London.

2 Sprague RL, Kalachnil JE (1991). Reliability, validity, and a total score cutoff for the dyskinesia identification system: condensed user scale (DISCUS) with mentally ill and mentally retarded populations. *Psychopharmacology Bulletin* **27**(1), 51–58.

3 Morrison P, Gaskill D, Meehan T, Lunney P, Lawrence G, Collings P (2000). The use of the Liverpool University Neuroleptic Side Effect Rating Scale (LUNSERS) in clinical practice. *Australian and New Zealand Journal of Mental Health Nursing*, **9**(4), 166–176.

Independent nurse prescribers in intellectual disability

The Department of Health and the Nursing and Midwifery Council state registered nurses with 3yrs post-registration experience may train to be nurse prescribers. Higher education institutions provide specific training courses with assessments, and the nurse has supervision by a medical practitioner. Independent nurse prescribers are now entitled to prescribe from the same formulary as medical practitioners.

- This allows nurses to prescribe any licensed medicine for any medical condition that a nurse prescriber is competent to treat, including some controlled drugs.
- It is essential that nurses are prescribing within their scope of practice and it has been negotiated appropriately with their employing authority.
- It is the responsibility of the individual nurse prescriber to be updated through continued professional development in accordance with the Nursing and Midwifery Council nursing regulations.

The nurse independent prescriber within the ID profession enables the nurse to provide holistic patient-centred care to improve patient outcomes and quality of life.

Occasions for prescribing in intellectual disability

People with ID often lack access to appropriate healthcare. They are also more vulnerable than average to a number of physical health problems, e.g. gastrointestinal disorders related to constipation, and UTI.

- For people with ID it can be more difficult to diagnose these conditions.
- Many clients are unable to articulate their complaints of illness because they may have communication problems or a deficit in understanding.

In these situations they may present signs of restlessness or behaviour problems, and their symptoms may be camouflaged. If these minor ailments are not treated they could lead to life-threatening situations. This is when it is important for the nurse to use their skills and knowledge during the assessment criteria, which is a fundamental part of nurse prescribing.

Prescribing in intellectual disability

In the instance of UTI it is essential that the independent nurse prescriber identifies and treats the cause with a course of appropriate antibiotics. The same principle applies if a client is constipated, the problem must be identified and the relevant treatment applied. This could be a laxative medication. Often ID individuals have other co-morbid health conditions such as mental heath, dementia, or epilepsy. Patients are often on several medicines (polypharmacy) for various states i.e. neuroleptic medication for mental health and challenging behaviour, and antiepileptic drugs for epilepsy. A number of these drugs have side effects that cause constipation.

Areas where nurses may work using nurse prescribing

Many practising nurse prescribers are based within an ID specialist multidisciplinary health and social team in the community or acute assessment settings. Subsequently they work alongside a medical practitioner who supports the nurse prescriber with their practice. Supplementary prescribing ethos is very useful for specific long-term health conditions. This systematic prescribing approach is applicable for ID using the process of an agreed patient specific CMP.

The advantages of nurse prescribing for people with intellectual disability

- Having a nurse available who is an independent nurse prescriber would be valuable for the service in the event a patient became ill and there was no medical practitioner accessible.
- Often the nurse has developed a therapeutic relationship with the patient. A reason for this is the nurse will see the patient more frequently than the doctor and have more time to spend in the consultation. Nurses may identify possible barriers or influence concordance i.e. lifestyle, work.
- The nurse can ensure that there is regular dialogue with the medical practitioners. Therefore it fosters better links with the doctor, and response to patient treatment intervention is more effective.
- Nurses can prescribe emergency medication in the event of crisis, i.e. minor ailments, prophylactic anti-epileptic, or antipsychotic drugs, enabling the patient to have a quicker response to treatment.
- The nurse can set up nurse-led clinics, enabling more autonomy in their practice.

Further reading

Allsop A, Brooks L, Bufton L (2005). Supplementary prescribing in mental health and learning disabilities. *Nursing Standard* **19**(30), 54.

Department of Health (2005). *Improving Health Services by Extending the Role of Nurses in Prescribing and Supplying Medication: Good Practice Guide*. Department of Health: London.

Beckwith S, Franklin P (2007). *Oxford Handbook of Nurse Prescribing*. Oxford University Press: Oxford.

British Medical Association & Royal Pharmaceutical Society of Great Britain (Regularly updated). *British National Formulary*. BMA: London.

Courtenay M, Butler M (2003). *Essential Nurse Prescribing*. Greenwich Medical Media: London.

Department of Health (2006). *Medicines Matters: a Guide to Mechanisms for the Prescribing, Supply and Administration of Medicines*. Department of Health: London.

Nursing and Midwifery Council (2008). *Standards for medicines management*. Nursing and Midwifery Council: London.

Prasher Vee P, Janicki MP (2002). *Physical Health of Adults with Intellectual Disability*. Blackwell Publishing: Oxford.

Mental health and emotional well being

Introduction

Mental health

Good mental health is integral to most definitions of health, which have for many years now highlighted the bio-psycho-social aspects to being healthy.

Mental health relies on an individual's positive sense of self. Good mental health affords us with the ability to cope with both positive and negative life events, includes the ability to develop and sustain relationships, self-purpose, to learn and adjust to new environments and situations, and interact with other people and the world around us.

Everyone has mental health needs and these are unique to each individual. When mental health needs go unmet, the individual is vulnerable to developing mental health problems.

Mental health problems

Mental health is concerned with human behaviour, which can be difficult to measure because of its subjectivity and varying behavioural norms that occur across cultures and societies. The term 'mental health problems' implies a presence of change and deterioration in an individual's functioning in areas such as cognition, emotions, thoughts, and behaviour, which have a negative impact on their overall functioning.

Classification of mental health problems

There is a range of symptoms that affect mental well-being. These can be clustered to form formal mental health diagnoses. The most widely recognized systems of classifying mental disorders, and guidelines for their diagnosis are:

- The ICD-10 Classification of Mental and Behavioural Disorders: Clinical descriptions and diagnostic guidelines (used in UK clinical practice)[1]
- DSM-IV TR: Diagnostic and Statistical Manual of Mental Disorders (Text revision).[2]

These manuals in turn group the different types of diagnoses into related sections, the example below is from ICD-10:

- Organic disorders—dementias, delirium
- Psychotic disorders—schizophrenia
- Mood disorders—depression, bipolar disorder
- Neurotic disorders—anxiety disorders, post-traumatic stress disorder
- Behavioural syndromes— eating disorders
- Personality disorders.

Both the ICD-10 and DSM-IV are commonly used with people with ID, although problems have been noted in their application because of a number of reasons, including: atypical presentation, poverty of experience, and ability of an individual to express themselves. This occurs across the range of abilities, but particularly in people with severe and profound ID. To address this, specialist diagnostic systems have been developed for this population:

- DC-LD: Diagnostic criteria for psychiatric disorders for use with adults with learning disabilities/mental retardation [3]

- DM-ID: A Clinical Guide for the Diagnosis of Mental Disorders in Persons with Intellectual Disabilities.[4]

These systems, however, are noticeable by their absence in general mental health settings, where most referrals will have a mild ID, in which ICD-10 or DSM-IV can be used.

Mental health and people with intellectual disabilities

Only over recent decades has it been accepted that people with ID can develop mental health problems just as the wider population. Studies have shown that people with ID are at increased risk of developing mental health problems. This vulnerability is thought to be due to the combination of developmental, biological, psychological, and social factors that people with ID are more likely to encounter in their lives.

The impact of mental health problems on people with ID can significantly affect quality of life, as the individual may not detect or understand changes, or indeed the significance of what is happening to them. It is vital that registered nurses in ID services have an understanding of mental health issues affecting the people they provide services to. Interventions need to be proactive, and include interventions and/or support aimed at promoting mental well-being, detection and assessment of mental health problems, knowledge of the range of interventions and services available, and relevant legislation.

1 World Health Organization (1992). *ICD-10 Classification of Mental and Behavioural Disorders: Clinical descriptions and diagnostic guidelines.* WHO: Geneva.

2 American Psychiatric Association (1994). *Diagnostic and Statistical Manual of Mental Disorders,* 4th Edn. APA: Washington DC.

3 Royal College of Psychiatrists (2001). *DC-LD: Diagnostic criteria for psychiatric disorders for use with adults with learning disabilities/mental retardation.* Gaskell: London.

4 National Association for the Dually Diagnosed (2007). *DM-ID: Diagnostic Manual–Intellectual Disability.* NADD: New York.

Promoting emotional well-being

In contrast to the promotion of physical health, the promotion of emotional well-being of people with ID has been given much less coverage and priority. Promoting mental health, or emotional well-being, involves 'any action that enhances the mental well-being of individuals, families and also communities'.[1] The activities that they identify can, and should, also be used for people with ID, but may need to be adapted.

People with intellectual disability are a vulnerable group

📖 Factors contributing to mental health (p.228) identifies the bio-psycho-social factors that contribute to this population developing high levels of psychiatric disorders (see Fig. 7.1).[2] In addition to these inter-related risk factors, there are further issues that need to be acknowledged.

Individual barriers—people with ID may lack the knowledge required of what to do when feeling unwell, and where to go and seek help.

Carer barriers—many people with ID are dependent on family carers to identify the symptoms of when they are unwell, and make a prompt referral to a GP. However, many of these carers may not recognize the early indications/triggers.

Societal barriers—stereotypical views that people with ID inevitably developmental health problems, and limited political willingness to provide supportive services that seek to promote and maintain recovery.

Professional barriers—primary healthcare professionals may have limited experience in working with people with ID, and have less knowledge about the needs of this population. They may also have less confidence, hold negative attitudes, may not have clear referral systems, be unlikely to use specific health screening tools, and also may have difficulty in communicating with people with ID.

These individual, care, and professional barriers may prevent the person with the ID from being proactive about seeking professional advice, and receiving adequate levels of support, early screening, assessment, and treatment.

Models of promoting emotional well-being

The Department of Health highlighted a two-stage model of promoting emotional well-being:[1]

Reducing risk factors—poverty, deprived communities, high unemployment, financial difficulties, poor educational opportunities, high crime rates, emotional/physical/sexual abuse, high stress levels, social exclusion, bereavement, family break-up, long-term caring, gender.

Increasing protective factors—quality environments, increasing self-esteem and empowerment, self- management skills, social participation.

Although it is impossible to prevent some psychiatric disorders from occurring, proactive measures are likely to have a significant impact on preventing the onset of mental health problems, and where mental health issues do arise, to reduce their severity, and reduce the potential for crisis management. Nurses should have a clear awareness and understanding of the risk factors that may predispose the person to develop mental health problems, and use this knowledge in the development of proactive and preventative individualized and group interventions.

A plan for promoting emotional well-being

- The increased use and development of targeted group-based programmes to promote mental health that focus on:[3,4,5]
  - promoting positive self-esteem and empowerment
  - developing the person's ability to make informed choices, promoting advocacy balanced with person-centred risk management
  - ensuring effective, receptive and expressive communication with individuals and groups, so people can speak up for themselves
  - providing environments where individuals feel safe and secure
  - ensuring and enhancing feelings of achievement and success.
- The promotion of mental health should become a routine component of assessment and care planning for every person seen. Identifying those most at risk by using early screening tools as appropriate, such as the PAS-AAD Schedules (see 📖 Screening of mental health problems, p.92).
- Informal and formal carers to receive health promotion information and training to identify warning signs earlier;[7] likewise people with ID should have access to health promotion material in a format that they can understand.
- Ensure optimal physical health, adequate leisure, and physical exercise by participation in more community and group activities.
- Develop positive relationships and friendships with peers, including positive family connections.
- Improve and facilitate access to primary and mental health services.
- Education, awareness, and support from specialists within the ID field to primary care and mental health services.
- Effective management of transition and loss.
- Develop specific relapse prevention plans for individuals who are particularly vulnerable, or in the stage of recovery from a specific mental health problem.

1 Department of Health (2001). *Making it Happen: A Guide to Delivering Mental Health Promotion*. Department of Health: London.

2 IASSID (2001) *International Association for the Scientific Study of Intellectual Disability Mental Health and Intellectual Disabilities: Addressing the mental health needs of people with intellectual disabilities*. IASSID. Available at 🖥 http://www.iassid.org

3 Devine M, Taggart L (2008). Improving practice in the care of people with learning disabilities and mental health problems. *Nursing Standard*, **22**(45), 40–48.

4 Hardy S., Essam V. and Woodward P. (2004) The Tuesday Group: promoting mental health. *Learning Disability Practice*, **7**(8), 20–23.

5 Moss S (2002). *PAS-ADD Schedules*. Pavilion Publishers: Brighton.

6 Moss S (2007). *Cha-Pas Interview Pack*. Pavilion Publishing: Brighton.

7 Black L, Devine M (2008). *Head Start: Promoting positive mental health for Children and Young People with a Learning Disability*. Positive Futures: Bangor. Available at 🖥 http://www.positive-futures.net

Promoting assertiveness

Being able to assert oneself is a skill many take for granted. Assertion is the ability to communicate confidently in a socially appropriate manner. When people are unable to assert themselves appropriately, either to get their needs met or perhaps to put across a point of view, this may lead the individual to compensate through other behaviours, e.g. withdrawal, aggression, or avoiding situations. The ability to assert is also context specific, in that people may lack assertion in certain situations but not in others e.g. at home or with friends, where assertion may not be an issue or problem. How people with ID react to situations may differ. It is likely that they will also encounter difficult situations through prejudice and being treated differently in a number of ways e.g. people being maternal, talking to family and carers rather than the person with ID, or being abusive and/or bullying. The individual's expectations in any given situation will be informed usually by their previous experience or preconceived ideas that may or may not be realistic. The way the person responds may not only be due to unrealistic expectations. For those with ID and/or mental health problems, the reaction may be more acute because of a number of factors, including thought disorder, poverty of experience, or inability to grasp the complexity of any given situation.

Developing assertiveness

Assertiveness training normally uses cognitive behavioural and self-help techniques. One of the aims is to identify the potential consequences, such as anger and aggression, and the process and stages that lead to the eventual display of these behaviours.

Assertiveness training is multifaceted, and is facilitated to:
- allow the person to respond in difficult situations in an appropriate manner
- build confidence and self-esteem
- prepare someone to engage in longer term treatment on a more equal footing
- replace maladaptive behaviours such as aggression.

Assertiveness programmes use a number of techniques:
- Repetition through:
  - role play
  - modelling.
- Using their own experiences to re-enact and learn from:
  - feedback
  - rehearsal.
- Homework to set goals to:
  - recognize areas to improve
  - practice classroom scenarios.

Assertion training can be facilitated in groups or individually, within a structured programme that will encompass educational issues around social skills, such as how we might conduct ourselves, how to handle feelings, coping with daily events, and then within these scenarios look at more positive ways of expressing feelings and needs. Other strategies that may be adopted include the individual having aids to complement the programme, such as a prompt card tailored to them. This might give guidance on how to cope in difficult situations, or it may be used to help the person practice difficult situations in a systematic manner.

Assertiveness training is designed to help the individual through positive and social reinforcement, to enable them not only to learn new skills but also to maintain them with the added bonus of increasing self-confidence, effectiveness, and self-esteem.

In seeking to support and enhance the assertiveness of people with ID, nurses should encourage and provide opportunities to practice communication skills that reflect the following:
• A positive solution focused orientation
• Make sure you listen to the other person
• Try to know what you want to say and say it
• Try to be direct but not rude
• Follow what is being said—in what context?
• Do not presume the outcome
• Make sure you are breathing calmly and try to recognize if you are becoming upset
• Focus on the event or task you want to talk about and not what you think about the person.

Primary care

Primary healthcare is the point of entry for the delivery of healthcare at the most local level of a country's healthcare system.[1] These services generally do not require a referral, and patients are able to register at one of a range of local services. Primary care is the gateway of access to the wider range of healthcare services.

Primary care and mental health

Primary care should be the first point of call for people with mental health problems, this generally being their GP. It is estimated that in the wider population, 40% of those seeing their GP have a mental health problem, and 20–25% of all appointments are concerning a mental health issue.[2] Primary care is able to offer a wide range of services to those with mental health needs including:

- Mental health promotion
- Advice and support
- Assessment
- Treatment
- Referral to secondary mental health services

Primary care services are pivotal in the government's plans to modernize and improve mental health care. In England and Wales this includes a dedicated standard within the National Service Framework, and the introduction of two new key posts:

- Graduate mental health workers are being recruited throughout primary care services. The role is to provide brief therapeutic interventions, such as CBT, to those with common mental health problems.
- Gateway workers have also been introduced, with their main aim being to ensure there are smooth pathways and interfaces between primary and secondary care.

Primary care is able to meet the needs of those presenting with a wide range of mental health problems, most commonly assessing and treating those with anxiety and depressive disorders. Those with more acute and complex needs or presenting with severe/enduring mental health problems, such as chronic schizophrenia or bipolar disorder, are likely to be referred on to secondary mental health care services.

Primary care, mental health, and intellectual disability

There is little research as to where people with ID get their mental health needs met, but care pathways for this group have tended not to mirror those in the wider population, with many people with ID experiencing difficulty in accessing services. The Disability Rights Commission held an inquiry into the health inequalities experienced by people with ID and/or mental health problems.[3] It found that people with ID have difficulty accessing primary care services, as information and appointment systems are often inaccessible. They were less likely to be offered health screening services (i.e. cancer) than those in the wider population. Difficulty was experienced in accessing health promotion services, especially access to exercise and advice on smoking, alcohol, and sexual health. Since this inquiry and other reports and policies were published, many examples of positive action can be seen. These include the introduction of annual health checks, hand-held personal health profiles, which include emotional well-being, training programmes for primary care professionals, and the development of nurse liaison posts.

With the government policy driving forward an agenda of inclusion, people with ID should be able to access primary care for their mental health, with or without the advice and support of specialist learning disability services. However, there is still some debate whether it would be better for people with ID to be referred on to secondary care services who may have additional expertise. It is important that professionals make decisions based on the overall best outcome for individual clients, and do not become blinkered by unquestioning adherence to new policy objectives or preference for previous systems of organizing care.

1 WHO - 🖳 www.who.int/en

2 Department of Health (2002). *Fast-Forwarding Primary Care Mental Health*. Department of Health: London.

3 Disability Rights Commission (2006). *Equal Treatment: Closing the Gap: A formal investigation into the physical health inequalities experienced by people with learning disabilities and/or mental health problems*. Disability Rights Commission: London.

Secondary care

Secondary mental health care services are generally provided by local NHS Trusts or Foundation Trusts. They provide community and inpatient services, meeting a wide range of mental health needs. Access to secondary mental health services is initially via a primary care referral, though once known to services, additional referrals through their GP are generally not required, and they may access secondary service directly, although the person's GP will be kept informed. There are a few services that are self-referral, such as walk in or emergency clinics.

Examples of secondary mental health care services

Community mental health teams (CMHT)

Throughout the UK community services are delivered locally in most areas through CMHTs. They can be accessed by any adult of working age, who has a severe and/or enduring mental health problem. CMHTs provide assessment, support and a range of treatment options. Teams are multidisciplinary and are often integrated with local social services. In some rural areas, CMHTs may see people with the full range of mental health problems. However many areas are now developing sub-speciality teams, which are described below. There are similar community mental health teams for children and adults:

- Child and adolescent mental health services (CAMHS)—<18yrs
- Community mental health team for older adults—>65yrs

Assertive outreach teams (AOT)

Some people with mental health problems present with complex needs, may be at a higher risk of relapse, or have a history of disengaging with services (e.g. substance misuse). AOTs are specifically designed to support these individuals, offering a more intense style of intervention. AOTs are interdisciplinary and offer an extended hours service, often 8am–8pm, although there is some variation among different services depending on local policies.

Home treatment/crisis resolution teams

These teams offer an alternative to hospital admission for those who are in the acute phase of mental illness. Treatment and support is offered in the least restrictive environment, normally the individual's home. They respond rapidly to people in crisis and can offer a wide range of support and interventions. They also facilitate early discharge from hospital, offering a home-based support package.

Early onset psychosis teams

Early onset psychosis teams are designed for young adults (generally 18–35yrs) who are experiencing a first episode of psychosis. Their aim is to provide an individually tailored package of care that will facilitate access to services, promote recovery, support people to adapt to their mental health problems, and reduce the likelihood of relapse.

Inpatient services

Most people receive mental health care in the community. A small minority, such as those either in crisis or experiencing a severe/acute episode, may need hospital admission, particularly where there is a risk to self or others. There are a range of inpatient services, which are generally separated by age range—child, adult, and older adult. It is also the intention that there should be separate clinical areas for men and women. Acute inpatient services are available throughout the country in each area and are often based on a general hospital site. They are staffed by nurses, with input from psychiatry, occupational therapy, psychology, and other professionals. Admission is voluntary wherever possible, but in some instances people may be detained under mental health legislation. Inpatient services work very closely with community services, trying to ensure a smooth transition home. A small number of rehabilitation inpatient services are available for those who need a longer period of admission, who are not acutely ill but present with complex and chronic needs.

Secondary care intellectual disability services

Most areas will have some type of community team for people with ID (some may only work with adults). They are multidisciplinary, offering packages of care to meet a range of health and social care needs. Though referred to as secondary services, access may not necessarily be through primary care but through self or carer referral. The extent to which mental health needs can be met within these teams is variable, as many are not resourced for this issue nor is it their focus. As the inclusion agenda becomes reality, these teams will develop a tertiary role, providing specialist support and input into secondary care services. Some areas have a community mental health team for people with ID.

Registered nurses working in ID services can make a valuable contribution to enhancing joint working with colleagues in secondary care, including:

- Identifying link nurses between the ID service and secondary care service
- Assisting with communication strategies
- Supporting a person-centred planning approach
- Working collaboratively with colleagues in mental health services to facilitate valid consent
- Developing training programmes for secondary care staff on meeting the health needs of people with ID
- Producing awareness and educational resource packs for secondary care services
- Supporting the development of joint protocols and care pathways to ensure smooth transition between services.

Tertiary care

Tertiary services are specialized health services that are provided by statutory or independent providers. These services tend to cover regional and/or national areas. They are for those people who need highly specialized care, and in regards of mental health, those with the most serious or complex needs that cannot be treated appropriately in local secondary services. The need for such services has been explored with service and policy reviews across the UK.[1,2,3,4]

As well as offering expert assessment and treatment, many tertiary services can fulfil wider functions that will support local services in their development, and provide an evidence base that will influence practice across other services. This knowledge can be disseminated in a number of ways including education and training, research, and consultancy. An example of such a service that provides this function is the Estia Centre in South London.[5]

There is much debate as to when a service is classified as a tertiary specialist, rather than a sub-specialist linked to secondary care services; identifying characteristics would include a separate management structure. Such services are, to a greater or lesser degree, self-financing, generating income from external organizations i.e. the commissioning or purchasing of beds. Some NHS and Foundation Trusts will provide secondary care services within their locality, while also providing similar care on a regional or national basis at a tertiary level e.g. forensic, challenging behaviour, and autism services.

Nursing roles within tertiary services

Nurses within tertiary services are employed increasingly in a variety of roles. These include working within specialist clinical inpatient settings e.g. forensic, or clinics for specific conditions such as autism or ADHD, and offer specialist assessment and/or treatment at a more senior level in some areas. Some regional services (e.g. The Estia centre[5]) will be used in other roles that promote collaboration through dissemination of specialist skills through training and consultancy, e.g. audit or service evaluation. They may also provide academic and skills based training programmes to local services, including adult mental health and residential services in areas such as ID awareness, risk assessment, or assessment and treatment strategies. The aim is to support these services to develop their own skills and knowledge base on the way to providing greater collaboration, and a more defined care pathway.

Specialist intellectual disability services

Specialist services are defined within the Specialized Services National Definitions Set: 21, which states:[6]

"Inpatient assessment, treatment and associated outreach for people with severe complex needs that cannot be managed by local assessment and treatment services including people with ID:
• who have severe challenging needs and present major risks to themselves and/or others

- and severe mental health problems, who cannot be addressed by general psychiatric services
- and ASD, with severe challenging and/or mental health needs."

These services should not be seen as a long-term option; however, these specialized services are sometimes required as an interim measure while local services are developed to accommodate an individual's particular needs.

Specialist mental health services

There is also specific mental health guidance, Specialised Services National Definitions Set: 22.[7] The type of services defined as specialist include forensic, Asperger's syndrome, and neuropsychiatry.

1 Department of Health (2001). *Valuing People: A New Strategy for Learning Disability for the 21st Century.* Cm 5086 HMSO: London.

2 Department of Health and Social Services and Public Safety (2005). *Equal Lives: Review of Policies and Services for People with Learning Disability in Northern Ireland.* DHSSPS: Belfast.

3 National Assembly for Wales (2001). *Fulfilling the Promises: Proposal for a Framework for Services for People with Learning Disabilities.* Learning Disability Advisory Group: Cardiff.

4 Scottish Executive (2000). *The Same as You? A Review of Services for People with Learning Disabilities.* Scottish Executive: Edinburgh.

5 The Estia Centre www.estiacentre.org [accessed April 2009]

6 Department of Health (2007). *Specialised Services National Definition Set: 21 Specialist learning disability services.* Department of Health: London.

7 Department of Health (2007). *Specialised Services National Definition Set: 22 Specialised mental health (adult).* Department of Health: London.

Prevalence rates

There are three main groups of prevalence studies into the rates of psychiatric disorders among people with ID.

- Studies that examined people with ID in hospitals—prevalence rates were 60–100%.
- Studies that examined people referred to community psychiatric clinics—prevalence rates were 60–100%.
- Community samples of adults with ID were 14–50%.

These studies clearly show that people with ID are significantly more likely to develop a psychiatric disorder compared with the general population.[1]

Similar international studies have reported that children and adolescents with ID living with their natural families were also more likely to have a psychiatric disorder compared with their non-disabled peers. Prevalence rates were 31–50%.[2] These figures contrast sharply compared with those reported for young people, 10–15yrs, without ID of 9%.[3]

Difficulties in obtaining accurate prevalence rates

Such discrepancies in obtaining accurate prevalence rates are a result of a combination of methodological difficulties, and issues pertaining to people with ID and third-party informants:

- Depending on the level of ID (i.e. mild or severe/profound), diagnosis may or may not be achieved
- For people with limited or no communication skills accurate diagnosis becomes more difficult
- How the information is gathered either from family/staff or from the person with the ID
- Methodological problems related to what is meant by a 'psychiatric disorder' or 'mental health problem'
- The type of classification system used to diagnose a psychiatric disorder (i.e. ICD-10, DSM-IV, or DC-LD)[4]
- The different assessment methods used to identify such clinical conditions (i.e. case records, screening tools e.g. PAS-ADD, PRIMA, REISS, and structured interviews)
- The reliability and validity of the screening tools used by frontline staff to identify potential cases
- Whether 'behavioural disorders' are included within the diagnosis.

Prevalence rates of specific psychiatric disorders

Affective disorder—a number of studies report that people with ID are more likely to develop depressive disorder compared with their non-disabled peers. As within the general population, women with ID were more likely to develop depression than men with ID.[5]

Anxiety disorder—people with ID have been reported as more likely to develop an anxiety disorder, adjustment disorder, and also post-traumatic stress disorder compared with the general population.[6,7]

Dementia—5–8% of the general population will develop a dementia compared with 15.6% of people with ID of 65–75yrs, 23% of 75–84yrs, and 75% of ≥85yrs.[8] For people who have Down syndrome, the prevalence rate of Alzheimer's disease is 8% in people of 35–49yrs, 55% in those of 50–59yrs and 75% in those of ≥60 years.[9]

Psychotic disorders—a small number of studies have examined schizophrenia in people with mild/moderate ID, and have reported that prevalence rates are 4 times higher than reported in the general population.[10,11]

Eating disorder—there is clear evidence of higher obesity rates in people with ID compared with the non-disabled population.[12] In addition other eating disorders are evident in this population: binge eating, pica, anorexia nervosa, bulimia nervosa, food refusal, and psychogenic vomiting. However, unlike the general population, no gender differences were found in these eating disorders.[13, 14]

Substance abuse—alcohol and illicit drug misuse in people with ID has been reported to be lower compared with the general population; although people with ID are at a higher risk to abuse such substances (see 📖 Substance misuse, p.244).[15]

Further reading

Bouras N (Ed.) (2007). *Psychiatric and Behavioural Disorders in Development Disabilities and Mental Retardation*. Cambridge University Press: Cambridge.

1 Deb S, Thomas M *et al.* (2001). Mental disorders in adults who have an intellectual disability, 1: prevalence of functional psychiatric illness among a 16–64 year old community-based population. *Journal of Intellectual Disability Research* **45**(6), 506–514.

2 Emerson E (2003). The prevalence of psychiatric disorders in children and adolescents with and without intellectual disabilities. *Journal of Intellectual Disability Research* **47**, 51–58.

3 Meltzer G, Gatward R, Goodman R, Ford T (2000). *The mental health of children and adolescents in Great Britain*. Office of National Statistics: London.

4 Royal College of Psychiatrists (2001). *DC-LD: Diagnostic criteria for psychiatric disorders for use with adults with learning disabilities/mental retardation*. Gaskell: London.

5 Lunsky S, Canrinus M (2005). Gender Issues, Mental Retardation and Depression. In Sturmey P (ed.). *Mood Disorders in People with Mental Retardation*, pp.56–68. NADD Press: New York.

6 Gitta MZ, Goldberg B (1995). Dual Diagnosis: Psychiatric and Physical Disorders in a Clinical Sample, Part 2. *Clinical Bulletin of Developmental Disabilities Programme*, **6**: 1–2.

7 Tsakanikos E, Costello H, Holt G, Bouras N, Sturmey P, Newton T (2006). Psychiatric Co-Morbidity and Gender Differences in Intellectual Disability. *Journal of Intellectual Disability Research* **50**(8), 582–7.

8 Parry JR (Ed.) (2002). *Overview of mental health problems in elderly persons with developmental disabilities*. NADD: New York.

9 McQuillan S, Kalsy S, Oyebode J, Millichap D, Oliver C, and Hall S (2003). Adults with Down's syndrome and Alzheimer's disease. *Tizard Learning Disability Review* **8**(4), 4-13.

10 Hemmings CP. (2006) Schizophrenia spectrum disorders in people with intellectual disabilities. *Current Opinion in Psychiatry*, **19**(5), 470–474.

11 Clarke, D. Schizophrenia spectrum disorders in people with intellectual disabilities (Chapter, 8, pp.131–142). In Bouras N. and Holt G. (2007) *Psychiatric and Behavioural Disorders in Intellectual and Developmental Disabilities* (2nd edition) Cambridge: Cambridge University Press.

12 Bhaumik S, Watson JM, Thorp CF, Tyrer F, McGrother G (2008). Body mass index in adults with intellectual disability: distribution, associations and service implications: a population based prevalence study. *Journal of Intellectual Disability Research* **52**(4), 287–98.

13 Gravestock S (2000). Eating disorders in adults with intellectual disability. *Journal of Intellectual Disability Research* **44**, 625–37.

14 Hove O (2004). Weight survey on adult persons with mental retardation living in the community. *Research in Developmental Disabilities* **25**, 9–17.

15 Taggart L, McLaughlin D, Quinn B, Milligan V (2006). An exploration of substance misuse in people with intellectual disabilities. *Journal of Intellectual Disability Research* **50**(8), 588–97.

Factors contributing to mental health

Fig. 7.1 shows that a dynamic interaction of biological, psychological, developmental, and social factors may contribute to the development of mental health problems in people with ID.[1]

Biological (examples)

- Behavioural phenotypes such as fragile X, Lesch–Nyhan and Prader–Willi, and a link with psychiatric conditions
- Strong link between people with Down syndrome and Alzheimer's disease
- Organic brain damage
- People with ID have higher rates of psychotic disorders, possibly linked with brain abnormalities
- People with temporal lobe epilepsy may also experience auditory hallucinations
- Difficulties in personal development that may arise secondary to sensory and physical impairments, or undesired effects of antipsychotic medication may also contribute to the development of a psychiatric disorder.

Psychological (examples)

- Impaired intelligence, memory deficits, and limited coping behaviours
- Poor communication and social skills
- Poor problem solving abilities and coping strategies
- Wanting to appear normal
- Low levels of self-esteem and disempowerment
- Higher levels of frustration, loss of motivation, and greater vulnerability of stress.

Social (examples)

- Most people with ID will experience more negative life events than the non-disabled population
- Higher levels of institutionalization, labelling, stigmatization, bullying
- Lack of choice and control
- Higher levels of separation and loss
- Greater loss in keeping friends/peers
- Limited social support networks[2]
- Many of the supports fail to fully understand the needs of people with ID and psychiatric disorders, and have little training in this area[3]
- Lack of opportunities regarding employment, education and recreational activities.

Risk factors in young people with intellectual disabilities

Young people with ID are also more likely to develop a psychiatric disorder compared with other young people as a result of a range of bio-psycho-social variables. Moreover, Emerson,[4] and Hassiotis & Barron,[5] have also identified a range of family and community variables that are also significant risk factors:

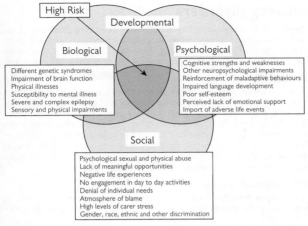

Fig. 7.1 Factors contributing to mental health problems in people with intellectual disability (reproduced from IASSID, 2001).[1]

- High levels of social deprivation/poverty
- Family composition (i.e. being brought up by a single parent)
- Poor mental health of primary caregiver/family history of mental health
- Presence of negative role models with less punitive child management practices/family in disharmony
- Negative life events (i.e. accidents, abuse, domestic violence, bereavement)
- Lower opportunities for employment, education, and recreation
- Excessive amounts of free time
- Limited relationships/friends
- Lack of meaning in life and routine/social exclusion.

1 International Association for the Scientific Study of Intellectual Disabilities (IASSID) (2001). *Mental Health and Intellectual Disabilities: Addressing the mental health needs of people with intellectual disabilities.* Report by the Mental Health Special Interest Research Group of IASSID to the WHO. 🖳 www.iassid.org [accessed April 2009].

2 McConkey R, Mezza F (2001). The employment aspirations of people with learning disabilities attending day centres. *Journal of Learning Disabilities* **5**(4), 309–318.

3 Bouras N, Holt G (Eds) (2007). *Psychiatric and Behavioural Disorders in Development Disabilities and Mental Retardation.* Cambridge University Press: Cambridge.

4 Emerson, E. (2003). The prevalence of psychiatric disorders in children and adolescents with and without intellectual disabilities. *Journal of Intellectual Disability Research*, **47**, 51–58.

5 Hassiotis A, Barron DA (2007). Mental health, learning disabilities and adolescence: a developmental perspective. *Advances in Mental Health and Learning Disabilities* **1**(3), 32–39.

Anxiety disorders

People with ID are exposed to greater risks of developing psychiatric disorders as a result of a dynamic interaction of physical, psychological, and social factors (see 📖 Factors contributing to mental health, p.228). Cumulatively, these risk factors will make the person more vulnerable to anxiety disorders.

Definition

Anxiety disorder is characterized by excessive, exaggerated worry about everyday life events. People suffering from an anxiety disorder may anticipate the worst and cannot stop worrying about their health, relationships, family, work, or other specific concerns. These excessive anxieties and worries are often unrealistic or out of proportion to the situation. Daily life becomes a constant state of worry, fear, and dread. Eventually, the anxiety controls the person's thinking, and interferes with their daily functioning (i.e. social activities, relationships, family, work).

Symptoms of anxiety

According to the ICD-10 the main symptoms reported are:
- **Somatic**—headaches, sweating, nausea, trembling, palpitations, muscle tension
- **Emotional**—excessive ongoing worry, emotional tension, crying, irritability, being easily startled
- **Motivational**—unrealistic view of problem, concentrating on difficulty
- **Thoughts**—a restlessness or a feeling of being 'edgy'
- **Behavioural**—including reduced appetite and sleep problems.

Types of anxiety disorders

Generalized anxiety disorder—the anxiety is not restricted to a specific event or situation but generalized to everyday life (i.e. free floating).

Adjustment disorder—a mix of both depressive and anxiety symptoms that has resulted from a specific life event (i.e. bereavement, change in living circumstances).

Post-traumatic stress disorder—a severe reaction to a specific life event/stressor (i.e. physical or sexual abuse, road traffic accident).

Panic disorder—recurring attacks of severe anxiety that are not attached to a specific event or situation; normally associated with intense feelings of having a 'heart attack' and 'doom'.

Obsessive–compulsive disorder—characterized by recurrent obsessions and compulsions, causing severe anxiety and repulsive thoughts, leading the person to undertake certain behaviours repetitively.

Phobia disorder—excessive anxiety is present whereby the person avoids the event or situation; even thinking about the event or situation can trigger intense worry and cause a panic attack. There are 3 types:
- Agoraphobia—fear of being in crowds or public places (i.e. shopping centres)
- Social phobia—fear of being noticed by other people and anticipating an extreme negative outcome occurring
- Specific phobia—restricted to specific events or situations (i.e. spiders, needles).

Prevalence

People with ID have higher levels of anxiety related behaviour and also anxiety disorders compared with the non-disabled population:[1] rates vary between 5% and 27%. Stavrakaki & Lunsky reported that people with ID were more likely to have a coexisting diagnosis of a generalized anxiety disorder, adjustment disorder, and a depressive disorder than their non-disabled peers.[2] These authors also report that people with ID can also experience post-traumatic stress disorder.

Symptom presentation

For many people with borderline/mild ID, they will show similar signs and symptoms of anxiety disorder as their non-disabled peers. In addition, other atypical symptoms may be displayed:

- Aggression/disruptive behaviours
- Agitation, irritability
- Obsessive compulsive phenomena (i.e. self-injury, obsessive fears, ritualistic behaviours, and insomnia)
- Greater likelihood of displaying more somatic/physical symptoms, and also appetite and sleep disturbance.

Assessment

Self-rating scales are widely used in general psychiatric practice; however, there is no reliable and valid method for assessing anxiety in people with ID. Recently, a number of specific screening tools have been developed for nurses to use with this population:

- PAS-ADD schedules[3]
- PIMRA[4]
- Glasgow Anxiety Scale[5]
- Yale–Brown Obsessive Compulsive Scale[6]
- Zung Anxiety Rating Scale: Adults Intellectual Disability Version.[7]

1 Deb S, Mathews T, Holt G, Bouras N (2001). *Practice Guidelines for the Assessment and Diagnosis of Mental Health Problems in Adults with Intellectual Disability.* Pavilion Publishing: Brighton, UK.

2 Stavrakaki C, Lunsky Y (2007). Depression, anxiety and adjustment disorders in people with intellectual disabilities. In: Bouras N and Holt G (Eds) *Psychiatric and Behavioural Disorders in Development Disabilities and Mental Retardation.* (Chapter 7). Cambridge University Press: Cambridge.

3 Moss S (2002). *PAS-ADD Schedules.* Pavilion Publishing: Brighton.

4 Matson JL, Kazdin AE. Senatore V (1984). Psychometric properties of the psychopathology instrument for mental retarded adults (PIMRA). *American Journal on Mental Retardation* **5**, 881–889.

5 Epsie CA & Mindham J (2003). Glasgow Anxiety Scale for people with intellectual disability (GAS-ID): development and psychometric properties of a new measure for use with people with mild intellectual disability. *Journal of Intellectual Disability Research* **47**(1), 22–30.

6 Feurer ID, Dimitropoulos A, Stone WL, *et al* (1998). The latent variable structure of the Compulsive Behaviour Checklist in people with Prader-Willi syndrome. *Journal of Intellectual Disability Research,* **42**(6), 472–480.

7 Lindsay WR & Michie AM (1988). Adaptation of the Zung self-rating anxiety scale for people with a mental handicap. *Journal of Mental Deficiency Research* **32**(6), 485–490.

Psychotic disorders

Definition

This grouping of psychosis brings together schizophrenia, schizotypal, and delusional disorders. They are generally characterized by the following two groups of symptoms:

- **Positive**—distortion of thinking (i.e. thought interference, insertion, withdrawal, broadcasting), perception (i.e. hallucinations, delusions), mood (i.e. rapid changes of highs and lows, incongruous, flattened), and behaviour (i.e. bizarre, impaired social functioning)
- **Negative**—apathy, lack of communication, social withdrawal, mutism, bunted mood.

Types of disorders

According to ICD-10 there are several different types of disorders within this grouping:

Paranoid schizophrenia—dominated by relatively stable, often paranoid delusions, usually accompanied by hallucinations, particularly of the auditory variety, and perceptual disturbances.

Hebephrenic schizophrenia—affective changes are prominent, delusions and hallucinations fleeting and fragmentary, behaviour irresponsible and unpredictable, and mannerisms common.

Catatonic schizophrenia—dominated by prominent psychomotor disturbances that may alternate between extremes such as hyperkinesis and stupor, or automatic obedience and negativism.

Simple schizophrenia—progressive development of oddities of conduct, inability to meet the demands of society, and decline in total performance.

Prevalence

A small number of studies have examined schizophrenia in people with mild/moderate ID, and have reported that prevalence rates are at least 3 times higher than reported in the non-disabled population: 3–3.7%.[1,2,3]

Assessment

Diagnosis is based on the presence of a number of complex and subjective symptoms, and thus a certain level of communication is needed to describe such symptoms (i.e. voices). Therefore, for those people with severe/profound ID with very restricted communication, diagnosis will be more difficult to obtain.

There are a number of screening tools designed specifically to aid nurses to assess a person's experiences of voices or disturbing thoughts; however, these will be helpful only for people with borderline/mild ID, with good communication skills:

- The Cognitive Assessment of Voices Schedule[4]
- The Hallucinations Rating Scale[5]
- The Delusions Rating Scale.[5]

Within the area of ID there are no specifically developed rating scales for nurses to use in relation to psychosis; however, within the PAS-ADD

Schedules a number of questions are set to collate some information about the person's thinking, perception, mood and behaviour.[6]

Difficulties in assessment

Deb et al. have offered nurses some advice in order to accurately assess psychosis in people with ID:[7]

- As sensory impairments are common in this population, these should be checked as they may aggravate symptoms.
- Some people with ID may have 'imaginary friends' which may be observed as a positive symptom of schizophrenia.
- As many people with ID may have limited communication, they may express themselves using behaviour that may appear odd or bizarre.
- People with ID may have difficulty recognizing their own thoughts, and therefore may attribute them to others.
- Some of the behaviours normally displayed by people with ID (i.e. marked apathy, paucity of speech, under activity, passivity) may represent the negative symptoms of this condition.
- Negative symptoms may be a consequence of medication and/or unstimulating environments.
- For many people with ID, they will have little control of their own lives, as carers and professionals supervise them.

1 Bouras N, Martin G et al. (2004). Schizophrenia-spectrum psychoses in people with and without intellectual disability. Journal of Intellectual Disability Research **48**(6), 548–555.

2 Hemmings P (2006). Schizophrenia spectrum disorders in people with intellectual disabilities. Current Opinion in Psychiatry **19**(5), 470–474.

3 Clarke D (2007). Schizophrenia spectrum disorders in people with intellectual disabilities (Chapter, 8, pp.131–142). In Bouras N. and Holt G. Psychiatric and Behavioural Disorders in Intellectual and Developmental Disabilities, 2nd edition. Cambridge University Press: Cambridge.

4 Chadwick P & Birchwood M (1994). The cognitive assessment of voices schedule: In Chadwick P, Birchwood M & Trower P (eds). Cognitive Therapy for Hallucinations, Delusions and Paranoia. Wiley: Chichester.

5 Haddock G (1994). The hallucinations rating scale. University of Manchester: Manchester.

6 Moss S (2002). PAS-ADD Schedules. Pavilion Publishing: Brighton.

7 Deb S, Mathews T, Holt G, Bouras N (2001). Practice Guidelines for the Assessment and Diagnosis of Mental Health Problems in Adults with Intellectual Disability. Pavilion Publishers: Brighton, UK.

Organic disorders

Both international classification systems (i.e. ICD-10 and DSM-IV)[1,2] clearly distinguish between two groups of psychiatric disorders based on a system of diagnosis:

- Organic disorders
- Non-organic or functional disorders.

This distinction between organic disorders and non-organic disorders is important as the causes for each of the two groups are different. The central clinical feature of most organic psychiatric disorders is impaired cognitive functioning. Cerebral dysfunction can, however, also cause organic mood states and personality change, as well as organic psychotic or neurotic states.

Organic disorders result from a cerebral malfunction of the brain caused by certain metabolic, toxic, or other cerebral pathogens/dysfunctions of the brain. Examples include:

- Anoxia
- Trauma
- Degenerative disease.

System of classification

A practitioner undertaking an assessment/diagnosis using ICD-10 and DSM-IV has to be fully aware of 3 facts when attempting to diagnose an organic or functional psychiatric disorder:

- A small number of psychiatric disorders are known to result from an organic cause such as brain injury.
- People suffering from any organic brain disorder can experience any psychiatric symptoms (i.e. hallucinations, delusions) as described by a person with a functional disorder.
- Many psychiatric symptoms can also be caused by the ingestion of psychoactive substances.

In making a diagnosis, both classification systems highlight that organic disorders are examined first and if appropriate excluded, before non-organic functional psychiatric disorder can be clearly identified.

Organic disorders

Within ICD-10 classification of psychiatric disorders there are a wide range of organic conditions, the following are some of the main organic disorders.

Dementia—there are a number of organic causes of dementia, which need to be identified clearly before a general diagnosis of dementia can be made. Some of these include cerebrovascular disease, Parkinson's disease, Huntington's disease, multiple sclerosis, epilepsy, hypothyroidism, vitamin B12 or folic acid deficiency, hypercalcaemia, and alcohol or drug misuse. Frontal lobe dementias can be caused by other brain diseases such as Pick's disease and Creutzfeldt–Jakob disease.

Delirium (acute and sub-acute confusional states) occurs more readily in older persons, acutely and chronically physically ill. Causes of delirium include septicaemia, urinary, chest, CNS and other infections, and cancer, cardiopulmonary, liver, renal, metabolic, autoimmune and other systematic physical health disorders. Delirium may also follow medication changes, and include medication toxicity, especially during anticonvulsant/psycho-tropic polytherapy. Delirium can also result from substance intoxication, substance withdrawal, and multiple aetiologies.

Other organic disorders listed in different categories with ICD-10 include:
- Psychoactive substance use
- Acute intoxication
- Harmful use
- Dependency syndrome
- Withdrawal state with delirium
- Organic affective disorder
- Organic anxiety disorder
- Organic delusional disorder: possible cause epilepsy, amphetamine intoxication
- Organic catatonic disorder
- Organic sleep disorders.

Further reading

Cooper SA, Holland AJ (2007). Dementia and mental ill health in older people with intellectual disabilities. In: Bouras N and Holt G (Eds). *Psychiatric and Behavioural Disorders in Development Disabilities and Mental Retardation.* (Chapter 10). Cambridge University Press: Cambridge.

McCarron M, Lawlor BA (2003). Responding to the challenges of ageing and dementia in intellectual disability in Ireland. *Ageing and Mental Health* **7**(6), 413–417.

Royal College of Psychiatrists (2001). *DC-LD: Diagnostic criteria for psychiatric disorders for use with adults with learning disabilities/mental retardation.* Gaskell: London.

1 World Health Organisation (1992). *ICD-10 Classification of Mental and Behavioural Disorders: Clinical descriptions and diagnostic guidelines.* WHO.

2 American Psychiatric Association (1994). *Diagnostic and Statistical Manual of Mental Disorders,* 4th Edn. APA.

Dementia (in people with intellectual disability)

While some studies report prevalence rates similar to the general population,[1] it is generally accepted that people with ID are at increased risk of earlier onset dementia. Compared with the general population, Cooper found that prevalence of dementia in adults with ID other than Down syndrome is 15.6% in 65–75yrs age group, 23.5% in 65–84yrs age group, and 70% in 85–94yrs age group.[2] For people with Down syndrome (acknowledged to be at even greater risk—see 📖 Older people with Down syndrome, p.134) estimates are that 15–45% of people with Down syndrome >40yrs have dementia,[3] considerably higher than general population rates of 4.3–10% in persons >6yrs.[4] Of dementias among people with ID, 50–60% are of the Alzheimer's type. Alzheimer's disease is an irreversible, progressive brain disease that slowly destroys memory and thinking skills. It is characterized by impaired memory and judgement, disorientation, impaired ability to learn and reason, high levels of stress, and sensitivity to the local and social environment.

The diagnosis of dementia in persons with ID relies on evidence of change from the person's previous level of functioning, and on meeting the following ICD-10 criteria:[5]

- Decline in memory
- Decline in other cognitive skills—thinking, planning, and organizing
- Clear consciousness
- Decline in emotional control, motivation, or social behaviour
- 6-month duration
- Exclusion of other disorders.

There is no equivalent to the MMSE in screening for dementia in persons with ID. Despite continued efforts, there is no agreed consensus on an optimal battery of test instruments; nor is there an established rapid assessment instrument with established cut-off scores.

Changes in personality, behaviour, and global day-to-day function, are often more relevant as warning signs than changes in cognition and memory. Identification of changes is more likely if there is frequent and early screening for such changes; recommendations are for annual baseline screening for persons with Down syndrome >35yrs, and for persons with ID from other aeteologies, >50yrs.[5]

Each person is unique and will experience dementia differently, yet clients and the services they need tend to fall into three groupings:

Group 1—some people may experience a relatively slow progression of dementia over 5–8yrs. While these individuals will require increasing supports, particularly in terms of staffing and some relatively low cost environmental modifications to their living spaces, they can often be maintained within their family unit, i.e. the home they have lived in throughout their decline. Retaining contact with familiar environments, family, and friends, is the optimal approach to service delivery for this group.

Group 2—for some people, while decline may not necessarily be compressed, they present, particularly at mid-stage dementia, with behavioural and psychotic features: night-time wakening, wandering, agitation, screaming, and visual and auditory hallucinations. Some behavioural issues may be addressed in existing settings with improved communication, programming, and environmental approaches. For others, dementia specific environments with specialist-trained staff will better respond to their additional care needs.

Group 3—for others, decline may be compressed and the person may progress to a stage of advanced dementia within a relatively short time, i.e. 1–2yrs. As dementia progresses, specialist nursing and palliative care will become increasingly important.[6]

ID services system has traditionally been focused on serving and maintaining people with ID in the community for as long as possible, and has been driven by a service philosophy that emphasizes positive approaches, skill acquisition, and increasing independence. The inevitable decline associated with Alzheimer's dementia challenges this programming philosophy, and there is a danger that with changing needs when dementia presents, service providers will seek to transfer a person to other, often more expensive, alternatives. This does not need to happen, as there are opportunities to support ageing in place, and a growing interest in understanding the role of specialized units for people with ID and dementia.[6]

1 Janicki MP, Dalton AJ (2000). Prevalence of dementia and impact on Intellectual Disability Services. *Mental Retardation* **38**, 276–288.

2 Cooper SA (1997). High prevalence of dementia among people with learning disabilities not attributable to Down's syndrome. *Psychiatric Medicine* **27**, 609–616.

3 Prasher VP, Krishnan VHR (1993). Age of onset and duration of dementia in people with Down's syndrome. *International Journal of Geriatric Psychiatry* **8**, 923–927.

4 Hoffman A, Rocca WA, Brayne C, et al. (1991). The prevalence of dementia in Europe: a collaborative study of 1890–1990 findings. *International Journal of Epidemiology* **20**, 736–748.

5 Aylward E, Burt D, Thorpe L, Lai F, Dalton A (1997). Diagnosis of dementia in individuals with intellectual disability. *Journal of Intellectual Disability Research* **41**,152–164.

6 McCarron M, Gill M, McCallion P, Begley C (2005). Health co morbidities in ageing persons with Down syndrome and Alzheimer's dementia. *Journal of Intellectual Disability Res* **49**, 560–566.

Psychopathology

Psychopathology is the term used to refer to the study of mental illness that includes the origins, development, and manifestation of mental disorder. Psychopathology is used to signify behaviours or experiences symptomatic of mental illness, even if they do not constitute a formal diagnosis.

Important factors, such as genetic causes of ID with specific behavioural phenotypes and associated health factors, e.g. hypothyroidism in a person with Down syndrome, physical health, and epilepsy should also be considered in the diagnostic assessment.

There is a range of models that can be adopted to study mental or behavioural disorders, and each of these includes three elements: aetiology, treatment aims, and treatment methods. Models of psychopathology comprise:

- Biological/medical
- Psychological
  - Psychodynamic
  - Behavioural
  - Cognitive
- Social cultural
  - Humanistic/existential
  - Family systems
  - Multicultural

Biological/medical models of psychopathology

This model focuses on studying signs and symptoms of disease, neurochemical abnormalities, brain defects, and possible genetic factors. It classifies psychopathology into diagnostic groups. Evidence of this model is based on a scan of biological markers (e.g. CT, PET) and their response to medication and disease treatments. Depending on the aetiology, treatment regimens may involve medication, ECT, and to a very limited extent neurosurgery. A variant of the medical model is the diathesis-stress model. This psychological theory explains behaviour as a result of biological and genetic factors, and life experiences (nature and nurture). It suggests that mental disorder is produced by the interaction of a predisposition to mental ill health, and a precipitating event in the environment, and this for example has been used to explain schizophrenia and bipolar mood disorder.

Psychological models of psychopathology

This model examines psychological actions e.g. early experiences, traumatic events, maladaptive learning experiences, and illogical thinking. Sigmund Freud was the first to formalize the psychoanalysis model, and this has influenced this approach ever since. In the psychoanalysis model, there is emphasis on the behaviour being seen as a result of an abnormal symptom; the importance of unconscious conflicts, early childhood experiences, and stages of psychosexual development are emphasized. There is a range of therapeutic approaches to treat disorder, including behaviour therapy. In this approach there is a concentration on the importance of conditional learning and classical conditioning, whereas cognitive therapy models focus

on thinking, and view abnormal behaviour and feelings as a consequence of faulty thinking. Rational–emotional behavioural therapy (developed by Dr Albert Ellis) views the relationship between events in a person's life as a direct consequence of emotions and behaviours.

Sociocultural models of psychopathology

This final model considers social and cultural influences on behaviour, arguing that these forces exert important influences. It views biological and psychological models as incomplete, because they do not also consider societal norms and expectations, subgroup influences, and family dynamics. Within family dynamics this model embraces a view that families can be a source of stress, can discourage change, and can encourage a member to be sick, and therefore the family as a whole should be the target of intervention. Suggested interventions include family therapy (see 📖 p.304), couples therapy, group therapy, and community interventions.

A combination of approaches

People with ID need to be able to access a combination of approaches, as more generally mental and behavioural disorders are probably better understood within a more comprehensive biological-psychological-social-developmental framework.

Further reading

Priest H, Gibbs, M (2004). *Mental Health Care for People with Learning Disabilities*. Churchill Livingstone: Oxford.

Casey PR, Kelly B (2007). *Fish's Clinical Psychopathology: Signs and Symptoms in Psychiatry*. 3rd edn. Gaskell: London.

Joseph S, Worsley R (2005). *Person-centred Psychopathology: A Postive Psychology of Mental Health*. PCCS Books: Ross-on-Wye.

Autistic spectrum disorders

An ASD is a lifelong developmental disorder, and although intervention might help to minimize the autistic symptoms or enable the individual to 'fully' participate in every aspect of daily life, some difficulties still remain. Differences in labelling have caused a lot of confusion among all concerned, as the ASD is also referred to as:[1]

- autism, childhood autism, autism spectrum disorder/autistic disorder
- pervasive developmental disorder, pervasive developmental disorder not otherwise specified
- autistic traits, atypical autism
- semantic-pragmatic disorder, childhood disintegrative disorder
- Asperger's syndrome; high-functioning autism
- DAMP.

All individuals with ASD will experience difficulties in the following areas, also known as the 'triad of impairments':

- social communication (verbal and non-verbal) and language
- social interaction
- social imagination, flexibility of thoughts, and pretend play.

Examples of characteristics or manifestations of ASD and challenges faced on a regular basis include:

- Stereotypic or repetitive behaviours in order to stimulate oneself (e.g. jumping, 'frogging', rocking, spinning, hand flapping)
- Resistance to changes in routine—a change of routine may cause an emotional reaction
- Limited interest in playing with others, lack of creativity; joining in the play only when the other person insists and assists them. Also unusual play with toys/things (e.g. spinning, lining them up)
- Busy environments can lead to emotional reactions and/or need to run away (e.g. strong or flickering lights, noise, and busy colours)
- One-way communication, odd language, talking about one particular topic (usually their special interests), echolalia (parroting), and difficulty in receptive language
- Difficulties in making or maintaining friends, limited understanding of unwritten social rules, difficulty to judge situations and outcomes
- Vulnerability, bullying, and no sense of danger
- Inappropriate laughing or giggling; no or intense eye-contact (gaze)
- Difficulties in multitasking
- Over-sensitivity or under-sensitivity to pain—either no emotions and notification of being hurt or overreaction to a gentle touch
- Using senses (smell, touch, and taste) to explore environment
- Unusual posture of the body or limbs.

Examples of associated difficulties and/or health problems:

- Epilepsy
- ADHD or ADD, problems with concentration
- OCD
- Gastrointestinal problems, acid reflux, problems with stool consistency
- Sleep disorders; food allergies
- Self-injurious behaviours/challenging behaviours

- Mental health problems (depression, psychosis, anxiety)
- Dis-disorders such as dyspraxia and dyslexia.

Some approaches to support people

In order for people with ASD to live as 'ordinary' and fulfilling lives as possible, there are many ways we can help them to cope with the world such as:

- Consistency in approaches (written guidelines on how to work with individuals for everyone to follow)
- Structure of activities (using visual schedules/symbols/pictures) or written direction/instructions for them to follow
- Clear and short sentences during a conversation
- Using pictures/symbols to help them to have control of their environment, give them a sense of direction (a toilet symbol on the door)
- Using reward systems for motivation
- Social stories (to help them to understand things in their way)
- No use of metaphors (people may make a literal understanding)
- Time to process information (sometimes repeating things a few times)
- Reduction of disturbing stimuli (e.g. flickering lights, too many pictures)
- Not putting too much pressure and/or demands on them at once
- Developing coping strategies (e.g. relaxation and breathing techniques)
- Teach them to understand unwritten social rules, relationships and social skills (what is/is not appropriate)
- Support them in gaining control over their lives
- Teach them meanings of facial expressions and emotions (a few tools developed by National Autistic Society)[2]
- Do not set tasks they cannot achieve.

Examples of interventions and approaches:
- TEACCH
- PECS
- Speech and language therapy/facilitated communication
- Music therapy
- ABA
- Lovaas early intensive behavioural therapy programme
- Son rise programme – early intervention
- Gluten and casein free diet.

1 Anderson M (2007). Autistic spectrum disorder. In: Gates B, Ed. *Learning Disabilities: Towards Inclusion.* 5th edn. Churchill Livingstone Elsevier: Edinburgh.

2 National Autistic Society website 🖳 www.nas.org.uk

Self-harm

What is self-harm?

Self-harm is any act that is deliberate, self-inflicted, and causes physical harm to the individual; its purpose is to relieve emotional distress. Self-harm is not a diagnosis *per se*. In mental health services, self-harm can be associated with a range of mental disorders. Types of self-harm include:

- Cutting
- Poisoning
- Burning
- Throwing self against an object
- Punching self

People self-harm for many reasons, including inducing a feeling of control over one's life, to relieve distress, or reduce feelings of guilt. Self-harm does not necessarily imply suicidal intent, as it is often used as a coping mechanism, a way to survive, and not as a method to take one's own life; however, possible suicidal intent should be considered in assessment (see 📖 Risk of suicide, p.548).

Self-harm and people with intellectual disabilities

There is little evidence to suggest the prevalence of self-harm (when associated with mental ill health) among people with ID. The assessment of self-harm should be considered at all levels of intellectual functioning, bearing in mind that presentation and mode of self-harm may differ across the spectrum of abilities. Nurses and other staff need to pay particular attention to assessing intent in people with ID. A person may carry out an act that appears insignificant, such as taking three sleeping tablets. However, the individual may lack the knowledge of what is a dangerous dose, yet they may be experiencing severe emotional distress and increase the dose on a future attempt. Another example is a person with ID who walks out into the road in front of oncoming traffic. Staff may believe this is due to a lack of road safety and overlook any suggestion of self-harm.

Management and intervention will differ from service to service, but should be based on a biological-psychological-social assessment (see 📖 Self-harm, p.546; 📖 Self-injury, p.550). On one end of the continuum, the focus is reducing opportunities to self-harm by removing from the environment objects to harm oneself, accompanied by one-to-one care. At the other end of the continuum, the focus may be on letting the person learn to be responsible for themselves through a harm minimization approach. Harm minimization approaches consider the actual harm that can occur from a person's current behaviour, and then considers how the threat of harm to the individual can be minimized by altering the environment and reducing access to opportunities for self-harm. In addition, a range of psychological treatments, e.g. problem-solving therapy and dialectical behaviour therapy, may be provided. Addressing the individual's social and relationship needs are also pivotal for a successful approach. Self-harm may also be in the context of mental disorders such as depression. In these cases the prescription of antidepressants will be indicated, as you would expect to see a reduction or discontinuation of the behaviour by treating the underlying condition in these circumstances.

Self-injurious behaviour and people with intellectual disabilities

The term 'self-injurious behaviour' is commonly used in services for people with ID. Its use can be confusing, as its meaning is somewhat different to that of self-harm. Self-injurious behaviour can include head banging and biting, or hitting oneself. Self-injurious behaviour is often associated with people with severe and profound ID, and is used as an intentional (and non-intentional) form of communication. For example it may be used to express feelings of pain or ill health, to avoid situations that the person does not understand or wish to be in, or to gain some form of interaction with those around them. Also self-injury may be present as a form of sensory stimulation for people with sensory impairments. In these instances, self-injurious behaviour is referred to as a type of challenging behaviour. Interventions will differ, and are based around supporting the person to engage in meaningful activities, developing relationships, and teaching the person new skills e.g. alternative forms of communication,

In a small minority of individuals, self-injurious behaviour is a characteristic of a particular syndrome; this is referred to as a behavioural phenotype. An example would be Lesch–Nyhan syndrome, where a striking feature is lip and hand biting.

Further reading

Self-harm: Recovery, Advice, and Support ▣ www.selfharm.org.uk

Self-injury ▣ www.selfharm.net

Substance misuse

There is debate regarding the prevalence of alcohol and illicit drug misuse in people with ID, as a result of methodological problems. Nevertheless, lower prevalence rates of substance misuse are reported compared with the general population; however, these figures may be under-estimated as they are based on only those people known to ID services.

Definition

According to ICD-10, 3 or more of the following must be present in the previous year to obtain a diagnosis of a 'dependence syndrome':

- A strong desire or sense of compulsion to use the substance
- Difficulties in controlling substance-taking behaviour
- A physiological withdrawal state
- Evidence of tolerance
- Progressive neglect of alternative pleasures
- Persisting with substance use despite clear evidence of overtly harmful consequences.

Aetiology

A clearer picture is emerging of the characteristics that place individuals with ID most at risk from misusing substances:[1]

Intra-personal variables—borderline to mild ID, young and male, co-existence of a mental health problem, low self-esteem, inadequate self-control/regulatory behaviour, cognitive limitations (i.e. illiteracy, short attention span, memory deficits, poor problem-solving skills, tendencies to distort abstract cognitive concepts, overly compliant dispositions), frustration.

Inter-personal variables—living in the community with low levels of supervision, poverty, parental alcohol-related neuropsychiatric disorders, presence of negative role models with less punitive child management practices, negative life events (i.e. neglect, abuse, bereavement), limited employment, educational and recreational opportunities, excessive amounts of free time, restricted friendships and relationships, lack of routine, loneliness, desire for social acceptance/method for 'fitting in'.

Assessment

Difficulties exist in assessing this population as a result of staff issues (i.e. a lack of skills/knowledge) and complex issues presented by the person (i.e. aggression, mental and physical health problems, offending behaviour). Furthermore, people with ID who misuse substances sometimes can be 'unwilling' or 'uncooperative' to fully engage in the assessment process—or may be labeled as such. Areas that need to be assessed include:

- Substance use patterns and impact
- Reasons for and knowledge of substance misuse
- Mental health
- Offending behaviour patterns
- Motivation to fully want to change and to engage in the process of helping.

Biological-psychological-social interventions

Biological—detoxification, psychopharmacology treatments, i.e. antabuse, naltrexone, methadone, and SSRIs.

Psychological—individual education (including anger management, relaxation training, challenging negative statements), modifications of AA & Twelve Step Programme, group therapy promoting feelings of acceptance/belonging using peer support, behavioural and cognitive approaches (i.e. assertiveness skills, distinguishing between positive and negative role models within substance abuse situations), motivational interviewing, relapse prevention programmes focusing on self-regulation of thinking and feeling, accepting past relapses, identifying the causes of relapse, and learning to prevent and interrupt relapses.

Social—social skills training (e.g. develop coping and refusal skills, self-monitoring skills, promote inter-personal communication, facilitate the expression of emotions, appropriately responding to criticism, engaging in realistic role plays), staff education, promotion of social support.

Advice to help people diminish substance abuse
- Target the person's intrinsic motivation to want to change and to engage in self-help, using the techniques of motivational interviewing.
- Offer education with more time flexibility, based on repetition and greater use of role-play
- Provide information leaflets about the harmful effects on people's bodies, minds, relationships and lifestyle in a user-friendly format.
- Address unresolved problems (i.e. bereavement, abuse, loneliness)
- Target specific offending behaviours
- Identify trigger factors of relapse.

1 Taggart L, Huxley A, Baker G (2008). Alcohol and illicit drug misuse in people with learning disabilities: Implications for research and service development. *Advances in Mental Health in Learning Disabilities* **2**(1), 11–21.

Responding to bereavement

Reactions to loss

Loss is a universal experience, which people respond to in many different ways. Reactions to death as loss can affect people in an emotional way (e.g. feeling guilty, profoundly sad or helpless), in a physical way (e.g. lacking energy, being lethargic, or having a hollowness in the stomach), and/or in a behavioural way (e.g. sleeplessness, crying, and restlessness). Most bereaved people seek the support they need from family and friends, but for a small percentage of people, the need for professional support (such as a bereavement counsellor or therapist) is required.

Intellectual disability and loss

The person with an ID may experience many more losses than the average person, because of the nature of the disability, and societal reactions to the person who may be perceived as being 'different' in some way. People with an ID do experience death and grief, but sometimes express it in ways that may be misinterpreted, or express grief a long time after the death, which may mean it is overlooked. People with ID may also be prone to multiple and successive losses as a result of the death of, for example, their main carer (mother or father), as illustrated in Fig. 7.2.

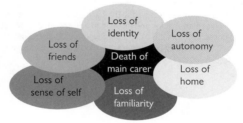

Fig. 7.2 Multiple and successive losses.

Often, when multiple losses are experienced, the raw realities of living (such as where the bereaved person will be sleeping that night) overtake the overwhelming sadness of death, and mourning the deceased may be delayed.

Factors affecting support

It seems that the more complex the ID, the less likelihood of being actively involved in loss and bereavement issues and associated opportunities. Subsequently, many people with an ID do not get the support they need following the death of their loved ones, and some may not even be told of the death, because of:
• difficulties in communicating effectively, which precludes meaningful reciprocal information and explanations
• challenges associated with cognition, and some people may struggle to understand complex and abstract concepts (such as death)

- limited attention span
- an inability to articulate feelings in a socially acceptable and meaningful way
- so much reliance on other people to help them to facilitate their loss
- the nurses supporting them, who may not feel comfortable talking about loss and bereavement
- the nurses supporting them, who want to protect them from the sad business of bereavement
- the nurses supporting them, who do not know how to offer appropriate bereavement support.

Such compounding issues can make bereavement and grief work difficult for this client population.

Disenfranchised grief

When a loss such as death cannot be openly acknowledged, publicly mourned, or socially supported, it often results in disenfranchised grief.[1]
- The relationship to the deceased is not recognized
- The loss is not recognized
- The griever is not recognized
- The circumstances around the death preclude involvement
- The way people have learned to grieve (or not) may influence involvement and coping styles.

These factors often result in the bereaved person being excluded from the rituals associated with death (such as attending the funeral or sending a wreath), and create additional problems for the bereaved by removing or minimizing sources of appropriate support. Groups likely to experience disenfranchised grief include children, elderly people, people with mental health needs, people with ID, and those with HIV and AIDS.

The nurse should remain open and honest with the grieving person with an ID. They should take every opportunity actively to include the person throughout the grief process and associated rituals. This helps to affirm the death and minimize the possibility of disenfranchised grief, which can lead to complex grief reactions and indicate the need for grief counselling or therapy.

1 Doka K (2002). Disenfranchised grief: New Directions, Challenges, and Strategies for Practice. Research Press: Illinois.

Planning with people and their families

Person-centred planning

What is person-centred planning?

The term person-centred planning means that the support for a person who has an ID is planned with the person themselves at the centre, as opposed to support being 'service led'. 'Person-centred planning is not just a collection of new planning styles'.[1] Historically, planning approaches for people with ID were goal orientated (set by the support service), and achievements were based on the individual's attainment of particular skills or completion of tasks.[1]

Person-centred planning is a fundamentally different way of regarding people who have ID. The person-centred planning process is aimed at exploring what is important to the individual and setting out how to act on this.[2]

The origins of person-centred planning

The development of person-centred planning reflects the journey services for people who have ID has taken. Historically, services were devaluing, provided within long-stay hospitals and institutions where service users were stripped of their own identities. Normalization theory lead onto O'Brien's 5 accomplishments, which prioritized the rights of people with ID with regard to community participation, respect, having a valued social role, making choices, and developing relationships.

After the closure of long-stay hospitals, professional dissatisfaction with 'individual planning' approaches grew, and whichever form the plans took they were predominantly service lead. The 'inclusion movement' was growing, where the concepts of equality and justice underpinned the philosophy of normalization and person-centred planning. The first person-centred planning approaches emerged in North America, between 1973 and 1986, and were embraced within UK services from 1979.

Valuing People defines person-centred planning as a 'process for continual listening and learning, focusing on what is important to someone now and in the future, and acting on this in conjunction with their family and friends'.[3] It defines person-centred approaches as ways of 'commissioning, providing, and organizing services rooted in listening to what people want, to help them live in their communities as they choose'.[3]

Where do I start with the planning process?

As stated above, it is an expectation in current service policy that people with ID who are supported by services will have a person-centred plan. A plan may be initiated simply because an individual does not have one, with an anticipated outcome that the individual's support will reflect their personal choices, and likes and dislikes. As a by-product of this, their support staff will get to know them better, friends and family become full partners, their capabilities are highlighted and strengthened, and a sense of commitment to the person and the listening and learning process is achieved.[2]

On other occasions a life event or transition may prompt the initiation of a person-centred plan, such as change or loss of a primary care giver, or moving from childhood to adulthood. Regardless of the reason or trigger for the plan, key questions are, 'Who are you and who are we in your life?

What can we do together to achieve a better life for you now and in the future?'[1]

Choice of tools (see 📖 Life planning, p.288)

There is a choice of tools available to use:

- ELP
- PATH
- PFP
- MAPS.

It is vital to note that the tool is only part of the process. Choosing the right tool is important, but the quality of the planning mechanism is much more dependent on the skill of the facilitator. Also, as the facilitator becomes confident and experienced with person-centred planning, they may pick and choose parts of various tools in order to tailor-make the plan to the individual's needs.

After the plan

The plan must be followed and reviewed. Understandably, a person's lifestyle choices will change over time, as do staff or carers, and the risk is that the focus person's hopes and dreams are extinguished overnight. This experience, repeatedly, would result in the person feeling hopeless and defeated by the service, as would the staff supporting the person, and their family and friends.

Further reading

Sanderson H (2000). *Person Centred Planning: Key Features and Approaches.* Joseph Rowntree Foundation: UK. Available at:
🖳 http://www.paradigmuk.org/pdf/articles/helensandersonpaper.pdf

1 Sanderson H, Kennedy J, Ritchie P, Goodwin G (2002). *People, Plans and Possibilities.* Joseph Rowntree Foundation. SHS, Edinburgh.

2 Sweeney C, Sanderson H (2002). *Factsheet—Person Centred Planning.* Bild: Kidderminster. Available at: 🖳 http://www.bild.org.uk/

3 Department of Health (2001). *Valuing People: A New Strategy for Learning Disability for the 21st Century.* HMSO: London, 11–16. Available at: 🖳 http://www.dh.gov.uk/en/Publicationsandstatistics/Publications/PublicationsPolicyAndGuidance/DH_4009681 [accessed April 2009]

Undertaking a nursing assessment

There is a range of person-centred planning frameworks for developing individualized plans for support with people with ID, such as those discussed in 📖 Life planning, p.288. Although such frameworks are not profession specific, nurses have a unique contribution to make in providing a nursing perspective in these discussions through the completion of a structured nursing assessment.

In undertaking an assessment, nurses should select an appropriate structured nursing framework on the basis of the initial information provided in the referral to them. All nurses need to be careful not to only use a specialist secondary assessment, such as those that are psychology based or medical based, without a comprehensive nursing assessment having been completed first.

Nursing assessment

A nursing assessment requires the systematic collection of information by a nurse, which is guided by a nursing framework and involves some or all of the following processes: the observation of the individual, questioning, active listening, data collection on physical/mental health, and physical examination.

The purpose of a nursing assessment is to gain comprehensive information on the current abilities and needs of the individual being assessed within a recognized nursing framework, and to establish priorities for nursing intervention.

Preparing for an assessment

- Prior to commencing a nursing assessment it is necessary to explain the process to the person with ID (and their carers if present)
- Provide opportunities for the person to ask further questions they may have about what the process involves
- Develop a rapport with the person with ID, sufficient for them to feel comfortable during the assessment process
- Obtain valid consent for the assessment to be undertaken and for information to be sought from other relevant professionals
- The preparation for a nursing assessment often requires more than one meeting with the person with ID, and family carers if they are actively involved in their care.

Conducting a nursing assessment

- Focus on the person and their current situation (including family circumstances)
- Select a structured nursing framework that identifies the areas to be considered within the nursing assessment
- Provide opportunities for person to demonstrate their abilities through day-to-day activities and where possible in a range of settings
- Undertake the assessment within an environment the person is familiar
- Avoid undertaking nursing assessments when people are distressed, if at all possible
- Provide positive feedback to the people involved during the process of the assessment

- Undertake the nursing assessment in manageable chunks, so that the person can maintain their concentration
- With the permission of the person with ID, seek information from other professionals/carers involved in providing support, in so far as it assists in the completion of the nursing assessment.

Recording and reporting
- All nursing assessment document and related care plans are legal documents and must be treated accordingly
- Record objective information on what was observed, heard and measured during the nursing assessment
- Write clear statements about what the person can do, before listing areas of need
- Avoid value judgements on behaviour observed, previous history and value-laden words such as 'vulnerable', 'aggressive', 'difficult'
- When identifying the abilities and needs of person clearly state the abilities and needs as expressed by the person with ID and those views expressed by other people
- Comply with the NMC requirements for reporting and record keeping.[1]

Identifying priorities for nursing action
- In discussion with the person with ID, review the information recorded and seek to identify their priorities, areas of strengths, and need
- Decide if further detailed assessment is required in relation to specific aspects e.g. physical mobility, epilepsy, mental health
- Review the areas of need identified and consider which of these may be responsive to nursing interventions (consistent with the nursing framework used for nursing assessment)
- Write a prioritized list of areas for nursing intervention, and share these with the person with ID. This will from the basis of the nursing care plans.

Further reading

Gates B (2006). *Care Planning and Delivery in Intellectual Disability Nursing*. Blackwell Science: London

Jukes M, Aldridge J (2007). *Person-centred Practices. A Holistic and Integrated Approach*. Quay Books: London.

---

1 Nursing and Midwifery Council (2007). *Record Keeping Factsheet*. Nursing and Midwifery Council: London. ▧ www.nmc-uk.org/aFrameDisplay.aspx?

Writing nursing care plans

Documented 'plan' for nursing actions

Nursing care plans provide details of the area of need, the objective of nursing intervention, the nursing interventions to be undertaken, and the date for evaluation of the nursing care plan. Nursing care plans are central documents to the organization of nursing interventions, have an important legal status, and provide the record for what care was meant to be delivered. Nurses should start to plan interventions from the priorities identified within the nursing assessment. The focus of nursing care plans must be consistent with the structured nursing framework used for assessment, and should be written within the headings used within the nursing framework.

Nurses often work within a wider interdisciplinary context and may be contributing to an overall interdisciplinary person-centred plan. In such situations they must remain cognisant of the fact that only a nurse can write a nursing care plan and they will remain personally accountable for the quality of the nursing care plan developed, delivered, and how this is documented, including any core care plan they sign without personalizing the content.[1] Therefore, an individual who has an overall person-centred plan, should also have nursing care plans that link to that overall plan. Nursing care should not be delivered without a nursing care plan in place except in emergencies, after which the care delivered and care plans, should be documented.

Area of need

Nursing care plans arise from the results of a nursing assessment, and must be able to demonstrate a clear link to the priorities identified within a nursing assessment. Nurses should clearly state the area of nursing needs within the wider context as it relates to the individual, for example: Eating and drinking—'Mary is underweight (providing her weight and BMI) and is at risk of pressure sores'. Nurses should not use short phrases or single words in outlining the nursing needs, such as 'restricted mobility' without providing the wider context and contributing factors.

Person-centred objectives

Objectives should start with the client's name, and written as a clear statement of:
- the skill/knowledge the person with ID is seeking to achieve (self-administer their own medication/eat 3 meals a day); this should not be stated as the objectives of the nurse
- the support they will need to do this (from pre-prepared blister packs/using adapted cutlery)
- the criteria that will be used to establish when the objectives have been achieved (for 5 consecutive days)
- a measure of success (without error/either by using a recognized instrument or self-reports from the person with ID and family carers
- a specific date for evaluation, rather than 'in 4 weeks' or the date for evaluation being described as 'ongoing'.

Objectives should be reviewed at interdisciplinary meetings when the individuals and their families are also present.

When nursing objectives have been agreed, nurses should ensure all necessary resources (staff, equipment) are in place before the care plan is commenced. Any delay in commencing the care plan should be recorded, and a rationale provided, as well as an unmet need and the appropriate person within the Trust notified.[1]

Nursing interventions

These should be written as clear action statements, which fully describe any actions required, e.g. provide information explaining the components of healthy eating in a format that is accessible to (client's name), or provide three 15min sessions of walking each week.

All nursing interventions to be undertaken should have the informed consent of the person with ID, and be based on best available evidence. Nursing interventions should be written in a format accessible to all staff who will need to read the care plan, and abbreviations should not be used in describing nursing interventions.

Recording amendments in nursing care plans

Nurses should keep an ongoing record of all nursing interventions provided and outcomes achieved. These notes should be cross-referenced by number or title to the ongoing nursing care plans. This will provide the necessary information for ongoing and summative evaluations. When the objectives of the care plan have been achieved, the care plan should be discontinued and this recorded. Any amendment to nursing care plans or interventions within these should be signed, dated, and time entered, together with a rationale for any change being recorded within the nursing notes.[1] Nursing interventions not written in the care plan should not be undertaken; if additional interventions are deemed necessary these should be added to existing care plans, or a new care plan developed in which the new need is identified.

Further reading

Gates B (2006). *Care Planning and Delivery in Intellectual Disability Nursing.* Blackwell Science: London.

Advocacy

Advocacy exists in various forms, and is fundamentally about speaking up:[1]
- for oneself as in self-advocacy
- with others in a group through collective advocacy
- through others in citizen or peer advocacy.

A basic definition of advocacy is speaking for oneself or on behalf of others.

Advocacy refers to a process by which people who use services, individually or in groups, make service providers or other people aware of their views and interests. It is important to make a distinction between advocacy and user involvement. Advocacy is about people who use services setting the agenda, not just about being consulted by professionals and organizations.

A crucial element of support is to assist people in gaining access to resources and information. In the case of a self-advocacy group, this might be access to a venue or a means of communication. An effective supporter helps to generate ideas and possible courses of action without controlling or making choices for the person or the group.

Independent mental capacity advocates

Recent legislation with important implications for people with ID includes: the Disability Discrimination Act 1995[2] (and 2005),[3] the Human Rights Act 1998,[4] Adults with Incapacity Act 2000 (Scotland),[5] and the Mental Capacity Act 2005 (England and Wales).[6] The effect in practice of the Mental Capacity Act 2005 is that capacity must be assumed. The Act (England and Wales) is founded on 5 key principles:[6]

- A person must be assumed to have capacity unless it is established that they lack capacity
- A person is not to be treated as unable to make a decision unless all practicable steps to help him to do so have been undertaken without success
- A person is not to be treated as unable to make a decision merely because he makes an unwise decision.
- An act done, or decision made, under this Act for or on behalf of a person who lacks capacity must be done or made in his best interests
- Before the act is done, or the decision is made, regard must be made to whether the purpose for which it is needed can be as effectively achieved in a way that is less restrictive of the person's rights and freedom of action.

In Scotland, the Adults with Incapacity Act 2000 applies.[5] This provides a 2-stage test for capacity. Firstly, it has to be established that a person suffers from an impairment of, or a disturbance in the functioning of, the mind or brain. Furthermore, it must be demonstrated that this impairment or disturbance results in an inability to make decisions.[7] Although Northern Ireland does not yet have equivalent legislation, specifically on capacity, the principles of informed consent apply in practice (DHSSPS 2003)[8] (see 📖 Consent to treatment, p.260).

The Act presumes that each adult has the right to make their own decisions and that individuals must be given all appropriate help before any conclusion is reached that they do not have the capacity to do this. Other principles of the Act (as well as presumption of capacity) are:

The right of the individual to be supported to make their own decisions—people must be provided with all the appropriate help before any conclusion that they cannot make their own decisions.

Unwise decisions—an individual is not to be treated as unable to make a decision simply because it is considered unwise.

Best interests—anything done for or on behalf of an individual without capacity must be in their best interests.

Least restrictive alternative—anything done for or on behalf of a person without capacity should be the least restrictive of their rights and freedoms.

The Mental Capacity Act 2005 states that the appropriate authority 'must make such arrangements as it considers reasonable' to enable persons (independent mental capacity advocates) to be available to represent and support persons who fall within the remit of the Act.[5] Sections 35 and 36 deal with the appointment and function of independent mental capacity advocates.

Functions of independent mental capacity advocates:
- Providing support to the person whom he has been instructed to represent ('P') so that P may participate as fully as possible in any relevant decision
- Obtaining and evaluating relevant information
- Ascertaining what P's wishes and feelings would be likely to be, and the beliefs and values that would be likely to influence P, if he had capacity
- Ascertaining what alternative courses of action are available in relation to P
- Obtaining a further medical opinion where treatment is proposed and the advocate thinks that one should be obtained (Mental Capacity Act 2005: Section 36).[6]

The Mental Health Act 2007 refers to the role of independent mental health advocates.[9] It places a duty on the appropriate national authority to make arrangements for help to be provided by such advocates.

Further reading

Department of Health (2001). *12 Key Points on Consent: The Law in England*. Department of Health: London.

1 Atkinson D (1999), *Advocacy: A Review*. Pavilion/Joseph Rowntree Foundation: Brighton.

2 The Disability Discrimination Act (1995). The Stationery Office: London.

3 The Disability Discrimination (Amendment) Act (2005). The Stationery Office: London.

4 The Human Rights Act (1998).

5 Adults with Incapacity Act (2000). Scotland

6 The Mental Capacity Act (2005). The Stationery Office: London.

7 Dimond B (2007). Mental capacity and decision-making: defining capacity. *British Journal of Nursing* **16**(18), 1138–9.

8 Department of Health, Social Services and Public Safety (2003). *Consent to Examination, Treatment and Care*. Department of Health, Social Services and Public Safety: Belfast.

9 The Mental Health Act (2007). The Stationery Office: London.

Patient advice and liaison service

The NHS Plan announced its commitment to setting up a patient advice and liaison service (PALS) in every Trust in England by April 2002.[1] PALS aim to provide information, steer users towards appropriate service, and resolve problems. According to the Department of Health the core functions of PALS are:[2]

- Be identifiable and accessible to patients, their carers, friends and family
- Problem solve promptly and efficiently
- Signpost patients to independent advice and advocacy, both locally and nationally
- Provide information about Trust services and health-related services
- Initiate change and improvement via its feedback mechanisms
- Link with other PALS
- Support staff throughout the organization to respond to patients.

For people who have ID, the PALS may be more difficult to access than for a non-disabled person. Abbott et al. point out that PALS may be underused by people who are already marginalized or demoralized.[3] Interestingly, the early findings of the National Evaluation of PALS did not specifically mention access difficulties or adaptations that may have been made for people with ID who intend to or need to use PALS.[4]

The Department of Health's preliminary report described case studies whereby people felt enabled and empowered having used PALS.[4] Outcomes have been very positive for people who have approached PALS with issues to address, such as with 'uncommunicative Trust systems' or complaints. It is believed that PALS effects and reduces the number of formal complaints, thus increasing public confidence, although the evidence has not been presented for this yet. Sometimes PALS is the last source of hope for some, yet people have still reported an improved experience of the Trust having accessed PALS. Abbot et al. suggest that people do need to go on to find independent advocates if inside problem solving does not remedy their issue.[3]

Some excellent examples of good practice can be taken from Ridgeway Partnership (Oxfordshire Learning Disability NHS Trust) with regard to ensuring PALS meets the needs of people who have ID.[5] When the PALS service was first created in 2002, two main consultants were drawn in to help plan the service (a person with experience of advocacy and a person with an ID). As a result of this the name was changed to LISTEN, and it was decided that a working group was needed to steer service development. The aims of the service have been summarized as: to listen, to provide information, and to help resolve concerns.[5]

A major feature of the work of the LISTEN service is that it aims to reach out to its service users, rather than assume its users will always seek the service out. As mentioned by Freelander, who set up a PALS service in a Mental Health Trust, the service user, their family/carer, or the member of the public may be in a state of stress, distress, or feeling powerless when they need or ought to contact PALS.[6] The success of the service is reliant on the interpersonal and problem solving skills of its facilitator/s. This is clearly valued, as positive customer surveys reflect the service user feeling reassured, listened to, and understood.[6]

LISTEN holds regular meetings, annual events and local team meetings. Aside from these activities, the LISTEN service acts just as any other PALS service in receiving and dealing with complaints. Most contacts are made from service users or their family, then public (which may include an advocate or neighbour), then staff.

Despite the number of activities that take place in one PALS service alone, it could still be felt that the service is underused. The early findings of the Department of Health's National Evaluation revealed vast differences in staffing, establishments, and budgets, as well as differences in how the PALS feedback within the Trust, and at which level of seniority.[4]

1 The Department of Health (2000). *NHS Plan. July 2000.* HMSO: London. ▣ www.dh.gov.uk/en/ Publicationsandstatistics/Publications/PublicationsPolicyAndGuidance/DH_4002960 [accessed April 2009]

2 Department of Health (2002). *Supporting the Implementation of Patient Advice and Liaison Services: A Resource Pack. January 2002.* HMSO: London. ▣ www.dh.gov.uk/en/Publicationsandstatistics/Publications/PublicationsPolicyAndGuidance/DH_4015493 [accessed April 2009]

3 Abbot S, Meyer J, Copperman J, Bentley J, Lanceley A (2005). Quality criteria for patient advice and liaison services: what do patients and the public want? *Health Expectations* **8**(2), 126–137.

4 Department of Health (2006). *Developing the Patient Advice and Liaison Service: Key Messages for NHS Organisations From the National Evaluation of PALS. October 2006.* HMSO: London. ▣ www.dh.gov.uk/en/Publicationsandstatistics/Lettersandcirculars/Dearcolleagueletters/ DH_4139498 [accessed April 2009]

5 Ridgeway Partnership (2006). Oxfordshire Learning Disability NHS Trust.

6 Freelander V (2004). My mental health. *Mental Health Practice* **7**(9), 28–29.

Consent to treatment

The Mental Capacity Act (2005)[1] provides the legal framework to protect people living in England and Wales who lack the capacity to consent, supporting and empowering people to make decisions for themselves. The Adults with Incapacity Act (Scotland)[2] provides the legal framework in Scotland; at the time of writing this book (August 2008) there is no equivalent in Northern Ireland, although clear guidance in *Consent to Examination, Treatment and Care* applies.[3]

Who needs to know about it?

Every person who works with, cares for, or needs to treat a person with an ID, because all care and treatment that is offered and/or provided to people with ID must always comply with the 5 key principles (see Fig. 8.1).

What are the five key principles?

- There must be an assumption of capacity
- All practicable steps are taken to support understanding
- The right to make what might appear to be an unwise decision
- Anything done for or on behalf of a person who lacks the capacity must be done or made in the best interests of the person concerned
- Least restrictive option (see 📖 Advocacy, p.296 for more detail).

Who should assess capacity?

This is the person wishing to undertake the care or treatment, and is specific to the decision in question. A number of different people will assess a person's capacity—the support worker assessing if the person agrees to have a bath, or the nurse with regards to administration of medications, or the doctor wishing to insert a PEG. It is recognized that a person may have the capacity to make some decisions but not all. If it is found that the person lacks the capacity to consent, treatment must be undertaken in person's best interests (see 📖 Making best interests decisions, p.264, and Fig. 8.2). Documentation relating to 'best interests' must be completed by the relevant members of the interdisciplinary team in conjunction with relatives. As a person's capacity to make decisions may vary depending on the actual decision, each decision must be considered separately, enabling people to be able to make decisions on one part of their lives but not on others.

Serious medical treatment

- This involves providing, withdrawing or withholding treatment that is likely to have serious consequences for the person.
- An Independent Mental Capacity Advocate must be instructed and involved if the person has no relatives or close friends, and the treatment involves serious consequences for the person.

New criminal offence

- The Mental Capacity Act introduces two new criminal offences of ill treatment and wilful neglect. These can include a failure to provide necessary care i.e. ignoring persons' medical or physical needs, failing to provide the healthcare needed, or withholding medications, food or drink.

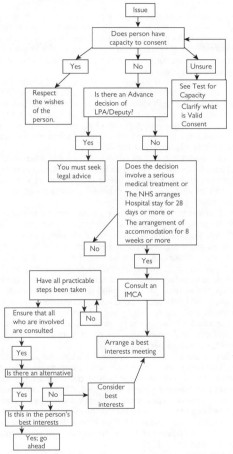

Fig. 8.1 Decision making pathway. Authors: Allyson Kent, Mike Hood (2007). This is an abbreviated version, a full colour version is available on request from allyson. kent@humber.nbs.uk

1 Department for Constitutional Affairs (2007). *Mental Capacity Act 2005 Code of Practice*, London

2 Adults with Incapacity Act (Scotland).

3 Department of Health, Social Services and Public Safety (2003). *Consent to Examination, Treatment and Care*. Department of Health, Social Services and Public Safety: Belfast.

Circles of support

"A circle is hard to describe; it's too simple" (Regina DeMarasse, Circles Network, 2005).[1]

A circle of support, sometimes called a circle of friends, is a group of people who meet on a regular basis with the ultimate aim of helping the focus person reach their dreams and aspirations in life. A circle might be created for a number of reasons—some people may be at risk of or experiencing social isolation, for others a circle may arise as a consequence of their person-centred plan.

The concept of circles of support was initiated in Canada, then spread through North America before arriving in the UK in the mid 1980s.[1] A circle of support is a markedly different idea to advocacy or befriending. An advocate or befriender may not naturally occur from the focus person's wider network, whereas one purpose of a circle is to 'draw together a group of people who are committed to helping someone they care about (or maybe love) to change his or her life.'[2]

Circles of support are not exclusively for people who have ID. They may be of benefit to any person who feels isolated, excluded or in need of support to realize or achieve a better life. For example, these include children or adults who are living in deprived circumstances, or those who have mental health problems.

Circles of support derive from truly person-centred principles. To this end the focus person is in charge, as they decide who can join the circle and which direction the energy of the circle is taken. Initially, a circle has a facilitator to get it started and to keep account of the action that is required to keep it working. Once formed, the circle meets regularly to assist the focus person to recognize their dreams and imagine their most desirable future. In order to help the dreams become reality, the members of the group 'realize their gifts and skills'. In addition, the circle helps to problem solve, and continues to build networks in order for the focus person to broaden their opportunities and achieve greater inclusion in their (chosen) community. Finally, a key ingredient is to have fun! It is expected that the facilitator withdraws once the circle is up and running, and fully operational for the focus person.

An important aim of a circle of support for a child or young person is to include at least one peer, often a peer who is non-disabled. Jay describes the merits of this to both the focus person and the non-disabled peers.[3] Jay recognizes that young people who have ID often miss out on the 'ordinariness' of growing up, and that advocacy is usually provided through adults. By involving non-disabled peers in the circle who have got to know the focus person, Jay professes that they have a different slant on life and 'are bound to have a closer and more accurate view of what young people want from life than an adult'.[3]

A circle may start small, even only 3 members. The members comprise family, friends, and community members, usually people who are not paid to be there. There may be a role for paid professionals, but the aim and focus of the circle must remain. As time goes on, the whole circle may not meet in its entirety each time. As the circle builds momentum, and gifts and strengths are identified, certain members may meet (always with the focus person) with respect to specific goals.

A circle of support is not the end result of a planning process, in fact once a circle has been formed further person-centred planning takes place. It is a planning style in itself, but it may also employ one or even a variety of planning tools, such as PATH or MAPS. Circles meetings usually take place monthly, more often in a period of crisis, and may last >2hrs. As an important aim of a circle is to have fun, celebrate, and enjoy being together, the meetings may take place in a whole variety of settings, such as the focus person's living room, in a pub, or in a café.

An expressed fear of a family carer might be that a circle is actually intended to replace or avoid paid support where it is needed. Circles Network (2007) insist that a circle of support is 'not a replacement for human services'.[4] Once a circle is formed, therefore, it must ensure that the focus person does not lose necessary paid support. One answer would be to ensure that a care/budget manager is involved where this fear is sensed, so plans can be made to develop or protect the focus person's paid support package. Also there might be concern that any efforts to befriend the focus person were tokenistic. However, the role of the facilitator is to ensure that everyone's gifts and skills are shared and used to work towards change.

1 Circles Network (2005). *Circles of Support*. Available at:
🖳 http://www.circlesnetwork.org.uk/circles_of_support.htm

2 Circles Network (2007). *Circles of Support: An Introduction to Person Centred Planning and the Values of Inclusion*. Circles Network: Rugby, UK.

3 Jay N (2007). Peer mentorship: Promoting advocacy and friendship between young people. *Learning Disability Today* **7**(3), 18–21.

4 Circles Network (2007). *Circles Network Impact Report*. Circles Network: Rugby, UK.

Making best interests decisions

The Mental Capacity Act (2005) provides the legal framework to ensure that anything done for, or on behalf of, a person who lacks capacity to consent is done in the best interests of the person concerned.[1] The decision maker is protected from liability if they ensure that the care/treatment is in the best interests of the person concerned (see Figure 8.2). Currently the legislation only covers England and Wales, and in Scotland, the Adults with Incapacity Act (2000) applies.[2] In Northern Ireland and Republic of Ireland, the separate guidance on *Consent to Examination, Treatment and Care* applies.[3]

Who is the decision maker?

The decision maker can be a number of different people, and is dependent on the decision in question i.e. for day-to-day actions, the decision maker would be the carer directly involved with the person. Where the decision involves medical or dental treatment, the decision maker would be the doctor or dentist responsible for carrying out the treatment or procedure. The Department of Health has produced a new consent form for best interests decision making for people who lack the capacity to consent. It is the responsibility of the decision maker always to ensure that the decision is in the best interests of the person concerned at that time.

What could I do to ensure that care and/or treatment is in the best interests of the person?

Support and encourage the person to take part, think about what the person would take into account if they were making the decision for themselves, try to find out the person's views by talking with others who know the person, review their past and present wishes and/or feelings, and do not make assumptions based on the person's age, appearance, condition, or behaviour. While there may be a number of possible outcomes, it is important that the decision maker and others involved are able to review the treatments in question to decide what is in the best interests of the person concerned at this time.

Best interests meetings

For major decisions with regards to healthcare, if the person is found to lack the capacity to consent, then a best interests meeting must be arranged and all relevant parties invited. These meetings may at times need to be arranged quickly, and it is therefore important to understand that only those people relevant to the specific decision in question need to be part of the best interests meeting. It is vitally important that an accurate record of events are made.

What if the decision involves serious medical treatment and/or a care home move?

An IMCA must be instructed, and invited to the best interests meeting if the person does not have any relatives or close friends.

What things must be taken into account when trying to work out what is in their best interests?

Locally best interests decision records will be available; these will provide guidance and evidence of how the decision was reached. If no agreement can be reached, legal advice should be sought within your own organization to seek Court of Protection ruling.

Best Interest Pathway

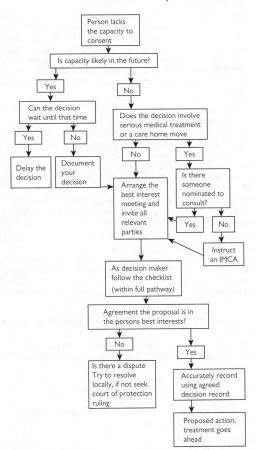

Fig. 8.2 Best interest pathway. Authors: Allyson Kent, Mike Hood (2007). This is an abbreviated version, a full colour version is available on request from allyson. kent@humber.nhs.uk

1 Department for Constitutional Affairs (2007), Mental Capacity Act (2005) Code of Practice, London, TSO.

2 Adults with Incapacity Act (2000).

3 Department of Health, Social Services and Public Safety (2003). *Consent to Examination, Treatment and Care*. Department of Health, Social Services and Public Safety: Belfast.

Vulnerability

The number of inquiries into ID services has highlighted the vulnerability of people with ID when receiving care and support from others. Increasingly the evidence is highlighting that people with ID are more susceptible to abuse than the general population. In recent years, abuse has been seen to occur within NHS services, independent sector provision, social care, and small community homes. A person's vulnerability can change over time, and may be dependant on a person's individual circumstances at any one time.[1]

What is abuse?

Abuse covers a wide range of actions, and could be:
- Financial e.g. theft, fraud, misuse of property, possessions, or benefits
- Physical e.g. hitting, inappropriate use of punishments, misuse of medications that make a person drowsy
- Sexual e.g. rape, sexual assault, sexual acts without consent
- Psychological e.g. threats of harm, restraint, intimidation, threats to restrict a persons liberty
- Neglect and acts of omission e.g. ignoring a person's medical or physical care needs, failing to provide health or social care, or withholding a person's medication or basic care needs.

It needs to be recognized that abuse is abuse and that all types of abuse are treated equally in the eyes of the law.

Neglect does not have to be a wilful act but can be a passive failure to respond to a person's needs. Each service should have local policy based on the protection of children and vulnerable adults, which reflects the national policies in this area (see 📖 Child protection, p.268, and 📖 Adult protection, p.270).

Why are some people with intellectual disabilities more vulnerable?

- Are more likely to be dependant on others for intimate care e.g. washing, bathing and toileting, which increases a person's vulnerability
- May have limited or poor communication skills
- Are more likely to have limited control over their lives
- May lack the opportunity to make choices
- Little understanding of the person's additional needs by others
- Are viewed negatively by some.

What can you do?

- Ensure that information is provided to people with ID in an accessible format
- Talk to people about their rights and how to keep themselves safe
- Always ensure the needs of the person are central to your thinking and your actions
- Think about what is in the best interests of the person (see 📖 Making best interests decisions, p.264)

- What do you think they (or their family or friends) would want for themselves?
- Put yourself in the 'shoes' of the person and imagine what it would be like receiving care and treatment that is being offered to the person
- Talk to your supervisor, line manager, or vulnerable adults protection services if you have concerns that a person is vulnerable.

The Mental Capacity Act (2005)—England and Wales[2]

This now provides the legal framework to protect vulnerable adults who lack capacity. Every person working within ID services must ensure that care and treatment complies with the 5 key principles of the Act at all times (see ☐ Consent to treatment, p.260, and ☐ Making best interests decisions, p.264).

Any person who has concerns with regards to suspicions of abuse should contact the relevant agency, e.g. the adult protection team within social services.

Under the Act there are two new criminal offences of ill-treatment and neglect. Ill-treatment and neglect are two separate sentences and anyone caring for a person who lacks capacity could be guilty of an offence if they ill-treat or wilfully neglect a person they are caring for and/or representing. People could receive a fine or imprisonment for up to 5yrs or both.

What does the NMC Code say?[3]

As a registered nurse you must protect and support the health of individuals, and act in such a way that justifies the trust and confidence the public holds in you. You are also accountable for your actions and omissions regardless of advice or directions from another professional.

What does this mean?

Do not keep your concerns to yourself. Remember this person may not be able to communicate, is dependant on others for assistance, and may not have anyone to look out for them.

Do something; becoming **aware** of an issue you have a **responsibility** and are **accountable** as a nurse to take action.

Further reading

Health Care Commission (2007). *A Life Like No Other*. Health Care Commission: London.

1 Davies R, Jenkins R (2004). Protecting people with learning disabilities from abuse; a key role for learning disability nursing, *Journal of Adult Protection*, **6**(2), 31–41.

2 Department for Constitutional Affairs, (2007), Mental Capacity Act (2005) Code of Practice, London, HMSO.

3 Nursing and Midwifery Council (2008). *The Code: Standards of Conduct, Performance and Ethics for Nurses and Midwives*. Nursing and Midwifery Council: London.

Child protection

Child protection is the process of ensuring the safety and welfare of children, protecting the child from physical, emotional, sexual abuse and/or neglect at all times.

Where are children at risk?

Children can experience abuse anywhere. This could be within their own home, at nursery, at school, or at after-school or out-of-school activities. Children with ID are particularly vulnerable, because of their difficulties in communication, their need for intimate care e.g. washing and toileting, and the provision of this care by a number of carers, which could be in schools or respite care facilities.

What are the different types of abuse?

It is important to remember that all types of abuse detailed below are abuse and are all equal under the law:

• Physical abuse includes hitting, slapping, shaking, burning, pinching, biting, throwing, or anything that causes physical injury, leaves a mark and/or causes significant physical pain.
• Emotional abuse can be difficult to identify, as there may not be any physical signs. It includes situations when shouting and anger goes too far, and when parents and/or others constantly criticize or threaten children so that their self-esteem and feelings of self-worth are damaged.
• Sexual abuse is any type of sexual contact that takes place between an adult and a person under 16yrs. Sexual abuse can also occur between a significantly older child and a younger child. This is called incest if it occurs between family members.
• Neglect occurs when a child or young person does not have enough food, clothing, love, medical care or supervision.

What should you do?

• Talk to a teacher, health visitor, community nurse, social worker or GP
• Talk to your clinical supervisor
• Talk to your local safeguarding/child protection team
• It is particularly important to ensure that events are recorded accurately, with dates and times to enable a clear record of events.

What will happen?

The local safeguarding/child protection team will decide if your concerns are serious enough for child protection procedures to be instigated.

If procedures are instigated:

• someone will contact the family and review if the child is safe to remain in their own home
• a child protection/safeguarding children case conference will be held.

If the team takes **no action** from your concerns, they may still intervene by offering the family extra support to ensure the risks of abuse and harm are minimized.

A Life Like No Other

This inquiry led by the Health Care Commission followed two formal investigations into NHS services that identified unacceptable and failing standards of care within services.[7] The audits undertaken by a number of people (each team consisted of 3 people, which included a family carer or a person with ID, a professional, and a member of the healthcare commission) only discovered a few services where the quality of care was good across all aspects of care.

The inquiry found a number of areas of concerns: there were 6 safeguarding concerns raised immediately within 5 organizations. A further 154 reports were written detailing a number of recommendations to each organization.

- Most services did not provide independent advocacy
- Inappropriate restrictions on a person's movements with the use of locked doors
- People had difficulties in accessing specialist healthcare services
- Procedures for the safeguarding of vulnerable adults was poor
- Lack of internal and external scrutiny within services.

What does the NMC code say?

As a registered nurse you must protect and support the health of individuals and act in such a way that justifies the trust and confidence the public holds of you.[8]

You are also accountable for your actions and omissions regardless of advice or directions from another professional.

New criminal offence

Under the Mental Capacity Act (2005),[4] in England and Wales there are two new criminal offences of ill-treatment and neglect. Ill-treatment and neglect are two separate sentences, and anyone caring for a person who lacks capacity could be guilty of an offence if they ill-treat or willfully neglect a person they are caring for and/or representing. People could receive a fine or imprisonment for up to 5yrs or both.

1 Department of Health (2000). *No Secrets*. Department of Health: London.

2 National Assembly for Wales (2000). *In Safe Hands*. National Assembly for Wales: Cardiff.

3 DHSSPS (2003). *Protection of Children and Vulnerable Adults in Northern Ireland*. DHSSPS: Belfast

4 Mental Capacity Act (2005). HMSO: London

5 Adults with Incapacity (Scotland) Act 2000.

6 Department of Health (2004). *Protection of Vulnerable Adults Scheme in England and Wales for Care Homes and Domiciliary Care Associations: A Practical Guide*. Department of Health: London.

7 Health Care Commission (2007). *A Life Like No Other*. Health Care Commission: London.

8 Nursing and Midwifery Council (2008). *The Code: Standards of Conduct, Performance and Ethics for Nurses and Midwives*. Nursing and Midwifery Council: London.

Care pathways

What is a care pathway?

A care pathway is an integrated, structured interdisciplinary care plan that outlines the care to be undertaken and the order that it should be delivered in. A care pathway is usually based on the best evidence, standards, or protocols available in relation to a particular clinical condition. A care pathway lays out a framework as to how care should be delivered appropriately, in the right order, and at the right time, and with the correct outcome for the individual. It must be remembered, however, that every nurse is required to consider how a care pathway relates to each individual in their care, and provide individualized care.

Different terms for care pathways

It has been identified that a number of terms are used interchangeably to describe a care pathway.[1] All the following terms have been used within the literature to describe care pathways:

- Clinical pathways
- Anticipated recovery pathways
- Multidisciplinary pathways of care
- Integrated care management
- Collaborative care pathways
- Care profiles
- Coordinated care pathways.

Implementing care pathways

The stages in developing and then implementing a care pathway are as follows:

- Appointment of a credible facilitator
- Identification of multidisciplinary team members
- Selection of topic
- Definition of problem or issue
- Review of evidence base, guidelines and protocols
- Audit of current practice
- Identification of users' views on current practice
- Consideration of local needs and constraints
- Development of the actual pathway documentation
  - Desired outcomes
  - Decision points
  - Procedures to follow
  - Outcomes and milestones to achieve
  - Detail of variance tracking
  - Detail of review
  - Detail of audit
  - Staff education
- Pilot of the pathway
- Review of pilot
- Amendment as required
- Implement pathway.

Variance tracking and analysis

Variance in a care pathway is the difference between the predicted outcome and the actual outcome. Thus if actual care varies from the care pathway this is recorded as a variance. It is apparent, therefore, that unexpected outcomes can be tracked. It is also apparent that if these unexpected occurrences happen in a number of cases, analysis can be undertaken, which may lead to new and improved pathways.

Benefits of care pathways

It is identified that care pathways:
- aid the use of local protocols and guidelines
- aid the incorporation of national policies, protocols and guidelines
- provide a framework for interdisciplinary working
- enable research based practice to underpin care
- promote team work
- enhance communication
- reduce the unnecessary variations in care
- ensure that people's care journeys are straightforward.

Barriers to developing care pathways

There are many barriers to developing pathways, including:
- Time
- Increase in meetings
- Education
- Evaluation
- True involvement.

It has also been suggested that the use of care pathways may overemphasize or medicalize the clinical condition at the expense of the individual.

Care pathways for people with intellectual disabilities

There are care pathways that are used within ID services, but there appears to be only a small amount of literature available. Care pathways that are detailed in the literature include:
- Crisis in challenging behaviour
- Oral healthcare
- Access to acute care
- Epilepsy
- Hearing impairment.

1 Powell H, Kwiatek E (2006). Integrated care pathways in intellectual disability nursing. In: Gates B (Ed). *Care Planning and Delivery in Intellectual Disability Nursing.* Blackwell Publishing: London.

Care programme approach

The care programme approach was introduced in 1991 to England, Wales and Scotland, and it is often described as the Government's cornerstone of mental health policy. It arose after a variety of inquiries concerning the follow-up care of people when discharged from psychiatric hospitals. This approach helps provide a framework for mental healthcare, and this could easily be translated into care of people with ID who may also have a mental health issue. Indeed, within forensic services, care is commonly coordinated and underpinned by this approach. It is a tool to prevent people from 'slipping through the net'; the process should enable people to be supported effectively in the community through an inpatient admission if necessary and discharge back into community.

Involvement of people with intellectual disabilities and their carers

The importance of involving users and carers has been stressed in successive guidance on the implementation of the care programme approach. Users should be involved in discussions about their proposed care programmes so that they can discuss different treatment possibilities, agree with the programme, and identify the outcomes. It is also important to involve relevant others in the development of the care programme. Carers often know a great deal about the user's life, interests, and abilities, as well as having personal experience of the person's mental health problems.[1] They may also provide much of the person's care.

Key components

The 4 key components or stages of the care programme approach are:[2]
- Systematic assessment of both health and social care needs
- Formation of care plan including identification of providers
- Appointment of key worker or care coordinator
- Regular review.

As well as involving the person and their carers, the development and implementation care programme should be an interdisciplinary activity.

Levels of the care programme approach

It should be noted that the person may move up and down the levels detailed below, as the mental healthcare needs change.

Standard care programme approach

This approach is suitable for people who require minimal social support, are relatively stable, and have low healthcare needs.

Enhanced care programme approach

This level is suitable for people who require medium/high levels of support and are less likely to remain stable. The person may also require further assessment, and it is likely that they will receive support from more than one professional, and the actual care plan will be more complex.

This level may also be required for people who have a severe mental health problem. They may also be unstable and volatile, and may pose a risk either to themselves or others. It is likely that the person requiring this level of support would also be unable to function socially. In this case the care plan will be detailed with arrangements for continual evaluation so that changes in the mental health status can be identified quickly. It is also imperative that the role of the differing professionals is identified within the plan in detail, and that the professionals communicate effectively.

Supervision register

This level of care programme is required for people who present a significant risk to themselves or others. The person is continually and actively followed up, and they may be placed on the supervision register.

Advantages of the care programme approach

The care programme approach:
- supports multidisciplinary working
- supports 'joined up' management
- encourages explicit roles
- enhances communication
- formalizes communication
- provides clarity for the person and their carers.

Disadvantages of the care programme approach

The care programme approach also has some disadvantages in that it may:
- increase bureaucracy
- increase stress for the person and their carer.

It may also lead to lack of control of confidential information, and it currently has no demonstrable evidence base.

1 Carpenter J, Sbarani S (2007). *Choice, Information and Dignity: Involving Users and Carers in Care Management in Mental Health*. The Policy Press: London.

2 Hepworth K, Wolverson M (2006). Care planning and delivery in forensic settings for people with intellectual disabilities. In Gates B (Ed). *Care Planning and Delivery in Intellectual Disability Nursing*. Blackwell Publishing: London.

Health action plans and health facilitation

The terms 'health action plan' (HAP) and 'health facilitation' (HF) origi-nated with the Department of Health White Paper *Valuing People*[1] (see 📖 Chapter 6, pp.139–212). These terms have since been endorsed with similar documents in Northern Ireland and are recognized good prac-tice elsewhere in the UK and Ireland.[2] This initiative was needed because there was growing evidence that people with ID had greater health needs than the general population, yet accessed health services less of-ten. Since 2005 all people with ID have been required to have a personal HAP. The responsibility for the HAP rests with an individual HF work-ing in partnership with the person with ID, primary healthcare providers, and GPs.

Helpful guidance regarding implementation can be found in *Action for Health—Health Action Plans and Health Facilitation*.[3] To address some of the challenges in implementing this initiative e.g. who should take the lead, in the UK a Primary Care Service Framework (2007) has been developed, which requires GPs to deliver a routine annual health check to their pa-tients who have ID (see 📖 Health checks, p.84).[4] Information that comes from these health checks can form the basis of the individual's HAP.

In practice, a HAP forms part of an individual's 'person-centred plan'. Essentially, it is an action plan initiated by the HF (in practice most likely in collaboration with others e.g. staff in a residential service). The HAP will normally include details about the individual's health under various domains:

- Oral health and dental care
- Fitness and mobility
- Continence
- Vision
- Hearing
- Nutrition
- Mental health needs
- Emotional, spiritual, and sexual needs
- Medication taken—side effects
- Screening tests results.

Following the health check, any interventions required can be put into action by the HF. For example, a dental appointment could be made for a man with ID who complains of a pain in his mouth, or for someone who had not seen a dentist in the last 12 months. It is important that all HAPs consider the person's lifestyle choice, culture, and values. Actions arising from the HAP should be agreed with the individual, and choices offered where practical (e.g. regarding treatment decisions). A copy of the HAP is held by the person with ID, so it should be written in an accessible format according to the person's need, in order that the individual can understand it. To ensure that health needs are closely monitored, it is recommended that a HAP is conducted at key points such as:

- Transition from education or young peoples' services
- Leaving home/moving into residential services

- Moving from one service provider to another
- Moving to an out of area placement
- If there has been a change in health status (e.g. following an illness)
- On retirement
- When planning transition for those living with older family carers.

Health facilitator

The role of the HF is to ensure that the actions arising from the HAP are followed up, and that the person gets the medical or other attention they need. Additionally the role may require liaison activities with GPs or other services, planning appointments for screening, or conducting further assessments. Exactly who undertakes this role varies from area to area, and depends on the nature of the service and the needs of the individuals. It may be a professional carer, or alternatively someone close to the person who is not paid to work with them (such as an advocate or friend). However any ID nurse with an interest in health needs should be well positioned to become a HF, with community ID nurses being particularly well placed for this activity.

More recently the Department of Health has endorsed the role of the 'strategic health facilitator'.[5] This is a broader role to be undertaken by a professional (e.g. an ID nurse). It concerns the need to overcome the barriers between primary and secondary healthcare and people with ID, and enable effective liaison with health staff in both these environments to improve the healthcare experience of people with ID. One way this may be achieved is through the proactive education of other professionals who have a responsibility for the care of people with ID (e.g. GPs). This role is considered critical to the effectiveness of local health and social care services for people with ID, as it aims to provide an interface between the strategic, operational, and the individual.

Further reading

Primary Care Service Frameworks - 🖥 www.primarycarecontracting.nhs.uk/204.php

1 Department of Health (2001). *Valuing People. A New Strategy for Learning Disability for 21st Century*. Department of Health: London.

2 Department of Health, Social Services and Public Safety (2005). *Equal Lives*. Department of Health, Social Services and Public Safety: Belfast.

3 Department of Health (2002). *Action for Health—Health Action Plans and Health Facilitation*. Department of Health: London.

4 NHS Primary Care Contracting (2007). *Primary Care Service Framework: Management of health for people with learning disability in primary care*. NHS PCC: London.

5 Department of Health (2007). *Health Action Planning and Health Facilitation for people with learning disabilities: Good Practice Guide*. Department of Health: London.

Care management, case management, continuing care

It is widely accepted that some individuals with an ID will have some element of a 'looked after life', and while not advocating that all individuals need professional intervention within their lives, it is necessary to acknowledge that lessons in support packages need to be learnt to ensure that individuals receive the care they need and deserve, 'Individuals should receive care, based on their unique need that is effective in its delivery and appropriate to their current situation'.[1] 'We have historically been more efficient in providing people for services that service for people.'[2]

While the notion of 'managing care' for individuals with ID is not new, the concept of specific 'care management' as we know it today, was first introduced in the 1989 Griffith Report. This became the template for the White Paper *Caring For People* in England,[3] with related documents elsewhere in the UK. One of the key objectives of the White Paper challenged services 'To make proper assessment of need and good care management the cornerstone of high quality care; packages of care should then be designed in line with individual needs and preferences.'[3]

From this it can be argued that a clear focus and definition of care management is to ensure that a specific, individualized package of resources is in place to ensure that the person's needs and wishes are met; it is not about fitting a person's service into a budget.

The contribution of care management has been defined as 'a dedicated person (or team) who organizes, coordinates and sustains a network of formal and informal supports and activities designed to optimize the functioning and well-being of people with multiple needs.'[4]

Essentially care management is a collaborative process—one which appropriately assesses, ethically plans, effectively implements, coordinates, and evaluates the holistic package of health and social care services required to meet an individual's needs.

As with all systems of care, there are inherent difficulties, e.g. care managers are often placed in invidious positions, particularly in relation to rationing and resource allocation/management. They frequently find themselves aligned to both the purchaser (i.e. the person in receipt of care) and the provider, entering into deliberations of 'best practice'.

Duffy describes how 'The role of the care manager is a particularly complex role. There is no final model of best practice; instead there are different interpretations".[5] What is widely accepted is that both nurses and social workers fulfill the criteria for care managers, and it is the employing authority that determines the focus of services provided. Within the joint Health and Social Care structures within Northern Ireland, many nurses have held active care manager posts.

It is important to acknowledge within this section long-term conditions and national service frameworks (NSF), as these both impact on a model of case management, and lead into continuing care. It is interesting to note that there is no specific NSF in England, Wales, or Scotland dedicated to people with ID (although one is being developed in Northern Ireland), but professionals often need reminding that all NSF apply to all citizens.

Case management

Not all people with ID have a 'labelled' long-term condition or need intensive case management; however this approach, whose origin is linked within healthcare, needs some exploration. It is recognized that for individuals who live with a long-term condition, their care becomes disproportionately complex and presents management problems for practitioners and the individual with the condition. Case management as defined by the Department of Health sets out to address this complexity: 'Case management is also the first step to creating an effective delivery system and implementing the wider NHS and Social Care Long Term Conditions Model'.[6]

Continuing care is not solely about health needs, and there needs to be an acknowledgment that effective social care is a facet of holistic healthcare and vice versa. It is well documented that people with ID have higher levels of unmet healthcare need, and therefore would benefit from such an approach, as outlined in continuing care strategies. There is no universally accepted definition—particularly where there has been concern that the term 'case' is derogatory—but there is some consensus about the main components of case management.[7] These are: screening or case finding, assessment, care planning and implementation, monitoring, reassessment, or review. Challis describes case management itself as: 'a specific job, a task within an existing job role within a single agency, a job or task within a joint heath and social work structure, an organizational process'.[8]

Further reading

Valuing People Support Team health resource pages:

🖳 http://valuingpeople.gov.uk/dynamic/valuingpeople118.jsp

1 Laverty H, Reet M (2001). *Planning Care for Children in Respite Settings: Hello! This is Me.* Jessica Kingsley: London.

2 O'Brian J, Lovett H (1992). Finding a Way Toward Everyday Lives. Pennsylvania Office of Mental Retardation: Pennsylvania, USA. 🖳 http://thechp.syr.edu/everyday.pdf

3 Department of Health (1989). *Caring For People.* Department of Health: London.

4 Moxley DP (1989). *The practice of case management.* Sage: Newbury Park, CA.

5 Duffy S (2002). *Care management and PCP.* Department of Health: London.

6 Department of Health (2007). *Case management.* Department of Health: London.

7 Hudson B (1993). *The Busy Person's Guide to Care Management.* Joint Unit for Social Services Research: Sheffield.

8 Challis D (1999). Assessment and Care Management: Developments Since the Community Care Reforms. In: Henwood M & Wistow G (eds.). *With Respect to Old Age*, pp.69–86. Research Volume 3, Cm 4192-II/3. The Stationery Office: London.

Service brokerage, direct payments, and self-directed support

Terms such as cash for care schemes, self-directed support, direct payments, consumer-directed support, cash and counselling, and personal budgets, are becoming more familiar to people with ID and their families in many countries of the developed world. Many people will be familiar with direct payments, whereby a person who is eligible for social care services can choose to spend their money themselves on meeting their needs. This idea is being taken further. One major demonstration project in England has been *In Control*,[1] a national organization that is helping local authorities to further transform traditional social care services to systems of self-directed support. This transformation is sometimes referred to as personalization; as outlined in the government documents *Our Health, Our Care, Our Say*[2] and *Putting People First*.[3] It shares many aims of the NHS about being more responsive, and enhancing choice and control. In the future, social workers are going to be spending less time on assessment and more on support, brokerage, and advocacy. Everyone eligible for publicly funded adult social care support will be awarded a personal budget, and person-centred planning approaches will put this in motion.

The essence of such schemes is that people with disability who are entitled to social care support know what is available to spend on meeting their needs, and that they and the people close to them have as much control as they want on how this money is spent. Evidence from the much studied direct payments schemes suggests that this way of working leads to greater satisfaction among people using social care services, to greater continuity of care, to fewer unmet needs, and to more cost effective use of public money (see the Care Services Improvement Partnership links).[4,5,6] People may wish to get support in different ways; one common way is to employ a personal assistant. Some people make arrangements themselves, others use the services of a support agency or support broker (often from the voluntary sector) to help with paperwork and other administrative matters, such as recruitment and checks on people's suitability.

Direct payments have been available in the UK for many years. Local authorities now have a duty to make them available. The legislation and regulations change frequently, but the websites provide updates and direct readers to further guidance and helpful sources of information.[4,5,6]

Nurses working with people with ID throughout the UK should ensure that they:
- are familiar with what is happening at local level so that they are able to help service users make the most of such new systems
- are confident in explaining the terms involved and know where are the local support agencies, what they do, and how to contact them
- keep up to date with the emerging evidence of what works and for whom
- know where people who are working as personal assistants can access training, e.g. around moving and handling, or they know the network that will have this information

- feel confident that they can raise concerns about possible mistreatment or neglect with local adult safeguarding services (contact the local council)
- help with communication needs if required
- keep alert to possible changes in such schemes, e.g. whether they include money to buy equipment, or to provide support to a person to enter employment
- are sensitive to possible difficulties and help people get timely or increased support
- they encourage people to think about whether their support plans are working well and they help people ask for a review if needs change or circumstances alter
- offer assistance or explanation, if required, with elements of the assessment that involve self-completion and self-assessment
- are aware of the circumstances in which support plans may be at risk of additional stress, e.g. at times of illness, when a condition deteriorates, or there are new elements of challenging behaviour
- are aware of the nature and extent of a person's support plan and work with it and the wider circle of support.

1 in Control - www.in-control.org.uk [accessed March 2009]

2 Department of Health (2006). *Our Health, Our Care, Our Say*. Department of Health: London.

3 Department of Health (2007). *Putting People First: A Shared Vision and Commitment to the Transformation of Adult Social Care*. Department of Health: London.

4 Directgov. *Direct Payments - arranging your own care and services.* www.direct.gov.uk/en/DisabledPeople/FinancialSupport/DG_10016128 [accessed March 2009]

5 Carers Scotland www.carerscotland.org/Policyandpractice/Research [accessed March 2009]

6 Citizens Advice Bureau. www.adviceguide.org.uk/nireland/family_parent/family_family_northern_ireland/community_care.htm#direct_payments [accessed April 2009]

Interdisciplinary teamworking

The need for interdisciplinary teamwork

Interdisciplinary teamworking is necessary in order to respond to the fact that no one profession has all the knowledge, skills and resources necessary to meet the increasingly complex and varied needs of all people with ID. Effective interdisciplinary teamwork can provide a way for services to deliver coordinated services that can be jointly planned and funded, which bring together people from a range of services, and prevent fragmentation of care packages within services that are increasingly becoming 'specialist', with at times quite exclusive referral criteria. Without effective interdisciplinary team working, there is a real possibility that people with ID and their families will encounter fragmented, uncoordinated, and at times competing services, providing conflicting advice and support.

Defining interdisciplinary teamwork

To move from being a group of people to become a team, it is necessary for the people involved to agree to work together, hold shared values, and all work collaboratively to achieve agreed goals and objectives. Interdisciplinary teamwork also requires team members to recognize their interdependence on each other if the objectives of the team are to be achieved. They need to work flexibly, challenging traditional divisions and stereotypes, and allocating work on the basis of the ability of people to effectively undertake it, rather than only on the basis of previous practices or professional titles. Together the members of an effective interdisciplinary team should be able to achieve more for people within ID than each of them working individually, put another way 'the whole should be greater than the sum of its parts'.

The requirement for nurses to work as effective interdisciplinary team members

All nurses are required to work as effective team members, it is not an optional extra for any nurse. Within the UK, the Nursing and Midwifery Council require all nurses to 'work with others to protect and promote the health and well-being of those in your care, their families and carers, and the wider community' and in doing so nurses must:[1]

• share information with colleagues
• keep colleagues informed when you are sharing the care of others
• work with colleagues to monitor the quality of your work and maintain the safety of those in your care
• facilitate students and others to develop their competence
• work effectively as part of a team
• work cooperatively within teams and respect the skills, expertise, and contributions of your colleagues
• be willing to share your skills and experience for the benefit of your colleagues
• consult and take advice from colleagues when appropriate
• treat your colleagues fairly and without discrimination
• make a referral to another practitioner when it is in the best interests of someone in your care.

Furthermore, when delegating any task to another person nurses must:
- establish that anyone they delegate to is able to carry out your instructions
- confirm that the outcome of any delegated task meets required standards
- make sure that everyone they are responsible for is supervised and supported.

However, nurses must also remember that despite the requirement to work collaboratively, the NMC also states that 'As a professional, you are personally accountable for actions and omissions in your practice and must always be able to justify your decisions'.[1] Therefore, nurses should always communicate their professional views effectively during interactions with other team members, and make it known to them and record in writing if they do not agree with any decisions proposed or taken within the team. If they have continuing concerns about a team decision they should seek advice from their professional supervisor, and if necessary directly from their registering body such as NMC or An Bord Altranais.

Supporting effective teamwork

There are a wide range of possible team structures and memberships; it is important, therefore, that decisions about team structures in ID services should be selected to match locally identified client needs. Effective teamwork does not just happen, it requires time and support to develop, with an investment of time and personal, as well as organizational, commitment. Teams work best when:
- Team development is facilitated
- People in the team want to be 'team members'
- The work of the team members is made positive and reinforcing[2]
- The value of 'conflict' is acknowledged (rather than suppressed or ignored), and appropriately channelled.

1 Nursing and Midwifery Council (2008). *The Code: Standards of Conduct, Performance and Ethics for Nurses and Midwives.* Nursing and Midwifery Council: London.

2 West M (2004). *Effective Teamwork: Practical Lessons From Organisational Research.* Blackwell Scientific Publications: London.

Interagency working

This section should be read in conjunction with 📖 Interdisciplinary team-working, p.282, as the key points about the need for effective communication, the professional requirements on nurses to work with other people, and the personal accountability of nurses made within that section also have relevance to interagency working.

Defining interagency working

Interagency working refers to people working collaboratively who are employed by or working in voluntary capacity for a number of different agencies that have different organization arrangements and separate management structures. Interagency working may occur at a number of different levels, ranging from formal structures such as those with transition planning for teenagers with ID, or those required for the management of people released from prison, or with forensic histories in which the remit of the group is clearly defined, as is the purpose of the meeting, which is formally chaired, with a record kept.

More often interagency working is in the form of a network based approach, in which people from a number of agencies are not within a formal team setting but working collaboratively, e.g. when people belonging to a number of other formal teams come together under the arrangements for developing a person-centred plan, planning leisure activities within a locality that could be made accessible to people with ID, or managing the support of a person with ID to access primary or secondary healthcare services. At times, interagency working can focus on wider strategic decisions related to policy making, and setting agreed priorities across organizations e.g. between health services, social services, housing, police and criminal justice services, focusing on a particular initiative such as support for people with ID at risk of crime.

Potential challenges in interagency working

When it works effectively, people with ID could potentially receive a flexible yet coordinated service in which people are clear about their roles, the interface between these, and the lines of communication. However, interagency working is not without challenges, and the difficulties with making it work effectively have been highlighted in inquiry documents, which sadly bear witness to the fact that when it goes wrong it can have catastrophic consequences, often for people most in need of protection.[1,2]

In particular, difficulties can arise when appropriate governance arrangements are not in place, the differing operational cultures (the tacit knowledge of how things are done in the team, 'practice wisdom', the unwritten rules and procedures) of agencies lead to events being viewed differently, e.g. a difference in opinion about the right of an individual to make their own decisions, and a concern over potential risk of exploitation or child protection issues being underestimated.

There is a risk that on other occasions the potential for interagency working is restricted due to priorities and/or budgets of separate agencies involved become competing, managers wishing to maintain autonomy, gain control or retain perceived hierarchical position, or are reluctant to share information that may show their organization in a poor light and wish to 'save face'.

In particular the need for effective sharing of information and a clear audit trail on how this was shared has been highlighted in several major inquires that investigated failures in interagency working.

Towards effective interagency working

Effective interagency working requires:
- The need for senior managers in each agency to be supportive of collaborative working between agencies
- The active involvement of people with the necessary knowledge and autonomy to make the necessary decisions, rather than people who will always have to refer back to their managers for further discussion (although this may happen from time to time in major decisions)
- A willingness to seek new solutions and ways forward for people with ID and their families, as this is the primary purpose for entering into interagency working
- Clear information on what each agency is prepared to bring to the joint venture in relation to time, people, budgets, and other resources
- Agreed procedures for managerial and professional supervision (if appropriate) of all staff involved within their respective agencies, which also consider their role in interagency working
- Clear procedures for highlighting concerns and resolving any differences of opinions or disagreements around decisions made, conflicts of interest, potentially including 'whistle blowing arrangements'
- A regular review of the arrangements for interagency working by the people involved and their respective managers.

Further reading

Nursing and Midwifery Council (2008). *The Code: Standards of Conduct, Performance and Ethics for Nurses and Midwives*. Nursing and Midwifery Council: London.

1 Department of Health (2003). *The Victoria Climbie Inquiry*. HMSO: London.

2 Department of Health (2004). *Harold Shipman's Clinical Practice 1974–1998: A Clinical Audit Commissioned by the Chief Medical Officer*. HMSO: London.

Commissioning

The *Commissioning Framework for Health and Well-being* aims to shift the focus of commissioning away from volume and price towards quality and outcomes.[1] So instead of commissioning a number of respite care beds, e.g. with an agreed contract with one provider of this service, local commissioners are thinking more about what will help to meet people's needs and wishes more individually. This might be for a holiday for one person, rather than respite, or it might be for a support worker to help another person go to a football match. In addition to this meaning of commissioning as tailor-made care or support, there is a wider effort to broaden the focus from health to citizenship; looking further than physical health problems to promote well-being, which includes social care, work, housing, and all the other elements that build a sustainable community. In the UK, local councils have often taken the lead in this, though in partnership with other public sector agencies.

World Class Commissioning is defined as the process of shifting away from traditional models of commissioning and creating world class clinical services and a world class NHS.[2] Drawing upon negotiating, contracting, financial, and performance management skills, world class commissioners are expected to shape local services and seek improvement in quality, safety, and choice. Commissioners are required to take an evidence-based approach, but as well as needing advanced knowledge management, analytical, and forecasting skills, they should be able to listen to and communicate with the local communities.

Joint commissioning between health and social care is particularly important for people with ID. Shared outcomes need to be agreed. The Local Government and Public Involvement Health Act 2007 places a statutory duty on upper tier local authorities and PCTs to produce a Joint Strategic Needs Assessment (JSNA). JSNA is a process to identify current and future health well-being needs in light of existing services, and to inform service planning, taking into account evidence of effectiveness. The need for careful commissioning was highlighted by recent reports of shortcoming in ID services.[3] These reports highlighted that significant problems that currently exist in commissioning of ID services are mainly due to a lack of awareness and understanding of the appropriate commissioning framework for people with ID, along with the setting of quality monitoring standards.

Nurses working with people with ID and their supporters should ensure that:

- they are familiar with local commissioning plans
- they are aware of and contribute to cross authority and regional commissioning plans
- people with ID and their supporters have information about local commissioning strategies, and that there are ways for people to influence these at all levels
- there are fair and transparent commissioning processes, and that providers of services have regular opportunities to share information with commissioners, e.g. at providers' forums
- commissioners have every opportunity to talk to people receiving services and to frontline workers.

In Scotland, the work of the Joint Improvement Team provides relevant material about commissioning and ID.[4] The All Wales Expert Advisory Group for Learning Disability Services offers a national forum for the development of evidence-based best practice. A web-based 'toolkit' for use by local health boards in carrying out needs assessments is available from the National Public Health Service for Wales.[5]

Further reading

The Valuing People Support Team funded by the Department of Health provides practical support and advice to the NHS, local government and independent sector on the delivery of the *Valuing People* policy including:

- A range of good practice support materials on the website
  ▣ www.valuingpeople.gov.uk
- A range of learning networks to support people leading change. These are regionally based.

DRC Formal Investigation Report: *Equal Treatment—Closing the Gap* and *Equal Treatment—One Year On* ▣ www.equalityhumanrights.com

Mencap Reports—*Treat Me Right!* and *Death by Indifference*
▣ www.mencap.org.uk

Primary Care Service Framework for Learning Disabilities
▣ www.primarycarecontracting.nhs.uk/204.php

UK Health and Learning Disability Network ▣ www.fpld.org.uk

1 Department of Health (2007). *Commissioning Framework for Health and Well-being*. Department of Health: London.

2 Department of Health (2007). *World Class Commissioning*. Department of Health: London.

3 Healthcare Commission and Commission for Social Care Inspection (2006). *Joint Investigation Into the Provision of Services for People with Learning Disabilities at Cornwall Partnership NHS Trust*. Healthcare Commission: London.

4 Scottish Joint Improvement Team— ▣ jit@scotland.gsi.gov.uk

5 National Public Health Service for Wales. *Learning Disability Toolkit for Local Health Boards*. http://www.wales.nhs.uk/sites3/page.cfm?orgID=719&pid=22753 [accessed April 2009]

Life planning

The life planning tools described in this chapter are person-centred in approach. Although the origins of life planning can be traced back at least two centuries in the UK and further internationally, *Valuing People* made it policy in the UK.[1]

ELP was developed by Michael Smull and Susan Burke Harrison originally to aid the planning process for people with ID who were moving out of long-stay hospitals. ELP is a very detailed planning tool that helps people to find out what is important to the person and what support they need to get a good quality of life. Helpfully, it also identifies what is working well and what is not working well for the focus person. Unlike other planning tools, it does not make provision for the individual's desired future, dreams, or aspirations, although a section could be added. ELP is an excellent tool for getting to know someone, and developing a service or team around them, especially when they do not use words to communicate. An ELP forms a useful support plan for an individual, but as with all planning tools it must be kept a live document, e.g. an individual's likes, dislikes, contacts, and routines will change over time, and their ELP must reflect this.

PATH was developed by Pearpoint, Forest and O'Brien, and it has the benefit of being suitable as a planning tool for both individuals and organizations. It is strongly focused, and starts by setting out the person's dream, then builds momentum, wit h timescales and action plans towards it. The initial planning meeting can be held in 1–2hrs, making the process 'short and sharp'. However, this might still be a challenging length of time for the focus person, and perhaps for some of the participants. The success of the PATH is heavily dependent on the commitment of the people who helped to bring it together, as it starts with the focus person's dream then works backwards from this, highlighting how and when each person is involved in the process. It requires skilful facilitation and energy from all involved. A PATH does not result in a daily support plan for the focus person, as it specifically addresses their dreams, aspirations and desires for a better future. PATHs are also useful tools to use with staff, staff teams, and even for business planning.

PFP or life building was developed by Mount and O'Brien, and enables a committed group of people to look at the focus person's life now, and what they would like in the future. It is geared at getting to learn more about the person's life (whereas PATH assumes this knowledge). The tool itself is designed to build on what is working well now and help the person move towards a desirable future. It does not create the support detail, which an ELP does.

MAPS is a planning tool developed by Snow, Pearpoint and Forest (with support from others). Originally it was used to help children with disabilities integrate into mainstream schools. It works on the basis that there are important lessons to be learned from looking at someone's past. It asks a series of questions about the person, their gifts and strengths, but also allows time to explore their fears and 'nightmares'. This is a very useful tool when planning very closely with families, as the tool is based on action plans that move away from the nightmare and towards the dream.

It is pictorial in design, which can make it a very accessible tool for people who do not read or who do not use words to communicate. It is less focused than a PATH, and less detailed than an ELP.[2] It requires careful and sensitive facilitation.

The largest scale and most comprehensive review of person-centred planning found that the most significant benefits for people who have ID were improved community involvement, contact with friends and family, and increased choice.[3] This report goes on to explain that the key determinants of success are committed facilitators, the personal involvement of the service user, and a person-centred, supportive environment being in place at the time of planning.

Circles Network warn against creating 'false hope' when initiating person-centred planning.[4] This does not mean that one should not elicit people's dreams and aspirations. However, when dreams become goals, reality must be sensed and facilitators must be open and honest about the seemingly difficult or impossible. The study by Robertson et al. claims that by clarifying the role of care managers and specialist practitioners in the policy and practice of life planning, access will be more equitable for people who have ID.[3]

As previously stated, life planning is not about a specific set of planning tools and their application in practice. Good quality and person-centred life planning is about selecting planning tools appropriately, and in some situations combining tools. It is important to understand that life planning is a continuous process, and should be reviewed and updated. This is emphasized by Heslop et al. describing it as a process not a single activity.[5]

1 Department of Health (2001) *Valuing People: A New Strategy for Learning Disability for the 21st Century*. HMSO: London. Available at: 🖳 www.dh.gov.uk/en/Publicationsandstatistics/Publications/PublicationsPolicyAndGuidance/DH_4009681 [accessed April 2009]

2 Sanderson H (2000). *Person centred planning - key features and approaches*. Joseph Rowntree Foundation: York. Available at 🖳 http://www.paradigm-uk.org/pdf/Articles/helensandersonpaper.pdf

3 Robertson J, Emerson E (2005). *The Impact of Person Centred Planning*. Institute for Health Research: Lancaster University, UK.

4 Circles Network (2007). *Impact Report*. Circles Network: Rugby, UK.

5 Heslop P, Mallett R, Simms K, Ward L (2002). *Bridging the Divide at Transition*. BILD: Worcester, UK.

Client held records

These are documents that are held by the person with an ID, and aim to articulate the individual and important aspects of a person's life in a way that is understood by the person, and informative and helpful to others involved in the person's care, e.g. the dentist, the doctor, or staff working within the acute hospital setting.

Types of client held records

There are a number of different client held records that you may find within your part of the country. Fundamentally they are documents that help the person with an ID and/or their carers to 'communicate with others' across the range of services that a person may come into contact with, e.g. staff working within the person's home, within assessment and treatment services, or within mainstream services. There is no set format, and people may have different sizes and designs dependant on the individual needs of the person. Some people use photographs or symbols to articulate their needs, while others may use a tape or video recording (CD/DVD).

Health Action Plans

Valuing People said that every person with a learning disability should have a HAP by June 2005.[1] People with ID have greater unmet healthcare needs than the general population, and the HAP can help the person to articulate simply their individual health needs. While *Valuing People* has offered guidance, there is no right or wrong way; nurses should be led individually by the person and what it is that they want.

There are important times when a HAP is helpful:[1]
- When a child is getting ready to leave school
- When a person is moving home
- When a person is going into hospital
- When a person is growing older and their needs are changing.

Person-centred plans

A PCP is a way of building a shared understanding of a person's life, their hopes and dreams, reflecting what the person wants in their life and their aspirations, it is not the wants of others, carers, or professionals. A PCP should challenge all to think about what they and/or society needs to do differently to meet this person's needs.[2]

Patient passport

A patient passport is a document that is used to support access into primary and secondary health services, seeking to reduce a person's vulnerability.[3] The passport provides details as to how the person normally presents e.g. 'I need help with eating and drinking'. This will help to reduce diagnostic overshadowing, when people think how the person presents is because of their ID not their illness. The passport makes a connection with those who know the person best i.e. parents/carers/community nurse/key worker, with those who know the person less, i.e. acute and/or primary care staff.

Communication passports

Communication passports is a tool that uses pictures and symbols to help a person communicate their needs to another person about their daily life and/or wants and desires.

What do the documents do?

- Empower people with ID—helps the person to articulate their own healthcare needs and understand their needs, what will be done, who is helping them, and when this will be happening. This ensures that professionals and carers work together with the person
- Improves communication—helping others to understand the important aspects of a person's life, or make contact with someone who knows them well, reducing the person's vulnerability while receiving help from primary and secondary care services
- Helps services to work together.

Challenges

- Well used by some people and services but not all
- The differences between the range of documents used make it difficult for people in primary and secondary services to use and understand
- Not everyone understands how to use them, which is frustrating for people and/or their carers, as they can take hours to do
- Duplication with other records kept within health services
- There are currently no links to the national computerized system available within the NHS.

Further reading

📖 www.vpst.org.uk—Review the many documents held within the *Valuing People* website on health.

1 Department of Health (2001). *Valuing People: a New Strategy for Learning Disability in the 21st Century*. Cmnd 5086. HMSO: London.

2 Helen Sanderson Associates 📖 www.helensandersonassociates.co.uk [accessed April 2009]

3 Kent A (2007). The patient passport: improving the patient journey through the acute hospital setting. *Community Connecting* **11**, 18–21.

Therapeutic interventions

Inclusive communication

What is it?

As discussed in 📖 Chapter 3, inclusive communication (sometimes called 'total communication') is achieved when we effectively provide information to others and demonstrate active listening to what it is they are telling us, *through whatever means they may use to do so.* Inclusive communication incorporates augmentative and alternative communication and is more likely to be effective because it starts from the premise that everyone communicates, and seeks to support people with communication difficulties both in understanding us and in telling us things. As such, it is fundamental to the delivery of person-centred services, and should form the foundation of all professional relationships with people with ID.

How do we do it?

Promoting understanding

- Be careful not to make assumptions about a person's level of verbal understanding or about their ability to hear what you say
- Consider how you are speaking, which words you are using and how much information you are presenting to the person at once
- Simplify your language (short sentences, easy words)
- Aim to use words the person is likely to know
- Present information in bite-sized chunks
- Repeat and rephrase as necessary
- Augment your speech with gestures, signs, written words, symbols, drawings, photographs, gestures, facial expressions, actions/mimes, vocalizations and objects.

Exactly how this is done in each interaction will depend on the assessed need of individuals we are communicating with. Nevertheless, it is worth considering what we could do unaided (just through our non-verbal signals and modification of the language we use) and also stockpiling a set of photographs, signs or other resources that are likely to be useful time and time again. Some AAC resources are suggested in 📖 Principles in using augmentative and alternative communication (AAC), p.66. A speech and language therapist may be able to advise you on how to use these both in a general sense, and with any particular individual. Furthermore there are various published materials available, for example:

- The British Institute for Learning Disabilities have a range of booklets on health topics that contain simple writing, backed up by clear line drawings[1]
- The *Hospital Communication Book*, which contains sound advice and photosymbols,[2] is useful for planned hospital visits and could be used in a variety of other healthcare settings. It is available to download for free[3]
- Use the NHS Photo Library when designing accessible information.[4]

Promoting expression

We must also recognize that people with ID may need support to use these same types of augmentative means of communication (or even alternative means) when interacting with us, especially where they have no speech, or where their speech is limited or not always easy to understand. People with expressive communication difficulties may carry their own AAC systems with them, but may require us to initiate their use. Similarly, people who know signs are unlikely to use these with us unless we also back up our speech with signs. It is a good idea to learn at least a basic vocabulary (e.g. yes, no, pain, nurse, doctor, medicine, injection, ill, happy, sad) and to practise using them, otherwise you will forget!

Inclusive means everyone!

Sometimes it is assumed that people with profound and multiple ID are not able to tell us anything. They may not have developed language but will use non-verbal means (e.g. vocalizations, laughing, crying, looking, posture, position, actions, or objects) to express themselves. Even though these signals may not be intended to deliberately signal a message, people who know them well (and/or who take the trouble to actively listen) will often be able to interpret the meaning. A good method is to ask family or key support staff how the person indicates 'like' and 'dislike'. Gathering examples of these allows us to draw out themes that can then be used to measure responses by that person to any new situation, thus ensuring we take their reactions (i.e. opinions) into account regarding what happens to them.

Communication strategies

ID services (and professionals) should aim to:
- have a communication strategy in place whereby various communication methods are used meaningfully across a range of services
- ensure that each person with communication difficulties has clearly presented, individualized communication advice (e.g. a communication profile) as well as their own communication passport and access to any appropriate AAC system or aid
- develop a resource base of AAC materials
- ensure that any information provided to people with ID is more accessible (i.e. with photos, drawings or symbols)
- have a systematic approach to communication training, linked into staff supervision and continuing professional development.

1 British Institute of Learning Disabilities - ▣ http://www.bild.org.uk/03books_health.htm

2 Photosymbols - ▣ http://www.photosymbols.com

3 Valuing People. *The Hospital Communication Book*. Department of Health: London. ▣ http://valuingpeople.gov.uk/dynamic/valuingpeople145.jsp

4 NHS Photo Library - ▣ http://www.photolibrary.nhs.uk/

Advocacy

Advocacy is associated with four types of representation—by self, by an unpaid person (such as a friend, relative or citizen advocate), by a paid person (perhaps a community nurse or social worker), or by an organization such as People First or Mencap. Gates has provided a topology of the various forms of advocacy,[1] however it should be remembered that the various types of advocacy are not mutually exclusive.

Self-advocacy

Self-advocacy is practised by many of us as individuals, but groups can provide a good setting for developing self-advocacy skills, particularly for people who are at risk of being devalued in society. Self-advocacy has great potential to enhance the lives of people with ID as they become more aware of rights, express needs and concerns, and assert interests. Self-advocacy has been described as the ultimate goal of all other forms of advocacy.[2] Definitions of self-advocacy often include 'speaking up for yourself', but making decisions, taking action, and changing things are significant components that self-advocacy groups have identified. According to Crawley, self-advocacy is 'the act of making choices and decisions and bringing about desired change for oneself.[3] Any activity that involves self-determination can be called self-advocacy. Self-advocacy is inclusive—all can be involved. 'Everyone can take part in self-advocacy at some level regardless of the severity of their disabilities'.[3] Self-advocacy involves the following skills:[4]

- Being able to express thoughts and feelings with assertiveness if necessary
- Being able to make choices and decisions
- Having clear knowledge of rights, and being able to make changes.

Other important components include: being independent, taking responsibility for yourself, getting things going yourself, being concerned for other people. Self-advocacy permeates and influences the person's whole life.

Citizen advocacy

Citizen advocacy refers to the supportive partnership that results when a volunteer develops a relationship with a person who is vulnerable to being disadvantaged through illness, age, or disability. It is important that advocates are 'valued people' (i.e. not themselves disadvantaged). Advocates form a close personal relationship with their partners, helping them to make choices and decisions. They work independently of services to uphold the rights of their partners as citizens. Citizen advocacy refers to the persuasive and supportive activities of trained, selected volunteers and coordinating staff working on behalf of those who are disabled/ disadvantaged and not in a good position to exercise or defend their rights as citizens. Citizen advocates are persons who are independent of those providing direct services to people with disabilities. Working on a one-to-one basis, they attempt to foster respect for the rights and dignity of those they represent. This may involve helping to express the individual's needs and wishes, helping them to access services, and providing practical and emotional support. The benefits of a partnership with a citizen advocate fall into two broad categories according to the nature of the needs met—expressive (human, emotional, and social needs) and instrumental (material needs).

Peer advocacy

Peer advocacy is individual support provided by someone who is also a member of a section of society that is in danger of being devalued or stigmatized. Thus, a person with ID could be assisted to articulate their needs and wishes by a peer who also has ID. The peer advocate is likely to have more insight into the experience of their partner than a non-disabled advocate would. A key difference between peer and citizen advocacy is that peer advocates are not 'valued persons' but people who are 'survivors of the system'.[5]

Professional advocacy

Professional advocacy has an important role to play in supporting the empowerment of clients.[6] This might involve introduction to a self-advocacy group or to an independent advocacy service. While the UK's professional body endorses nurses taking on an advocacy role,[7] it has been stressed that ID nurses should only advocate on a client's behalf after 'careful consideration of the issues involved'.[8]

Collective advocacy

Collective advocacy is about user representation. There is an important nuance here between advocacy and user representation. Self-advocates represent their own interests; citizen advocates uphold the rights of their partners. User oganizations cannot represent each individual's views but they can promote the cause of minority groups, including people with an ID, by raising public awareness and lobbying policy makers on their behalf. Key organizations that help to further the cause of people with ID include: Mencap, People First, BILD, Values into Action, and SCOPE.

1 Gates B (1994). *Advocacy: A Nurses' Guide*. Scutari Press: Middlesex.

2 Atkinson D (1999). *Advocacy: A Review*. Pavilion/Joseph Rowntree Foundation: Brighton.

3 Crawley B (1988). *The Growing Voice: A Survey of Self-Advocacy Groups in Adult Training Centres and Hospitals*. CMH: London.

4 Clare M (1990). *Developing Self-Advocacy Skills*. Further Education Unit: London.

5 Brandon D (1995). Advocacy—*Power to People with Disabilities*. Venture Press/BASW: Birmingham.

6 Kay B, Rose S, Tumbull J (1995). *Continuing the Commitment*. Department of Health: London.

7 UKCC (1998). *Guidelines for Mental Health and Learning Disabilities Nursing*. United Kingdom Council for Nursing, Midwifery and Health Visiting: London.

8 Jenkins R, Northway R (2002). Advocacy and the learning disability nurse. *British Journal of Learning Disabilities* **30**, 8–12.

Multisensory rooms

The concept of multisensory rooms began in De Hartenberg, Holland in 1975. The idea of providing a specialized sensory environment in which the patient could be actively or passively involved grew because of a positive response to an initial introduction to the approach. The Dutch term for this form of sensory intervention is Snoezelen (pronounced *snooze len*), a contraction of two words meaning 'to sniff' and 'to doze'. The term Snoezelen is used today only as a trade name for a company supplying sensory equipment in the UK, otherwise the term 'multisensory room' is used.

What is the role of the multisensory room?

We gain information about the world around us by using all of our senses together in order to make our world clearer and to enable us to:

• understand the environment
• understand ourselves
• communicate with people.

Multisensory rooms are specifically designed environments, which enable people with ID to experience a wide range of sensory stimuli for therapy, learning, relaxation, and enjoyment. The concept is to stimulate the tactile, visual, auditory, olfactory, and gustatory senses, which can be manifested through sound and visual effects, tactile experiences, vibration, use of aromas and music, all in many combinations and variations. The result is an environment in which the patient can completely relax or interact with and control all elements of the room, thus enabling people with varying degrees of ID to change and influence their environment in a positive way.

Who uses the room?

Multisensory rooms are used by people with ID of all ages, and all levels of cognitive and physical ability. Assessment of the patient/client is vital if rooms are to be used to their full potential. Nurses should be aware of the specific care needs of their patients as certain situations could prove to be more ineffective than therapeutic. For example, light projection may prove to be painful for a patient presenting with a visual impairment such as cataracts, which could well subsequently present in challenging behaviour for those patients who are preverbal or non-verbal.

Multisensory rooms are found in a wide variety of settings, e.g. hospitals, schools, resource centres, residential units, and private houses. The room should be accessible to all users and should therefore be relatively easy to operate. The equipment should have clear instructions, and staff training should be provided to ensure that they are confident to apply the technology and to ensure that the equipment is used in a safe and appropriate manner.

Multisensory environments

The multisensory white room combines the use of light and sound, together with neutral-coloured walls and comfortable furniture, to create an environment that can help to calm, relax, and offer gentle stimulation. The multisensory white room was traditionally introduced to adult services to meet the stimulatory needs of people with profound and multiple ID. However, with experience, the room has proven to be an invaluable resource for relaxation and anxiety management for people with dual diagnosis.

The multisensory dark room is typically designed to empower individuals with profound multiple ID and severe ID, using hi-tech interactive equipment against a dark backdrop to promote visual and auditory skills training.

The physical activity environment is designed to promote mobility and expression in a bright, soft, colourful, interactive environment.

Switching systems and LED lighting projection may be used to offer a multisensory experience within a jacuzzi or pool environment to enhance the therapeutic benefits of water therapy.

Further reading

Ferguson D, Young H (2000). *Exploring Multi-sensory Rooms: A Practitioner's 'Hands-on' Guide.* Spacekraft: Shipley, West Yorkshire.

Hirstwood R, Gray M (1995). *Practical Guide to the Use of Multi Sensory Rooms.* TFH Special Needs: Worcestershire.

Sensory integration

What is sensory integration?

We are all familiar with the senses of touch, smell, hearing, taste, and sight. There are other important sensations such as the pull of gravity, our movement, and the awareness of our bodies in space. Our nervous system receives, filters, organizes, and uses motor and sensory information to provide information to our brains to make sense of all of this. This neurobiological process is known as sensory integration. Sensory integration is necessary for us to interact with our environment.

Sensory integration begins in the womb as the main sensory systems mature: the vestibular system responds to gravity and movement, and the proprioceptive system receives input from muscles and joints. When these systems interact with tactile sensation (the sense of touch), the process of sensory integration takes place. Sensory integration develops when, as children, we explore sensations and body movement by touching, rolling, hugging, crawling, jumping, and climbing. Sensory integration is necessary for motor coordination and motor planning.

Dysfunction in sensory processing

Sensory integration serves two main functions: it protects us from over stimulation and helps us to interact with and learn from our environment. Children whom we suspect of having sensory dysfunction may present with the following signs:

• Overly sensitive to touch, movement, sights or sounds—withdraws when touched; avoids certain textures, clothing and foodstuffs
• Under reactive to sensory stimulation—seeks out intense sensory experiences such as body spinning, or falling into objects; may appear oblivious to pain or body position
• Unusually high/low activity levels—constantly on the move or may be slow to get going and tires easily
• Co-ordination difficulties—may have poor balance, may have difficulty learning a new task that requires motor coordination, appears awkward, stiff, or quite clumsy
• Delays in academic achievement and/or activities of daily living—may present with difficulties in handwriting, using scissors, tying shoes, buttoning and zipping clothing
• Behavioural issues—may be impulsive or distractible, may have difficulty adjusting to a new situation or following directions, may get frustrated, aggressive, or withdraw from activity when they experience failure, may appear bored or unmotivated.

Formal tests can be conducted to determine deficits, but observations of a child's normal daily life are needed to provide a complete assessment.

Sensory integration therapy

The treatment concepts related to sensory integration come from a body of work developed by A Jean Ayres PhD in the 1950s and 1960s. Professionals, usually occupational therapists, following assessment, can design a 'sensory diet' to help make life more manageable for the individual with sensory dysfunction. This incorporates an observation of developmental levels, which will determine whether sensory–motor processing is impaired.

As well as providing sensory integration therapy to children, the professional may also work with families, training them to replicate therapy in a natural environment. Sensory integration therapy may present as play, as this is traditionally how children learn and develop. Activities are chosen carefully to stimulate development in deficient areas. Although parents and carers can perform many of these activities at home with the child, professionals are trained to identify and address areas of special need.

Behavioural interventions

Behavioural interventions are based on behavioural principles, which suggest behaviours (the observable things individuals do) are learned and maintained by reinforcing events or stimuli. These reinforcing events are usually termed 'positive reinforcement' that involves an individual learning a particular behaviour as they are exposed to a pleasant event after the behaviour. Positive reinforcement may be physical, social, emotional, or sensory. The other main type of reinforcer is negative reinforcement, which is often misunderstood as punishment. This is not a true understanding of this in behavioural terms. Negative reinforcement involves an individual indulging in a particular behaviour in order to avoid some negative impact. It should be noted that 'reinforcement' increases behaviour, whereas punishment reduces behaviour, although perhaps only in the presence of the 'punisher'. By far the most frequently used behavioural interventions are based on the use of positive reinforcement.

Use of behavioural interventions

Behavioural interventions can be used in two main ways to help people with ID.

- To help individuals develop new skills—to facilitate their learning and to promote development and social functioning.
- To decrease behaviours that an individual may indulge in that are troublesome or may cause themselves or others difficulties.

These types of behaviours are sometimes referred to as challenging behaviours as they present a challenge for services as to how they respond to them.

Interventions

Interventions should be based on a number of guiding principles and these are outlined below. Over-arching these principles is the need to work in collaboration with the person with ID and their families to bring about positive change. Some view behavioural principles as manipulative, but they should be viewed as a means of positive development of an individual who needs guidance and support.

Assessment

Baseline measurements of behaviours should be made to facilitate the success of interventions and for evaluation. Behaviours have a function for the individual who expresses the behaviour and an assessment should be undertaken to determine this function. An ABC (antecedents, behaviour, consequences) approach is useful to assess behaviours.

Antecedents are events, stimuli or occurrences that are observed to take place before behaviours, and these may be prompts or stimuli that lead to or cause the behaviour. A physical assessment to rule out any physical causation of the behaviour is always necessary.

Behaviour refers to an accurate record of the actual behaviour that takes place in exact terms, and also a record of the frequency that the behaviour occurs; it should also involve detail of the impact of the behaviour in terms of severity for the individual, other people, or the environment.

Consequences are outcomes, or what happens after the behaviour takes place. Consequences are important, because these are often the reinforcers that maintain or lead to increases in the behaviour in question.

Plan

Based on assessment of the behaviours function and an ABC analysis, a written plan of the interventions to take place should be established. This plan should include:

- A clear description of behaviour to be focused on that needs to be reduced and what the goals of the intervention are
- What the intervention involves and who is to undertake the intervention—this is liable to be a therapist but family members or staff in the individual's residence need to be involved in implementation.

Implementing interventions

This might involve any or a combination of the following interventions:

- Removing, altering or facilitating avoidance of antecedent causative stimuli and avoiding positive reinforcements that cause or maintain the behaviour; providing the individual with the reinforcement before they indulge in the challenging behaviour; using positive reinforcements identified to teach the person other behaviours to replace the challenging behaviour; using positive reinforcements identified to teach the person other behaviours that are incompatible with the challenging behaviour.
- Facilitating diversion from the challenging behaviour by encouragement of physical activity, music, art, social interactions or other activities.
- Helping the individual find alternative ways to achieve the function that the challenging behaviour has for him/her, e.g. this may involve teaching the individual how to communicate more effectively.
- Making necessary changes to the environment that may be stimulating the behaviour, and teaching family members, residential, day-care or school staff the interventions to promote consistency, as interventions will fail without this.

Evaluation

Evaluation should involve:

- Re-recording of baseline behavioural measurements and comparison at set times following interventions, and evaluation of the impact of the interventions for the individual and others
- Reviewing the process and consistency of interventions, and how staff and family are coping
- Agreed goals/targets set for expressed times should be measured against specified outcomes
- As well as agreed times for outcomes, evaluation should be ongoing during the day-to-day implementation of interventions.

It should be expected in the early stages of an intervention that the challenging behaviour will increase and escalate before improvement is evident, which is a common phenomenon in behavioural therapy. However, if no improvement takes place or the behaviour worsens, the therapist needs to remain open to the use of alternative interventions.

Family therapy

Family therapy developed from the 1950s as clinicians struggled to make progress in individual therapy. They were looking for alternative ways to work with people presenting with complex difficulties, such as schizophrenia or anorexia.

Family therapy is based on some core beliefs:
- Each family is a system that contains sub-systems e.g. parents, sisters or brothers, and is itself part of other systems e.g. community, schools, workplaces, culture, and race
- The behaviours of each individual impact on other members of the system on an ongoing basis. Therefore, if one family member changes an aspect of their way of interacting with another person, this will result in a change in the relationship.

In the area of ID nursing, family therapy can be used in any of the areas in which it would be used in any other family, where there is a specific difficulty, e.g. schizophrenia, anorexia, or bereavement. Some families may have difficulties in adapting to the changing stages of the family life cycle.[1] In some instances it may not be the person who has ID who is the referred person, but the therapist should be sufficiently skilled to ensure that they (the person with ID) have a voice in the session and their views are heard. An example might be where the family or an ID nurse, who knows the person, is asked to 'help' the therapist to communicate with the person.

Traditionally there were three main models of family therapy. These were the strategic model, structural model, and the systemic model (the Milan Model).

Models have continued to evolve and new models have been developed, such as narrative therapy.

Theoretical models have also been influenced by post-modern ideas such as feminism, constructivism, social constructionism, linguistics, and the influence of culture. Many therapists have incorporated these ideas into their practice. This section provides an introduction to the Milan Model and illustrates how it works. This model is widely used in the UK.

The Milan Model

In the 1970s, four psychiatrists in Milan, following the work and writings of Bateson[2] and Watzlawick[3], developed a process of family therapy, which was to become known as the Milan Model of family therapy.[4] In the 1980s the group split. Palazzoli and Prata continued to develop strategic ways of working with families, while Cecchin and Boscolo developed the model in a different direction by travelling throughout the world, consulting, teaching others, and learning from their experiences.[5]

A session in the Milan Model is made up of five segments:
- The pre-session discussion
- The main interview
- The mid-session discussion
- The message to the family
- The post-session discussion.

The original model had the therapist in the room with the family, while the consulting team sat behind a one-way mirror and observed the interaction. This has now developed to a more transparent way of working, where, if the team is behind the one-way mirror, they join the family during the mid-session break and reflect on their understanding of the relational difficulties in front of the family in an open and respectful way.[6] The idea behind this is to introduce 'difference' (this is where the family are encouraged to view the difficulties from alternative perspectives, including each family member's and the therapist's) to the family's view of their story or narrative. It is also important that the 'difference' is sufficient to cause the family to feel safe enough to consider it and not so different that it causes the family to reject it immediately.[7] Following this the family then comments on the reflections.

There are three guidelines for therapists.

Hypothesizing is the discussion of ideas in the therapeutic team, in a conversation, which takes place prior to the therapist joining with the family. These ideas are about what might be happening in the family that has led this family to seek help for the identified patient. Hypotheses should be systemic in nature and should not be blaming of any one individual in the family. Unlike scientific hypotheses, family therapists do not aim to prove or disprove them; rather they view them as more or less useful.

Circularity is the idea that all behaviours and interactions within the family are systemic in nature, and are both influenced by and influence other's behaviour. It also covers the way in which questions asked of the family are constructed. They are composed in such a way as to elicit information about the relational aspects of the family.

Neutrality refers to the stance of the therapist, and is a position from which each member of the family should feel equally engaged and listened to. No one member of the family should feel blamed for the difficulties that the family is experiencing.

Although nurses may follow a model of family therapy, it must be emphasized that in order to provide the best possible care for the family, many different theories, techniques, and skills may need to be drawn upon in order to respond to a family's needs. In some situations, the ID nurse may collaborate to ensure the person with ID has their views heard.

Further reading

Burnham J (1986). *Family Therapy: First Steps Towards A Systemic Approach*. Routledge: London.

Carr A (2006). *Family Therapy: Concepts, Processes and Practice*, 2nd edn. Wiley: Chichester.

1 Barr O, Gates B, Eds. (2007). *Learning Disability: Towards Inclusion*, 5th edn. Churchill Livingstone: Oxford.

2 Bateson G (1972). *Steps to an Ecology of Mind*. Ballantine: New York.

3 Watzlawick P, Beavin J, Jackson D (1967). *Pragmatics of Human Communication*. Norton: New York.

4 Palazzoli MS, Boscolo L, Cecchin G, Prata G (1980). Hypothesising - Circularity - Neutrality: Three guidelines for the Conductor of the Session. *Family Process* **19**:3–12.

5 Cecchin G (1987). Hypothesising, Circularity and Neutrality Revisited: An Invitation to Curiosity. *Family Process* **26**(4):3–12.

6 Andersen T (1991). *The Reflecting Team: Dialogues and Dialogues about the Dialogues*. Norton: New York.

7 Mason B (1993). Towards positions of safe uncertainty. *Human Systems* **4**:189–200.

Touch

Jackson has suggested that nurses perform four types of touch:[1]
- Instrumental (e.g. bathing, giving injections)
- Expressive (e.g. empathic promotion of compassion and understanding)
- Systematic (e.g. deliberate manipulation of soft tissue, such as massage)
- Therapeutic.

The primary goal of the nurse should be to evaluate the patient's response towards the touch interaction and to be aware of what touch could convey. Understanding the use of touch could provide the nurse with a potent therapeutic tool with unexplored potential.[2]

Touch as a communication tool

Aromatherapy and multisensory massage

Aromatherapy is defined as the use of essential oils, obtained from plants, to promote health and well-being. Aromatherapy is mainly used to help people relax; however, aromatherapy is also used for stimulation, to promote concentration, and to build communication.

Massage can be used purely for relaxation and to improve health, with the introduction of massage tools e.g. electric massager, the activity can be identified as sensory stimulation accompanied by oil, lotion, or cream.

Tactile defensiveness

The cause of tactile defensiveness is neurological, causing the individual with ID to perceive tactile sensory input as extreme and uncomfortable; the ability of the CNS to process tactile sensory input is distorted, causing the individual great discomfort. The CNS must rely on 5 sensory nerve receptors in the skin to keep it informed about its environment—these receptors are light touch (surface), pressure (deep), temperature (hot/cold), and pain. It is possible for one type of receptor to be sensitive and the other to be 'normal'. This explains why someone may tolerate light touch, but dislikes firm hugs, or why someone dislikes hair cuts—the discomfort experience can be compared with the experience of trimming your fingernails too close, the raw sensation experienced can be highly irritating. Sensory integration techniques may be valuable in the process of attempting desensitization.

Deep touch pressure

Deep touch pressure (DTP) involves hugging, stroking the skin, or swaddling. Whereas light touch pressure (LTP) involves superficial stimulation e.g. tickling or stroking. LTP arouses the sympathetic nervous system, leading to increased pulse rate and respiration, whereas DTP is calming and leads to a reduction in pulse rate and respiration. DTP may be beneficial for those with ASD who are over sensitive to sensory stimulation, or for people with acute anxiety.

Touch in the multisensory room

Tactile experiences can be ignored somewhat in the multisensory room. The sense of touch is vital to our survival and one of our best modes of communication. We learn about our sense of touch through experience; like all the senses, we keep our sense of touch in trim by using it all the time. The multisensory room may be a place to experience tactile objects and panels. We can highlight them with projectors, fibreoptics and other lighting equipment.

Consent

Prior to any nursing intervention or therapeutic practice the nurse must gain patient consent. Consent is particularly relevant when using touch as a therapeutic medium. Consent should be obtained through a local consent policy, and documented accordingly.

1 Jackson A (1995). Alternative update. *Nursing Times* **91**(8), 61.

2 Gale E & Hegarty JR (2000). The use of touch in caring for people with learning disability. *British Journal of Developmental Disability* **46**(2), 97–108.

Complementary and alternative therapies

Terminology

The most commonly used term is either complementary and alternative medicine (CAM) or 'integrated healthcare'. Complementary approaches refer to a broad set of healthcare practices that are generally used to complement existing healthcare. The term encompasses therapies such as:

- Therapeutic touch and massage
- Relaxation and meditation
- Visualization and aromatherapy
- Reflexology and iridology
- Yoga and kinesiology.

Background

As many as one-fifth of the population have used some form of CAM.

Why are people turning to CAM?

- Instigated by clients or consumers with a desire and demand for more choice in treatment and failure of conventional healthcare and medicine to treat and/or find a cure for some long-term and terminal health conditions
- Healthcare practitioners, in particular nurses, who want to enhance individualized patient care.

Research and literature

- The most popular complementary therapy used with people with ID is aromatherapy and/or massage
- Evidence predominantly refers to their use in general hospital and clinical practice areas
- Information on the use of complementary therapies in ID settings is limited in comparison, and comprises mainly anecdotal evidence and/or case studies
- Research evidence is emerging to suggest that some complementary therapies may be effective and have therapeutic impact.
- There is disagreement as to appropriate research methodologies to best evaluate complementary therapies.

Potential therapeutic benefits

Touch

The basis of many CAMs is touch, and this can be used to:

- communicate encouragement, concern, emotional support and warmth
- help the person to have contact with the social world, to receive information and to convey it.

Aromatherapy and/or massage can create and provide a stimulating atmosphere that makes use of both touch and smell.

Relaxation

The structured use of therapeutic touch can result in:
- improved levels of relaxation
- reduced anxiety
- improved mood
- reduced challenging behaviour
- increased sensory awareness and communication.

Client–therapist interaction

Client-centred work is central to the practice of CAMs. This allows the practitioner to:
- provide the client with one-to-one attention and establish close inter-personal contact, as well as using touch as a social and therapeutic medium through which positive regard can be communicated.

Client choice and empowerment

- People with ID can make informed and valued choices to give consent to treatment including complementary therapies. It is possible to gain an understanding of how non-verbal communication signs (e.g. facial expression and body language) communicate a 'language'. Makaton signs and symbols can also be used.

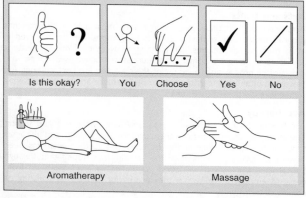

Fig. 9.1 Examples of Makaton signs and symbols. Reproduced with permission from Gates B (2007). *Learning Disabilities: Towards Inclusion*. 5th edn. Complementary therapies in learning disability settings. Chapter 23 p 490. Churchill Elsevier: Edinburgh.

Art, drama, and music

The arts are organized as expressions of ideas, feelings, and experiences in images, music, language, gesture, and movement. They provide for sensory, emotional, intellectual, and creative enrichment, and contribute to the individual's holistic development. Art opportunities enable the patient to explore alternative ways of communicating with others. It encourages ideas that are personal and creative. A robust arts programme in the care setting is life enhancing and is invaluable in stimulating creative thinking. Attempts at artistic expression are valued, self-esteem is enhanced, spontaneity and risk taking are encouraged, and difference is celebrated. Art opportunities encompass a range of activities in the visual arts, music and drama. These activities and experiences help the patient to make sense of the world, to question, to speculate and to find solutions, to deal with feelings, and to respond to the creative experience.

Sensory art

Art in healthcare may take the form of sensory art, where the medium used is carefully selected to stimulate the senses of the artist while producing a valued and valid art piece. It is vitally important to recognize the contribution of the artist at this cognitive ability level, as therapeutic benefit could be compromised by the enthusiasm of a dedicated enabler.

Arts and crafts

Arts and crafts continue to provide a substantial part of the patient's programme. A fairly sophisticated arts programme can be observed in many modern day facilities. Silk painting, weaving, card making, pottery, and scrap booking are some of the current art activities on offer, with artists often progressing to exhibiting their work in local art galleries. Art pieces are often used to contribute to the cosmetic and therapeutic environment of the patient themselves.

Art therapy

Art therapy focuses on how the patient/client is thinking and feeling. The therapist and the patient then explore the feelings and thoughts together by either talking and/or by enhancing further what has been developed during the course of the session. It is hoped that through this process the patient will come to understand and move on from personal emotional issues that they are having difficulty articulating or coming to terms with.

Drama

Drama offers an integrating approach for people with ID that holistically addresses their learning needs—it can increase their ability to relate to others more effectively.

The appeal of drama to people with ID is that they are caught up in situations that are both fun and intriguing. They are engaged in active learning, in contexts that are live, dynamic, and likely to be remembered. Drama can be used as a tool to help patients recollect past experiences.

Drama therapy

Drama therapy refers to those activities in which there is an established understanding between the client and the therapist, where the therapeutic goals are primary and not incidental to the ongoing activity.

Music

Music is a highly motivating activity for many people with ID. It can help to elicit responses from individuals whose interest is often quite difficult to arouse. The elements of music sessions are usually made up of listening, observing, singing, performing, and composing.

Music therapy

Music therapy is the use of sound and music within an evolving relationship between a patient and a therapist to support and encourage well-being. In a typical session, the music therapist and the person with ID create music together. They establish a relationship through which the individual can communicate their thoughts and feelings in a safe and supported environment.

Intensive interaction

Intensive interaction is a good way to get to know the people we interact with and to support them in developing social and communication skills. It also assists them to open up to the world, and let people get to know them better—their desires, needs, aspirations and personality, and what makes them happy or unhappy. This form of interaction is mainly used with people with complex needs, severe or profound ID, and ASD who also have ID. It could also be applied when interacting with, or teaching people with other disabilities (physical) and impairments (visual, auditory or sensory).

The approach and principles are based on the parent–baby interaction. Adults respond to a baby's actions and this gives them meaning, and this builds and strengthens their confidence in interaction at a later stage of their lives and relationships. It also helps them to understand the basic principles of communication, especially unwritten rules like taking turns, eye-contact, consideration to others, and non-verbal communication (e.g. facial expression and gestures).

When interacting, always consider yourself and your abilities, as these are the key points to successful interaction:

- Do you feel confident in imitating people's actions and noises?
- Does it come naturally to you or do you need training?
- Are your voice, face and body language tense or natural when interacting with these people?
- Do you understand the person's abilities and level of understanding?
- Do you need support?
- Are you comfortable and relaxed in the environment the interaction is taking place in?
- Do you know the person and his/her behaviours well?
- Are you enjoying yourself?
- Can you give full attention to the person?

The principles of the adopted caregiver–baby interaction used in the interaction include:

- Having time for the interaction with that person
- Talking at his/her level of understanding
- Having a good time together and enjoying each other's company
- Responding to people's actions and giving them meaning
- Imitating or copying their noises, expressions and behaviours
- Letting them take the lead
- Creating a relaxed and enjoyable environment
- Giving them space and time to respond, permitting pauses
- Building on the actions and interactions by trying new things
- Developing a repertoire of the actions to ensure familiar pattern and routine that can be repeated frequently

People we interact with need our full attention and creativity. We need to follow their actions and messages, and use these in games as well as using available equipment to keep them interested and surprised. These people may have short attention span or be easily bored, but by using the above they might enjoy it and try to test us or surprise us too.

This will allow them to learn skills needed for communication that is interactive, and perhaps transfer the skills to a different place or taking them to another level.

Useful and practical tips for successful interaction:

- Be accurate and objective in your observations—learn their language by paying close attention to what they are doing, and focus on even the smallest stimuli (e.g. changes in breathing, gentle teeth grinding, nails digging and eye gaze), and once you have learnt their way of communication, choose appropriate way to interact (familiarity, acceptance and non-threatening behaviours are keys to success).
- Make sure you are aware of all their impairments and not only their disability—sensory difficulties, problems with vision, hearing or fine motor skills may be undiagnosed or even be unable to process received signs. You need to take those into consideration when planning the interactive activities or use of equipment, tools or materials in order not to make them distressed.
- Always wait for a response or their initial signal that they are ready to interact—overloading may cause a negative effect.
- Develop a good rapport—mutual trust and their full attention is always important for a successful interaction.
- Use their signals and ways of communicating—when introducing something new make sure the person is ready because if they are not, they may get upset or display negative behaviours.
- Use their interests in equipment and materials, and their abilities to enhance the interaction further (e.g. musical instruments, musical toys and sensory materials), and make it more enjoyable.
- Listen to them and copy their behaviours as precisely as possible at the beginning, add something new or different at a later stage—if you try to teach them from the beginning rather than follow, you may lose their trust and they may retreat into themselves. They also may be testing you and change their ways to see if you are listening/ concentrating.
- Make sure the environment is appropriate and keep distractions to a minimum; sometimes you may need to adjust your movements or use something to catch their attention (e.g. tap in the rhythm of their rocking, sit in front of them and rock with them), and finally use a minimum of language.

Further reading

Caldwell P, Stevens P (1998). *Person to Person: Establishing contact and communication with people with profound learning disabilities and whose behaviour may be challenging.* Pavilion: East Sussex.

Nind M, Hewett D (2001). *A Practical Guide to Intensive Interaction.* BILD: UK.

▣ www.intensiveinteraction.co.uk – information on intensive interaction

Hydrotherapy

Hydrotherapy has many benefits for people with a variety of disabilities and impairments—recovering from surgeries and injuries, long-term and short-term conditions, pains in joints and back, and other problems. Hydrotherapy pools are usually equipped with special equipment, are easily accessible as they have special hoists, slings and rails around the pool, and are shallow. Hydrotherapy pools are used for any type of physiotherapy as well as a gentle exercise, or for those who cannot access public swimming pools for a number of reasons. Hydrotherapy pools are not really suitable for cardio-type exercises, such as aerobics or swimming distances, as they tend to be too warm and are not very big.

Physiotherapists usually create an exercise plan that is suited to a person's needs—they are based on an individual's assessments and type of difficulties. These exercises, however, should be carried out by the physiotherapists themselves or people who have had special training and know how these exercises must be carried out. If the exercises are not implemented correctly, they may not be as effective and may cause potential damage, pain or distress to the person, and affect their overall hydrotherapy experience.

The benefits of hydrotherapy for people with disabilities and impairments include:
- Pain reduction—the environment offers warm water and a warm atmosphere, which can have a positive effect on a person's overall physique (mainly joints and muscles) as the pressure from their body weight is counteracted by the water. Sometimes they may try new exercises and moves that may relieve overall pain.
- Pleasurable and a relatively calm environment—this may reduce their anxiety levels, relieve stress and relax them, which might lead to an increase of social interaction.
- Improvement of overall physical well-being—e.g. relaxation of the muscles and strengthening of weak muscles reduces load on joints and spine, improved circulation, reduced muscle spasm, increased mobility, improved posture and balance, reduced weight (regular exercise), relieves strain on internal organs that could be caused by a person's limited mobility (e.g. people in a wheelchair), and improved breathing.
- Improvement of mental health well-being—enjoyable and fun, might help people gain control over their body, increase self-confidence and independence, and provide a secure and safe environment.
- Multisensory experience—e.g. water temperature, visual effects, sounds, feel of water on the skin, different types and textures of equipment, floating sensation of water, and smells.

There is equipment available, specialist or otherwise, that is used during hydrotherapy. The equipment is either recommended by a physiotherapist or is used to enhance the overall experience for a person. The equipment used might include:
- Specialist hydrotherapy chairs
- Hoists and slings

- Soft or specialist tubes/noodles with or without handles and Velcro, and of a different lengths and thickness
- Arm bands, swim rings and swim vests
- Agua body belts and wrist bands
- Specialist support braces
- Specialist exercise kits (e.g. hydrotherapy hand bar weights and flotation devices)
- Swim floats, loungers and boards
- Toys, soft play balls, inflatable animals and beach balls
- Goggles and swimming caps
- Music and/or special effects (e.g. light displays and bubbles).

Before taking people for hydrotherapy:

- Be prepared that some people may feel emotionally drained after hydrotherapy—offer emotional support and understanding.
- Hydrotherapy could be tiring for some individuals—be aware of their limits as they may not be aware themselves. Some people may display negative behaviours.
- Always take drinks and snacks with you.
- Have enough staff with you, usually 1:1 ratio is optimal. This depends on the individual's disability, risk assessment and behaviours.
- Be aware that hydrotherapy is relatively expensive.
- Be aware that there is no physiotherapist available, only a pool supervisor, for health and safety purposes when hiring the pool privately.
- Do not perform any exercises with the individuals if you are unsure or untrained in their safe practice, to prevent any damage or pain.
- Do not rush people to enter the pool, sometimes they may not feel like going into the pool due to the temperature or unwanted sensory stimulus (e.g. strong smell). Offer alternatives (e.g. bring the water to them in a bucket and play with it, ask them to sit by the pool and dip their hands or feet into the pool).
- Contact the hydrotherapy pool before you visit and let them know if you require any specialist equipment. It might not be available.
- Make sure that all the individuals going to the hydrotherapy pool have risk assessments including manual handling.
- Bring people's favourite toys and/or equipment with you if possible.
- Some people may need goggles, as the chemicals in the water may be irritating and cause distress.

Further reading

Harry's Hydro Charity (2008). *What is Hydrotherapy?* Available from: http://www.harrys-hydro.org/hydrotherapy.htm. [Accessed 15th March 2008].

Longfields Association (2004). *Service-user Facilities, Activities and Opportunities.* Available from: http://www.longfieldsassociation.org.uk/facilities.htm. [Accessed March 2009]

Kellogg JH (2007). *Outlines of Practical Hydrotherapy.* Kessinger Publishing: USA.

Eidson R (2008). *Hydrotherapy.* Delmar Learning: Canada.

Conductive education

CE was developed in Hungary by Professor Andreas Peto, who worked with children with motor disorders that resulted from a damaged CNS. In 1952 the first National Institute of Motor Therapy was opened.

CE has been used for people with cerebral palsy; however, its teaching style also seems to benefit people with neurological and motor related disabilities, and difficulties that include spina bifida, Multiple sclerosis, Parkinson's disease, developmental delays, dyspraxia, and those recovering from cerebral vascular accidents (strokes). The purpose of CE is to provide the necessary support and instruction required to gain or regain control of their bodies.

The benefits of CE include:
- Helping people to regain their lost skills
- Building their confidence and ability to problem-solve
- Reinstating their independence
- Improving their and their care givers quality of life
- Increasing mobility
- Overcoming difficulties with fine motor skills
- Reducing dependence on equipment
- Helping to improve coordination, communication and attention.

Programmes are developed and mainly implemented by specifically trained conductors and their assistants. Care providers and family members are involved in this intervention, and are taught how to support people in their care so that they might practice their acquired skills successfully. Every programme is condition and age specific, and is based on an individual assessment done by the conductor.

When supporting people in this programme never;
- set people up to fail
- set tasks that cannot be achieved
- do tasks too fast
- reward only the results (reward the effort as well)
- demotivate people
- leave a person unsupervised for an extended period of time
- perform the tasks without being specifically trained.

CE is an intensive life-long, day-to-day learning process, so it is important for people to be kept motivated through visual representation of their achievements. A person (other than the conductor) who is assisting a client with CE needs to be aware of the key points of CE:
- Developing a good rapport and trust among all involved
- Creating a good learning environment
- Working in groups as people learn and support each other with problem solving in achieving day-to-day tasks (groups are usually condition, age and skills matched) and everyone in the group is involved
- Providing guidance through tasks
- Providing a structured programme (including play to make it more interesting and creative) and timescale
- Offering guidance to perform the task rather than doing it for them
- Each task needs to be tailored and made to suit the individual's needs

- Linking together movement, speech and thought (e.g. I roll from left to right side—the whole group has to repeat this then perform the task using a count)
- Understanding people's conditions and how these can have an impact on their learning and lives
- Planning support and identifying any required equipment
- Emotional security.

The skills learnt through CE could include:
- Development of daily living skills (dressing, drinking, and potty/toilet training) as well as experiencing the world through play, and communicating about hobbies and other interests
- Coordination and improving posture and weight-bearing
- Eye exercises
- Breathing exercises
- Writing skills
- Facial expressions
- Playing with others or peers
- Social skills.

Elements of CE

- The conductor—a trained professional who designs and delivers the programme
- The programme—carefully planned, usually takes a whole day and is intense
- The tasks—what the group/person need to learn
- Intention (including the use of rhythm)—method of learning and encouraging people to use speech
- The group—a team of people matched together according to their abilities and age. This encourages them to learn from each other.

Further reading

Bairstow P, Cochrane R, Hur J (1993). *Evaluation of Conductive Education for Children with Cerebral Palsy – Final report (Part 1)*. HMSO: London.

Brown MR (2006). An insight into the benefits of conductive education. *Nursing and Residential Care* **8**(3), 122–125.

Rozsahegyt T (2006). Careful planning and routine are key to development. *EYE (Early Years Educator)* **August**, 52–54.

▣ www.conductive-ed.org.uk—information on CE.

▣ http://www.nice.org.uk/—NICE (The National Institute for Health and Clinical Excellence)—information about services.

TEACCH

Treatment and Education of Autistic and related Communication-handicapped Children

TEACCH was developed in 1966 from work of Eric Schopler and colleagues. It was established that autism is not caused by bad parenting but that it has neurological origin. The effective treatment also emerged from their research that highlighted the importance of parents' presence as co-therapists.

Structured teaching using principles of TEACCH is widely used with people with communication difficulties, and especially those with ASD, and not only when teaching them new tasks and helping them to understand what is required of them, but also to become more independent and effective in their environments (home, school, community). The intervention is a lifelong approach and takes into consideration the persons' strengths and difficulties. The developed programme considers the person and his/her functions as it is, and supports them to develop their skills as much as possible. Before the programme is developed it is important for a person developing it to:

- Understand the ASD or the communication problems of the individual (e.g. manifestations, impairments, strengths, and characteristics) to understand behaviours and learning styles
- Assess the person's abilities, get to know them better—their skills, needs and interests in order to make the programme effective
- Involve people in their lives (parents, cares, siblings, teachers, assistance, professionals) as they help to maintain and develop it further, and to provide information about the person
- Consider the learning environment, the task(s) to be taught and how these will be achieved (e.g. task organization, physical organization, teaching methods, reinforcements, cues), as consistency and clear instructions are important, and discuss all plans with the person who the programme is aimed at (a communication aid might be needed)
- Attend TEACCH training to learn the principles, aims, skills, and strategies needed for successful delivery.

Difficulties and strengths presented by individuals with an ASD or communication difficulties may be demonstrated by changes in behaviour and include:

- Communication—non-verbal and verbal expression (not having the essential language) and/or not understanding what is required of them (difficulties in receptive language)
- Organization—inability to organize oneself and being easily distracted
- Processing of information (cognitive processing difficulties)
- Sequencing—not understanding what follows or what happens next; this may occur due to poor memory and transfer of skills from one situation/environment/task to another—difficulties in generalizing
- Resistance to change in routines and going back to familiar things, activities or behaviours.

When using the TEACCH techniques always consider the following.[1]

Organization

- Appropriate environment (e.g. lighting, space, noise levels, organization, exits, distractions, colour of walls, use of dividers, smells, materials)
- Visual cues—for associating the activity/task to a place (e.g. a picture of hand washing on the wall above the sink, a toilet picture on the toilet door)
- Clear organization and structure of the tasks/activities
- Identifying specific areas for specific tasks (e.g. playground, kitchen)
- Accessible teaching materials (e.g. in a tray with their name and photo)
- Clear boundaries and transition area identified (where the schedules are placed).

Schedules

- A sequenced visual timetable marking clear beginning and end of activities to be clearly visible
- Tailor made to a person's cognitive ability and experiences
- Use—objects of reference, pictures, photos, symbols, numbers, words, diaries, own writing, ticking technique, magazine pictures
- Presentation—a key ring (to take out), vertical or horizontal (with a person's photo or name)
- Time—beginning and end to be clear e.g. use egg timer, a clock (digital), colour coding (on the paper clock), hour glass.

Teaching approach

- Use verbal prompts (clear, consistent, key words only, sequenced—first do this and then do that)
- Use gestures—e.g. pointing while talking to enhance the understanding, make sure the person follows what is being shown to them
- Use non-verbal prompts—visual cues, written instruction, schedules
- Use physical prompts—hand over hand approach, guide their hand, let them model you, demonstrate first and let them to copy you
- Use prompts for certain situations—what to say in certain situations (e.g. goodbye when leaving), provide reassurance and use rewards and find motivators, always address the behaviour at the time.

Further reading

Hanbury M (2005). *Educating Pupils with Autistic Spectrum Disorders: A Practical Guide.* Paul Chapman Publishing: London.

▣ www.nas.org.uk—information about TEACCH.

▣ www.teacch.com —TEACCH autism programme.

---

1 Schopler E, Mesibov G (1995). *Learning and Cognition in Autism.* Plenum Press: New York.

Gentle teaching

GT is a therapeutic approach to work with people with ID. The approach is characterized by:

- the unconditional valuing of others
- placing relationships at the centre of learning and development
- incorporating a non-aversive strategy that aims to promote complex, meaningful relationships between client and carer
- the values of respect, equity and mutual change
- viewing people as social beings
- using specific techniques and procedures to facilitate change.

Definition

The central tenet of GT is that all human beings need to participate in reciprocal, loving relationships, and to participate with others in activities that comprise daily life.

Application of gentle teaching

The success of GT is determined by the extent to which parties involved in a relationship move towards a more functional form of interaction. The practical application of GT focuses upon four key areas.

Gathering information

The focus of gathering information is to identify how best to begin the process of engagement:

- How does the person participate?
- How does the person communicate?
- How does the person relate to others?

Introducing participation through the use of activities

GT sees activities as opportunities for engaging people and should:

- be simple and easily broken down into steps, and have repetitive sequences
- call for the use of materials and be done in a variety of places
- require active participation and two-way interaction
- have built in mini-breaks.

Finding the 'entry point'

Within each sequence of repeated steps in an activity, the GT practitioner observes the person's non-verbal cues closely to identify the 'entry point'. This is the point that the person finds interesting or attractive e.g. they may increase eye contact, or change facial expression when that point occurs. The person is more likely to engage in the activity at this stage than at any other.

Dealing with behavioural difficulties through 'defusion'

Defusion describes a strategy used by GT practitioners to manage behavioural difficulties within the context of shared participation in activities and relationships. It is used to provide emotional and physical safety for both the person with ID and the practitioner. It involves the following:

- Demands being placed on the person are reduced or removed
- Mini-breaks are introduced to allow the person some time to relax

- The practitioner gradually recommences the activity, seeking an entry point
- The focus is shifted from the person's behaviour to the calm, predictable safety of the shared activity.

Success of gentle teaching

Some criticisms have been levelled against GT.

It is ineffective at reducing behavioural difficulties and that this is proven by research

The focus and purpose of the GT approach is quite different from behavioural ones, concentrating on the whole person and relationships rather than on specific behaviours. Research evidence to date demonstrates some success for GT, particularly in the areas of:

- communication
- relationships
- skill building.

It is potentially 'aversive'

It may be potentially distressing to people:

- who experience difficulties engaging in relationships (e.g. those on the autistic spectrum)
- whose behavioural difficulties are motivated by a desire to escape interaction.

The central tenets of GT are not operationally defined

The Caregiver Interactional Observation System (CIOS) and the Person Interactional Observation System (PIOS) were developed as a measurement tool by practitioners to code the dyadic variables of interactional change. However, attempts to replicate these variables under research conditions have failed to find any significant differences in therapeutic effect between GT and other interventions.

GT uses behavioural techniques

GT evolved out of behavioural approaches and has adopted some of their techniques e.g. positive praise, ignoring behaviour, shaping, extinction, reinforcement, fading, errorless learning, physically redirecting self-injury, restructuring the environment, maintaining normal conversation, using physical and visual cues.

Further reading

O'Rourke S, Wray J (2000). Gentle teaching. In: Gates B, Gear J, Wray J, Eds. *Behaviour Difficulties: Concepts and Strategies*. Ballière Tindall: London.

Polirstick SR, Dana L, Buono S, Mongelli V, Trubia G (2003). Improving functional communication skills in adolescents and young adults with severe autism using gentle teaching and positive approaches. *Top Lang Disorders* **23**(2), 146–153.

Sanderson H, Harrison J, Price S (1992). *Aromatherapy and Massage for People with Learning Disabilities*. Hands On Publishing: London.

Hegarty JR (2000). The use of touch in caring for people with learning disability. *The British Journal of Developmental Disabilities* **46**(2), 91:97–108.

Anger management

Anger management applied to people with ID draws on a range of techniques. These techniques are designed to enable people with ID to cope better with their anger, and the potential aggression that may develop from it. The techniques are generally of a cognitive behavioural nature (see 📖 Cognitive behaviour therapies, p.324), although some techniques are not. The techniques applied should be based on the cognitive ability of the person or people who could benefit from the technique(s), and the nature of their anger.

It is generally accepted that cognitive behavioural methods of anger management are best suited for use with people with a mild to moderate degree of ID, as the success of these approaches is underpinned by the ability to communicate and reason at a relatively high level. Novaco has proposed that anger is an emotion that has three components:[1]

- Physiological
- Behavioural
- Cognitive.

Novaco and more recent theorists have advocated that anger management plans should be built around these three areas. In very broad terms the techniques recommended for each component of aggression are:

- physiological—involving environmental management and relaxation techniques
- behavioural—involving the person recognizing how anger causes them to behave aggressively or inappropriately and to develop more acceptable coping skills
- cognitive—involving restructuring of distorted thinking that leads to anger.

Readers are advised to consult further reading for more detail. In order for anger management to work preparatory measures should be undertaken:

- Thorough assessment of the anger and it's consequences for the individual and others
- Self-report questionnaires and interviews
- A thorough exploration of the individual's history, to include carer's views, triggers of anger, and environmental issues
- Functional analysis and communicative function of the anger
- The level of communication of the individual and their methods of communication.

Anger management techniques are normally developed during a series of structured facilitated sessions, the aims and methods of which are:

- To develop an understanding of anger and aggression
- Individual and group reflections on the development of anger and it's consequences
- Developing coping skills that can help manage situations that have previously caused anger, and to generalize these to other anger provoking contexts
- Teaching relaxation techniques.

Participants are encouraged to reflect on the sessions and their developing anger management skills by use of a reflective diary/self-report, which can be discussed in the sessions. Depending on the cognitive and communication level of participants, pictures, charts, pictorial rating scales, role-play and 'traffic light' systems can be used.

For people with more severe ID and sensory impairments, it is recognized that the cognitive and some of the behavioural aspects may not be useful, and therefore physiological techniques should be encouraged, including:

- Aromatherapy
- Reflexology
- Hand massage
- Multisensory rooms
- Music therapy
- Hydrotherapy
- Art therapy.

The role of the intellectual disability nurse

The cognitive aspects and anger management programmes are often facilitated by clinical psychologists; however, nurses are often involved with such groups. More specifically nurses are likely to be involved with the assessment process and supporting individuals with behavioural and physiological aspects of anger management.

Further reading

Gulbenkoglu H, Hagiliassis N (2006). *Anger Management: An Anger Management Training Package for Individuals with Disabilities*. Jessica Kingsley Publishers: London.

1 Novaco RW (1975). *Anger Control: The Development and Evaluation of an Experimental Teatment*. DC Heath: Lexington.

Cognitive behaviour therapies

CBT is based on the assumption that individuals construct a world view that may be at variance from reality. These personal constructs, which are also known as schemata, are developed and maintained through everyday experiences, and they are a coping mechanism, which help people understand their own behaviour and that of others. If events (often during childhood) and behaviours are consistently negative and emotionally damaging, then the individual can develop profoundly negative constructs and resulting behaviors, such as self-injury. These constructs have been called self-defeating beliefs and errors in thinking. These distorted errors in thinking and resulting behaviours are often subconscious processes over which individuals have little control. It is often the case that individuals have little or no insight into their cognitive thought processes. CBT allows for the individual through a skilled therapeutic intervention to bring previously subconscious thought processes to a conscious self-aware level. This can then lead to exploration of these thought processes and the development of a more accurate and healthy world view. Given that subconscious negative self-constructs can develop due to persistently negative life experiences, it is reasonable to suggest that some people with ID are very likely to have developed negative self-views resulting from the often damaging ways in which they have been treated. It is therefore evident that some people with ID could benefit from CBT. The benefits of CBT include:

- The opportunity to deconstruct negative self-views
- It is a humanistic intervention
- It is holistic and pursues personal growth
- It offers an understanding of seemingly irrational behaviours.

It shifts the focus from an emphasis on behaviours and symptomology to an understanding of the damaging nature of causative factors, which can then be addressed.

CBT is a well accepted and widely used intervention in mental health services. It is less commonly used with people with ID, and this is because it:

- requires and presupposes that an individual engaging in CBT has the cognitive ability to do so; this will potentially preclude a significant number of people with ID
- demands compliance with what the therapist and others may agree to be an acceptable world view rather than a real understanding of how a person with cognitive impairments makes sense of the world
- necessitates the individual being actively engaged in the process.

This section should be understood in conjunction with 🕮 Counselling and psychotherapies, p.328, as there are significant links and common themes between the two. CBT is relatively simple to explain but a complex intervention to implement. It is recommended, therefore, that readers consult the further reading.

Further reading

Turnbull J (2000). Cognitive behavioral interventions. In: Gates B, Gear J, Wray J, Eds. *Behavioural Distress, Concepts and Strategies*. Ballière Tindall: London.

Support associated with loss and bereavement

Supporting the person with an intellectual disability

Just because a person has an ID, it should never be assumed that they cannot grieve. Nurses should recognize the need to give them extra consideration because of their disability. Death never occurs in a vacuum but within a social context, and that social context in which they are being supported may be crucial in helping a person with an ID to deal with their grief in a constructive way.

Facilitating grief

Nurses need to educate people about the impact of loss and its potential effects, using naturalistic opportunities such as events happening in the media or portrayed on the television. If nurses helped people with ID to learn about loss and bereavement, actively participate in the grief process, and facilitated grief in a constructive way, then the need for specific therapeutic interventions would be minimized. Health and social care professionals need to remember that:

* Fundamentally everyone has a right to know when someone close to them dies.
* Introducing, and talking about, difficult news needs to be undertaken in conjunction with a familiar carer whenever possible.
* Accurate information needs to be conveyed in a simple manner and given in a consistent way, and active listening is the key to personal support.
* Information may need to be clarified in a way that the person understands, repeated often and reassurance regularly offered.
* Grieving individuals need an invitation to talk, which includes acknowledging the pain they may be feeling, recognizing the need for a safe, quiet space and privacy, and providing ongoing constructive support.
* Individuals may find it difficult to articulate their feelings in a coherent manner. Picture/story books might help them to recognize and explore their feelings with support.
* It may take time for the grieving person to accept the reality and finality of the loss, therefore accurate record keeping is essential for future ongoing support. Grief work takes time, and everyone grieves in their own unique way.

Creative approaches

Some people with an ID may have communication challenges; they may feel uncomfortable with support that relies on dialogue alone. Therefore, the nurse needs to be creative in the bereavement support process, using pictures, photographs or artwork as a means of facilitating expression. Many people with ID lack personal heritage and history, and the development of a life-story book is an excellent way of recording events in a tangible, accessible, and meaningful way. Similarly, the creation of a memory book around a particular person who has perhaps died or moved on, captures vital information in an accessible and visual format.

Responding to disenfranchised grief

Disenfranchised grief is described in 📖 Responding to bereavement, p.246 and according to Doka, ways of minimizing the chance of this occurring with people with ID include:[1]

- Acknowledging and legitimizing the loss, actively listening to the bereaved person, and being empathic, trying to imagine how the person may be feeling, and helping the person to make sense of what has happened
- Encouraging the constructive use of ritual (such as visiting the grave or memorial), sharing fears and anxieties, exploring spiritual needs and support, offering options for mutual support (such as group work), and bereavement counselling.

Those who may need therapeutic interventions

Although most people generally deal with their grief in their own way without the need for therapeutic interventions, some people with an ID may need to be referred for specific bereavement interventions. People who may need additional help include those individuals who:

- are unusually angry or who profoundly miss the deceased
- have a restricted social support network[1] and people who are assessed as not coping[2]
- are excluded from the funeral or who have not been told about the death for some considerable time after the event.

Impact of offering support

Working with loss and bereavement can affect professionals in different ways. It may make some recall friends and family who have died, it may make them think about current losses, or even dwell on the potential for loss and death in the future. Nurses should remember to look after themselves, and that a healthy carer provides healthy support. Recognizing and acknowledging this difficult time with senior managers is important. Clinical supervision is one way of accessing support during such difficult times, as is peer support and counselling.

1 Elliott D (1995). Helping people with learning disabilities to handle grief. *Nursing Times* **9**(43): 209–13.

2 Read S (2007). *Bereavement Counseling for People with Learning Disabilities: A Manual to Develop Practice*: Quay Books: London.

Counselling and psychotherapies

Psychotherapy and counselling applied to people with ID encompass a vast range of theories and potential approaches. Because of this the reader is strongly advised to pursue the recommended further reading at the end of this section. Although there are many available counselling and psychotherapeutic approaches available, they all, in essence, share a common theoretical basis, and they all share the same potential benefits. This section will therefore briefly outline some key approaches and their shared origins, and then outline the key common benefits. Psychotherapeutic approaches are based on the belief that individuals can experience errors in thinking that are emotionally damaging and can result in distressed states of behaviour (see 📖 Cognitive behaviour therapies, p.324). Common errors in thinking include:

- Arbitrary inference—drawing negative conclusions without supporting evidence
- Selective abstraction—focusing on negative detail rather than an overall view
- Over generalization based on a single negative occurrence
- Magnification and minimization—over emphasis on the importance of a negative issue
- Absolute dichotomous thinking—things are perceived as entirely all good or bad as well as catastrophizing
- Mind reading—belief that others have negative thoughts about you
- Blaming—assumption that someone must be to blame
- Emotional reasoning—e.g. 'if I feel this way then so must everyone else'
- Heaven's reward—dismay at unrewarded virtue
- Desensitization—people avoid experiencing the external world to dull emotional pain
- Deflection—avoiding contact with others to avoid emotional abandonment
- Introjection—being ruled by feelings of 'should' or 'ought' so that the individual's needs are neglected
- Projection—attributing to others what cannot be acknowledged by the self
- Retroflection—the process of turning things back against oneself.

Approaches to allowing the individual to explore and address the often subconscious processes listed above have common themes, but there are several major therapeutic approaches. CBT has been outlined in 📖 Cognitive behaviour therapies, p.324; other recognized approaches include:

Cognitive analytical therapy (CAT)—this stems from a belief that coping strategies that are often dysfunctional develop as a form of self-protection, and this allows for the potential to develop less damaging coping strategies.

Rational emotive therapy (RET)—this is based on the premise that humans have tendencies to irrationality and the potential to change, and therefore it is about confronting irrational beliefs to make positive changes.

Treatment approaches may vary between the different methods of psychotherapy and counselling, but they are likely to include the need for a thorough assessment that might involve:

- A thorough exploration of the individual's history
- Functional analysis to include known triggers of distress
- Arousal levels, patterns of behaviour and current coping strategies
- Psychological questionnaires and interviews, and identification of errors in cognition
- The level of the individual's motivation to change and their ability to follow a treatment plan.

Treatment might include:

- Giving information and developing understanding of specific disorders (e.g. paranoia)
- Social skills training involving role play and re-enactment of past triggers
- Learning relaxation techniques and problem solving, and challenging errors in thinking
- Modeling and cognitive distraction (e.g. visualization)
- Testing out coping strategies within a controlled environment
- Self-report methods and desensitization to stressful situations
- Guided fantasies and dream work, and brainstorming solutions.

The common benefits of psychotherapy and counselling

A criticism of psychotherapy and counselling in relation to their application to people with ID is that many within this client group are not of a sufficient cognitive level of ability to benefit from them, because of issues of communication, understanding, and engagement with the process; however, many people with ID will benefit from some of the common benefits of psychotherapy and counselling, which are:

- The building of a relationship based on trust, genuineness and mutuality, in which the individual feels listened to and understood
- The development of a working alliance in which the individual and therapist feel they are working in partnership to achieve shared goals
- Support and reassurance, and the development of insight
- The development of healthy and adaptive responses via the implicit reinforcement of appropriate behaviour and responses.

The ID nurse will not usually be engaged in these approaches as they are undertaken by trained psychotherapists and counsellors; however, many nurses undertake post-qualification training courses so that they can engage in this important area of care.

Further reading

Wilberforce D (2003). Psychological approaches. In: Gates B (Ed), *Learning Disabilities: Toward Inclusion*, 4th edn. Churchill Livingstone: London.

Appropriate use of medication

Psychopharmacology

Psychopharmacology refers to the effects of drugs on mental illness and mental function. Within the field of ID the use of psychotropic drugs (medication that affects the mind) is a contentious issue, particularly concerning the use of such drugs to manage behaviour rather than for the purposes of therapeutic intervention. Consequently, the reader is referred to recent guidelines outlining good practice standards in this area: *Using medication to manage behaviour problems among adults with learning disabilities*.[1] However, it is important to acknowledge that medication has a vital and important role to play in the therapeutic treatment of many individuals with mental health issues. Nevertheless, it is also important to understand that medication is only one component of a holistic therapeutic plan, which must also consider psychological, educational, and social interventions in the pursuit of remission and recovery.

Types of psychotropic medication

A range of different medications are used by in people with ID who have mental health problems, including:

- Antipsychotics—a group of drugs used to treat psychosis; they may also be used to sedate people who are agitated or aggressive
- Antidepressants and mood stabilizers—a group of drugs used in the treatment of mood disorders such as depression or bipolar disorder
- Anxiolytic medications—a group of drugs used to treat anxiety disorders or reduce symptoms of anxiety.

Side effects of psychotropic medication

The use of psychotropic medication has been found to induce a number of severe and irreversible side effects, and it is essential that nurses have adequate knowledge and systems in place to identify such adverse effects early. These side effects include:

- Memory impairment
- Anticholinergic effects (i.e. dry mouth, constipation, urinary retention and confusion)
- Dyskinetic movement disorders (i.e. involuntary repetitive writhing or jerking movements)
- Neuroleptic malignant syndrome (i.e. fever, severe muscle rigidity, altered consciousness, automatic arousal, death)
- Pseudo-Parkinsonian symptoms (i.e. unsteady gait, bent posture, expressionless face and tremors).

Professional guidelines for appropriate use of medications

There are a number of professional guidelines regarding the appropriate use of medication. Whether the medication is used to target a specific physical problem or to address challenging behaviour and/or mental health problems, these should be fully adhered to (see 🕮 Medicines management, p.208).

Guidelines for appropriate use of medications for nurses

Considering the frequency of use of psychotropic medication in this population, alongside the potency of this medication, and the difficulties that people with ID encounter with regard to self-reporting effects and side effects, it is crucial that all staff working in this field apply rigorous standards of good practice. These are outlined below.

Good practice in the use of psychotropic medication

- Ensure adequate education and training of all staff involved in the administration of psychotropic medication
- All staff involved in the administration of psychotropic medication must have up-to-date knowledge of the expected side effects of each drug administered
- Side effect rating scales should be used to systematically identify the onset of side effects for psychotropic medication (e.g. LUNSERS)
- Extreme care and close monitoring is necessary during periods of reducing medication or withdrawal
- The capacity of the individual to provide informed consent should be assessed, and appropriate information given to the person and carers in a easy read format/information leaflets[2]
- It is important that the administration of psychotropic medication can be justified from a best interest's perspective
- Ensure that there are clear parameters specified around the use of PRN (as necessary) medication
- Ensure regular monitoring and review of treatment efficacy, and the need for continued use, as part of the bio-psycho-social model of intervention.

Further reading

Nursing and Midwifery Council (2008). *Standards for Medicines Management*. NMC: London.

1 Deb S, Clarke D, Unwin G (2006). *Using Medication to Manage Behaviour Problems Among Adults with Learning Disabilities*. University of Birmingham.

2 ⌨ The Elfrida Society: ⌨ http://www.elfrida.com/ [accessed April 2009]

Supporting people in mainstream health services

General practitioners

General practitioners, or GPs as they are generally known, are considered to be gatekeepers to primary care services. Across the UK, all British citizens are entitled to the services of an NHS GP. People can register as patients with any local NHS surgery, providing they live in the practice catchment area, and if that practice has vacancies. It is through registering with an NHS GP that people gain access to the full range of NHS services within that area.

Education

GPs are qualified medical doctors, having completed at least 4yrs post-graduate experience and a postgraduate training in general medicine. Some GPs specialize in particular aspects of medicine, within surgery settings. Most GPs work as independent contractors to the NHS, being responsible for providing adequate buildings and teams of staff to deliver a wide range of healthcare. They may do this individually or as shared part-ners in bigger practices. These teams may also include other GPs, working on a sessional or temporary basis.

Role in practice

PCTs in England, local health boards in Wales, regional health boards in Scotland, and Local Commission Groups in Northern Ireland are all responsible for the commissioning, planning, and delivery of high quality primary healthcare services to the local population. In order to treat NHS patients, GPs must have their name and details registered on a primary medical performers list. Every PCT, and their equivalents across the UK, are responsible, and must ensure that GPs have the right qualifications, skills, and experience to work in the NHS. The PCTs and equivalent struc-tures in other countries are responsible for monitoring and checking that these skills are kept updated.

An average GP has ~1800 patients registered with their practice. Of these patients, about 36 can be expected to have ID. Most patient consul-tations take place at the surgery and, less frequently, during home visits. Out-of-hours care is often provided by the primary care organizations, although there are indications in England that this may soon change, with practices being open for longer unsocial hours. GPs, with other practice staff, record their patient consultations on electronic clinical systems, using Read codes. At present electronic recording systems vary from practice to practice across the countries. Current negotiations are exploring the pos-sibility of standardizing these.

GPs are paid under a UK wide GP contract. Within this contract is a quality outcomes framework (QOF). The aim of the QOF is to provide additional financial rewards, based on a points system, for offering GPs better management of chronic disease. The QOF is voluntary, although most practices choose to take part. The QOF is subject to an annual review. In 2006/2007, QOF points were introduced for the development of a practice ID register. Further standards were set within the specifica-tions for direct enhanced services in 2007 (🖳 www.pcc.nhs.uk).

In meeting the specific health needs of people with ID, a national call has recently been made for all GP practices to provide regular health checks to people with ID.

GPs and people with intellectual disabilities

GPs are responsible for the day-to-day medical care of people with ID who live in the community. People with ID have been found to visit GPs less frequently than the general population, or other vulnerable groups. A number of barriers have been identified as affecting a GP's ability to provide an effective primary care service:

- A lack of basic and postgraduate training in the skills of working with this population
- A lack of experience in working with the ID population, associated with reduced confidence
- Limited skills in communicating directly with people with ID
- Limited knowledge on the specific health needs of the ID population
- Constraints associated with limited time for appointments
- Difficulties in physical examination
- Diagnostic overshadowing (reports of physical health being viewed as part of the ID, therefore not investigated or treated).

A number of solutions have been proposed to address these barriers:

- Compulsory training for GPs in ID issues at undergraduate level, and availability of postgraduate refresher courses. This should be delivered by community ID staff, in collaboration with self-advocacy organizations
- A coordinated approach to sharing information, and closer working relationships between community ID teams and primary care services
- Having a named GP within each practice to take the lead on the health issues of people with ID.

Further reading

DRC (2006) *Closing the Gap*. Equality and Human Rights Commission: London.

MENCAP (2007) *Death by Indifference*. MENCAP: London.

Royal College of General Practice. ⌕ www.rcgp.org.uk

Health visitors

Health visitors within the UK are also known as public health nurses. The term 'family health nurses' is used in Scotland, and although the term 'public health nurse' is used in the Republic of Ireland, the role of these nurses also includes work undertaken by District Nursing services within the UK. Health visitors were originally employed by local authorities to meet the public health needs of new mothers and their children, and the role was developed to reduce infant mortality and improve maternal health. Health visitors are now employed, in general, by NHS Trusts, and are expected to offer a whole family approach in their work. The main focus of their role is in public health, helping people to stay healthy, and the prevention of ill health.

Employed by NHS Trusts, or their equivalents, health visitors are usually attached to, and based within, GP practices. Other work bases include children's disability teams or, increasingly, children's or family centres.

Education

As registered nurses or midwives who have an additional qualification in health visiting (now at degree level), their role is wide and varied. Health visitors support children, parents, and families within their own homes and communities.

Health visitors usually work within heath visiting teams that comprise staff of different levels of knowledge, interests, and expertise. Health visitors also work in partnership, and across a wide number of other teams and agencies. These may include education, social services, acute and specialist health teams. Most health visitors also work closely with midwives in preparing parents for the birth of their children.

> ### Areas in which health visitors may support families with young children
>
> - Child growth and development
> - Recognition and management of common infections
> - Managing teething, sleeping, eating, toilet training, anger or behaviours that parents find challenging
> - Breastfeeding, weaning, healthy eating
> - Safeguarding children
> - Home safety
> - Postnatal depression
> - Child or family bereavement
> - Domestic violence.
>
> ### Health visitors support families with young children by:
>
> - Home visiting
> - Coordinating local child immunization programmes
> - Organizing and running baby clinics
> - In some areas they deliver portage (child development) programmes in partnership with families
> - Running health promotion groups e.g. breast feeding, parent support, parenting courses, home safety courses
> - Non-medical prescribing.

Within the UK every family with a child under 5yrs has a named health visitor. Increasingly health visitors describe themselves as offering a whole family approach to their work. In reality, however, the way in which health visitors work, and the focus of their role, is extremely variable within, and across the UK. This variation may result from the need to prioritize locally to meet government targets e.g. immunization, child protection, health promotion initiatives.

Health visiting and people with intellectual disabilities

Health visitors work with and support all families with children, including those with ID, based on their assessed individual needs. The health visitor is often the professional that detects an early delay in child development, referring the child on for specialist assessment and support. In these situations, child and family support is usually offered by the health visitor, in partnership with interdisciplinary children's disability teams, and they often work closely with school nurses, social workers, and community paediatricians. This support may continue after the child reaches school age, but has usually finished by the time the child is 14yrs, the age that planning for child transition to adult services usually starts. For many families the child will become the responsibility of the school nursing services by their 5th birthday.

Increasingly people with ID are becoming parents themselves. The need for health visitors to develop expertise in working with parents with ID has been highlighted.[1] The need for health visitor training in this area has been requested, along with the need to develop policies across community care services to define the parenting support role to this population.

Further reading

Community Practitioner and Health Visitor Association
http://www.amicus-cphva.org/

Sines D, Appleby F, Frost M (2005). *Community Healthcare Nursing*, 3rd Edn. Blackwell Science: London.

---

1 DH/DfHS (2007). *Good Practice Guidance on Working with Parents with a Learning Disability*. Department of Health: London.

District nurses

District nurses are a UK wide resource; within the Republic of Ireland this role is undertaken by public health nurses. Working predominantly with people within their own homes, they are central to the care of people with acute conditions, and chronic diseases, and the provision of palliative care within their own homes and other community settings including residential homes and health centres. District nurses are usually based in GP practices or health centres, and have a key role in integrated delivery of care, working in partnership with a range of different agencies.

Education

District nurses are usually registered nurses, having completed a 3yr training in the adult branch of nursing, gaining the qualification of registered general nurse (RN Adult/RGN) or earlier equivalent (SRN). An increasing number of district nurses have also completed a post-registration degree level course in district nursing. In addition they may have attended many other condition-specific courses equipping them with the skills to manage a wide variety of different nursing needs. Specific additional training courses may include, care assessment and coordination, nurse prescribing, chronic disease management (e.g. COAD, asthma, diabetes, stroke care), care of the dying, and Doppler training (assessment and training of leg ulcer care).

What are the key principles of district nursing?

- To provide a high-quality service to people in their own homes
- To promote and maintain independent living
- To facilitate and ensure a coordinated approach
  to hospital discharge and subsequent care in the community
- To reduce hospital admission and readmission rates by supporting parents and carers at an early stage of ill health
- To operate a public health, preventative, healthy lifestyle approach
- To operate an evidence-based approach to clinical practice
- To promote user involvement in service planning
  and evaluation.

Delivering services

District nurses are based predominantly in health centres, and within geographical boundaries of GPs, with whom they share a common patient population. District nurses visit people within their own homes, including residential care homes, or provide services in health centres. In their nursing role they provide direct care to patients, as well as supporting family members, or paid carers in their caring roles.

Most district nurses work as members of a district nursing team. These teams comprise a number of qualified healthcare/nursing assistants that work a range of different hours, covering a 24hr period. Many localities also have district nurses working within more acute services such as intermediate care teams and 'hospital from home' type services that seek to prevent hospital admission or support earlier discharge.

District nursing teams are also often members of wider integrated care teams. These teams work across professional boundaries, preventing duplication of roles, promoting the need for good communication and partnership working. Membership of integrated teams is wide and may include:
- GPs
- Health visitors
- Practice nurses
- Care home staff
- Allied health professionals (e.g. physiotherapists, occupational therapists, podiatrists)
- Social workers
- Community mental health nurses
- Community ID nurses.

District nurses and people with intellectual disabilities

District nurses will meet people with ID in their working roles, but they may not have training in the specific health needs of the population, or the knowledge of local service provision. This is an area of work where nurses in ID teams should use their knowledge and skills to work collaboratively with district nurses to meet the healthcare needs of people with ID.

District nurses may develop and support healthcare for people with ID in the following ways:
- Identify patients with ID on home visits to other family members. Check and ensure they are included on practice ID registers and any practice health checks
- Offer and deliver health screening/health checks for patients with ID who will not attend GP visits
- Identify unmet needs of patients with ID and refer to specialist ID services for intervention
- Identify older family carers. Refer on to social services for carers assessment, or to access carer's support
- Assist people with ID to understand and take control of their healthcare, by teaching them about their physical condition using accessible information.

Further reading

Barrett A, Latham D, Levermore J (2007). Defining the unique role of the specialist district nurse practitioner. *British Journal of Community Nursing* **12**(10), 442–448.

Sines D, Appleby F, Frost M (2005). *Community Healthcare Nursing*, 3rd Edn. Blackwell Science: London.

Community children's nurses

Community children's nurses (CCNs) work with children of all ages, who have a wide range of complex health conditions, and who are living at home. Their main role is to enable sick children with acute and chronic illnesses or disabilities to remain in their home or familiar environment. The delivery of nursing care to children at home, or in nurseries and schools, often enables children to remain within their families, to continue to attend normal daytime activities and reduce the disruption to routine of everyday family life. CCNs are employed and funded by a range of different organizations, including children's integrated trusts, charitable trusts, and primary and acute NHS trusts. CCNs usually work as specialist services in support of other services helping children with complex physical healthcare needs, and therefore do not work with all children.

There is considerable variation in the services provided by CCNs, influenced by factors such as:

- A different picture of children's needs across geographical localities
- Local service priorities and funding
- Varied skills and resources including hospital provision and access to nurse training.

Education

Qualified CCNs are generally registered children's nurses, having the RN (Children's) or former qualifications such as RSCN (Registered Sick Children's Nurse) qualification, with an additional community nursing qualification. Children's nurses may also have qualifications in other branches of nursing, health visiting or midwifery, as well as clinical skills or specific condition management training. Qualified CCNs often work in mixed skill teams, which may include nurses with a range of different skills and levels of experience. This may include CCN assistants.

Role in practice

Key roles of community children's nurses

- Long-term support for children with complex health needs
- Support and care for children requiring palliative and terminal care
- Support and care for children with cancer
- Support for children that are tube fed or require intravenous therapy
- Wound management, including at times removal of stitches and staples
- Management of children, and educating carers on severe allergy
- Care of children on home traction, including escort support
- Management and support for children with chronic skin conditions
- Management and monitoring of chronic disease e.g. diabetes, epilepsy, cystic fibrosis, muscular dystrophy
- Management and support of chronic medical conditions e.g. constipation, Crohn's disease
- Provision of specialist equipment and supplies for home care
- Monitoring of medication and adjusting as required
- Child protection.

CCNs generally work as members of teams. They may work from either hospital or community office bases. Much of their role requires liaison with other agencies:

- GPs, paediatricians, consultants, and other doctors
- Health visitors, school nurses, community ID nurses, and community psychiatric nurses
- Dietitians, physiotherapists, and occupational therapists
- Social workers and home care staff
- Specialist hospital and hospices, including any outreach workers
- Home support workers, who may be supervised by them.

In addition they work in close partnership with parents, carers, and siblings in the provision of education, information, and support.

Policies on referral for treatment by CCNs vary in different areas. These usually include anything from a medical only referral ranging to an open referral process. Parent's consent is usually required before a referral is accepted.

CCNs and children with intellectual disabilities

CCNs are often directly involved in the care of children with ID, who have complex physical healthcare needs. To deliver a coordinated approach to treatment and prevent duplication, CCNs often work in close partnership with ID nurses. A strong focus of their role is on promoting and supporting independence, although they also work closely with families. Effective collaborative working is essential in order to provide effective services, and coordinated support and advice to children and their families.

Further reading

Royal College of Nursing (2000). *Children's Community Nursing. Promoting Eeffective Teamworking.* RCN: London.

Sines D, Appleby F, Frost M (2005). *Community Healthcare Nursing*, 3rd Edn. Blackwell Science: London.

School nurses

The health of children in schools is a high government priority in all countries of the UK, with the focus of all school healthcare being to improve the health of all school-age children.

The key health concerns regarding school children

- Exercise
- Obesity
- Healthy eating
- Emotional health and well-being
- Sexual health
- Smoking
- Drugs and alcohol
- Immunization status
- Home and community safety
- Child safety.

Education

School nurses are registered nurses who have completed nurse education in the general, children's, mental health, or ID areas of nursing. In addition some of them may have completed a post-basic registration specialist practitioner nursing qualification.

School nursing role

Since the development of the school nursing service in 1908, the role has changed considerably. Periodic medical inspections have mostly been replaced by a health promotion focus to the role, with less emphasis on routine medical examination, although medical inspections are often still provided for children with complex health needs, and for children at risk. All schools have a named school nurse and medical officer linked with every school or a group of schools.

A number of different approaches exist to address school healthcare. Central to these is the role of the school nurse and the wider school healthcare team. This team may include community medical officers and community dental services. The school nurse role is gradually changing from that of individual child screening and child health monitor to that of a school public health practitioner. The focus of the role, however, can vary considerably to meet the above priorities across different parts of the country. School nurses may also have a clinical role to meet the different and enhanced needs of children with physical impairments and mental health difficulties.

What are the key roles of a school nurse?

- Supporting children with medical needs such as asthma, diabetes, epilepsy, mental health issues
- Clinical interventions such as gastrostomy feeds, catheter care
- Administration of immunizations and prescribed medication
- Training school staff on the management of health conditions
- Carrying out preschool developmental screening
- Promotion of healthy living, including sex education
- Team working within the schools to help develop health protocols
- Assessment of the school health needs/school health profile
- Responding to health inequalities
- Working across sectors to address wider threats to health e.g. crime reduction, housing, transport
- Working with parents and carers in the meeting of health needs
- Children protection.

In addition there are a number of whole school approaches to health. These include the National Healthy Schools Programmes in England, and the Healthy Schools Programme in Wales and Northern Ireland.

The key aims of healthy schools programmes

- To support children and young people in developing healthy behaviours
- To help raise pupil achievement
- To help to reduce health inequalities
- To help promote social inclusion.

School healthcare, and children and young people with intellectual disabilities

School nurses and community nurses for people with ID should work in partnership when planning the children's transition to adult services, and there should be good, clear communication between children and adult services. Planning for adult services, which are significantly different to childrens services, can commence anytime after the age of 14years. A good HAP, to which any nurses working with the child should contribute, will help direct adult services to meet identified needs.

Further reading

Sines D, Appleby F, Frost M (2005). *Community Healthcare Nursing*, 3rd Edn. Blackwell Science: London.

Midwives

Midwives support women and their partners through the period of pregnancy, labour, and the early postnatal period. Midwives work within hospital and community settings, meeting the individual needs of women, their partners, and babies.

Education

Midwifery training takes 3yrs. It requires education at university to degree level, with a variety of placements within hospitals and community settings. Within their training, midwives have to work with and support women throughout the process of pregnancy. This includes caring for newly pregnant women, monitoring the woman and her baby throughout pregnancy, preparing them for childbirth, delivering babies, and caring for mothers and their babies in the newborn stage, known as the postnatal period.

Midwives may have followed a direct entry route or have previously been a registered nurse. Men or women can apply to start training. Midwives have to register with the Nursing and Midwifery Council on the midwifery register, before they can practice.

Midwives are currently in short supply, so there is an increasing number of spaces for training available. There are also a number of incentives to try to encourage nonpractising midwives to return to the role.

Role in practice

Midwives are, in general, employed by NHS trusts; however, small numbers of midwives practice independently. NHS midwives offer free maternity care. Independent midwives usually charge for their services. Midwives work across hospital and community settings.

Midwifery services are accessed by registration with a GP. Midwives are generally GP attached, therefore, as with other GP attached staff, cover a geographical locality. Midwives frequently work across a number of different GP practices, therefore may work from a central health base, children's center, or hospital. There is no national uniformity of base. Midwives are, however, expected to work across professional boundaries and in partnership with other staff working with the woman. Other staff may include social workers, physiotherapists, health visitors, GPs, children's centre staff, or specialist nurses, including community ID nurses. A teamworking approach is provided to ensure women, their partners, and babies, receive care based on individual need.

Where possible, midwives offer a named midwifery service, to help promote consistency of care. Midwives meet with women, and their partners, at regular intervals throughout pregnancy. Women carry and look after their own maternity records, to aid accurate communication, for all working with the woman.

Midwives visit women and babies within a range of environments. All new mothers and babies are visited by midwives in their own homes, on the day after discharge from hospital, or after birth. Regular home visits will continue by the midwife, where necessary, for up to 28 days after birth, or until discharged by the midwife, to the care of a health visitor.

Midwives and people with intellectual disabilities

Midwives may need to address issues relating to ID, in a number of significant areas.

What issues may midwives encounter relating to intellectual disabilities?

- Discussion and support regarding prenatal antenatal screening or testing scanning that might identify a baby with a condition associated with ID
- Breaking the news and helping parents interpret and come to terms with the result that their newborn baby has a condition associated with an ID
- Supporting a woman with an ID, and her partner, throughout the pregnancy, labour and early postnatal period.

The manner and skill in which news regarding ID is shared with parents is crucial. In addressing the above issues, midwives require a good understanding of a number of issues. These include the ethics of scanning, knowledge on the range of scanning methods available, and the efficacy of the results. In addition, they need to know where to access current knowledge on the range of conditions associated with ID, and contact details of parental support services for particular conditions. Effective counselling skills are also required.

Government strategies promote the requirement that all parents should access locally primary and acute service provision. Parents with ID may require the same, different, or increased service provision, to get their needs met. A number of issues have been identified to help midwives meet the needs of parents with ID.[1] These include, to:

- have local policies, protocols and guidelines in place for working with parents with ID
- identify the ID at an early stage, refer to, and work in partnership with staff in the local CLDT
- complete an early and thorough assessment
- ensure all information is clear, is in an accessible format and consistent
- use models, videos, and pictures when available
- allow longer times for appointments
- offer consistency of midwife and other support personnel.

Further reading

Royal College of Nursing (2008). *Pregnancy and Disability. A Guide for Nurses and Midwives*. RCN: London.

1 Williams L (2006). Learning Disability and Parenting. *MIDIRS Midwifery Digest*, **16**(3), 315–317.

Maternity services

Maternity services are an important part of the range of health services available to members of the general public, and are located within primary care, in health centres and GP services, and within maternity units linked to general hospitals.

Maternity services are provided by GPs, midwives (see 📖 p.344), and obstetricians, and may also include ultrasonographers (who undertake ultrasound scans). In a small number of services, the care of mothers and their partners may be provided by midwives, when it is anticipated that the pregnancy and birth will be uncomplicated; these units are sometimes referred to as 'midwifery-led units'. Health visitors often have a role to play in supporting new parents, and usually meet with prospective parents during antenatal preparation.

Supporting inclusive maternity care

Recognizing the desire for parenthood

It is now recognized that some people with ID wish to be parents, and therefore will require access to maternity services. People with ID, as prospective mothers and fathers, should have equity of access to maternity services.

Supporting consent to examination, treatment and care

During contact with maternity services, prospective parents will be provided with a lot of new and unfamiliar information and choices, on things ranging from choices of antenatal screening, various examinations that may be necessary, and their plans for the birth of the child. Nurses within ID services would work collaboratively with their colleagues in maternity services to facilitate informed decision making, and to ensure that the requirements for consent to examination, treatment, and care are fulfilled (see 📖 Consent to treatment, p.260, and 📖 Vulnerability, p.266).

Developing agreed communication links

Nurses within ID services can have an integral role in supporting people with ID in accessing services, through providing information about local services, and encouraging people to consider their needs for antenatal care and education (see 📖 Parenting groups, p.348). They should also develop clear communication links with midwives in their local services, and work collaboratively with them to support people with ID in making effective use of local maternity services.

Within each locality, identified nurses from within ID services could become the link to a designated midwife within maternity services. They could meet on a regular basis, once every 2–3mths, to discuss the strengths each of them and their respective colleagues could bring to supporting women and men using maternity services.

Developing accessible information

Nurses and midwives could share examples of good practice, such as accessible information, and revised protocols that are effective in making services accessible for people with ID can be identified and shared across ID and maternity services (see 📖 Providing information, p.62). It is important to remember when developing accessible information that this may also be useful with other people who have difficulty in understanding written English.

Establishing recognized links between local ID and maternity services will also provide a clear point of contact if any concerns or emergencies involving people with ID arise within maternity services.

The suggestion of links between designated people within ID and maternity services is not to support a designated midwife for people within ID who are expecting a baby, as this may place unnecessary restrictions on the choice of midwife; rather it is to support the development of nurses and midwives could be resource people for other professionals within the services which are seeking to support people with intellectual disabilities.

A balanced approach

It is important that a person's choice to have a baby is respected; however, if there are any indications that an assault, abuse or exploitation has occurred these should be discussed openly with the person, and considered within local policy guidelines under the protection of vulnerable adults.

While some people seek to become pregnant, nurses within ID services, as well as midwives and health visitors, should also be alert to the risk of exploitation and abuse of women with ID that would result in a pregnancy. Staff should also remain alert to the possibility of the exploitation or abuse of men with ID by women who wish to become pregnant. Therefore, it is important to engage in discussions with women and men with ID who are about to become parents.

Irrespective of the origins of the pregnancy, if the woman's decision with capacity is to continue with the pregnancy, they will need to have supported access to maternity services.

Further reading

Parents with intellectual disabilities:
🔲 www.intellectualdisability.info/lifestages/ds_parent.htm

Parenting groups

For most parents with ID, parenting is a struggle, and is made all the more difficult by social and economic pressures that are known to undermine the coping abilities even of non-disabled parents. Attitudes have changed in recent years; however, becoming a parent if you have an ID is not easy. People with ID are more likely to be parenting with limited support from family and friends, but with extensive involvement from statutory services. Without support within the early days of parenting and for a sustained period of time, it is unlikely that the child will be able to remain with a parent who has ID.

What can help parents with intellectual disabilities?

Training and adequate social support through family, friends, and initiatives such as Sure Start, makes it more likely that parents will succeed, but often this involves agencies and services working very closely together as few agencies have the skills and long-term finances to support families where the parent has ID. Parents are more likely to succeed if services work with a person's individual strengths, rather than their inadequacies as a new parent. Research shows that families need support from the time the baby is born for a number of years, with extra support again at specific times, e.g. during toddler years, going to school, puberty, and adolescence.

Parenting groups

These are groups that are set up to support new mums and dads with all aspects of parenting. Sometimes these can be led by health visitors or by working in partnership with specialist ID services, with involvement from an ID nurse or psychologist.

What will the groups talk about?
- What it is like to be a parent
- How to keep your child healthy
- What to do if your child becomes ill
- How to keep your child safe
- Helping your child develop
- Managing difficult behaviours
- Other issues initiated from concerns raised by parents.

The groups will also provide the opportunity for parents to talk and learn from each other and make friendships. These groups can provide ongoing support to people to review skills learnt, and to support the maintenance of skills in the longer term.

Evidence from research shows that parenting is more successful using a combination of methods—group work alongside individual work within people's homes, showing people how to perform tasks with time to practice new skills in a supportive environment.[1]

The groups can support parents to learn together from each other as well as from the health visitor or ID nurse. It is vital that the facilitators of the parenting group are skilled in working with people with ID, and are able to adapt to the individual ID of people within the group. It is important that the facilitators of the group are able to develop trusting relationship, whereby parents feel safe to ask questions and seek support when they need it without fear of reprisals, e.g. their children being taken into care.

Further reading

Kent A (1999). Helping parents with learning disabilities to parent. *Florence Nightingale Study Tour*, report available from Florence Nightingale Foundation. 🖥 http://www.florence-nightingale-foundation.org.uk/

Tymchuk A (2000). *Nurturing Program For Parents With Special Learning Needs And Their Children.* Family Development Resources: Park City, UT.

Department of Health (2007). *Good practice guidance on working with parents wit a learning disability.* Department of Health: London. 🖥 www.dh.gov.uk/en/publicationsandstatistics/publications/publicationspolicyandguidance/DH_075119

1 McGaw S (2000). *What Works for Parents with Learning Disabilities.* Available from 🖥 http://www.barnardos.org.uk/wwparwld.pdf

Dentists

Oral and dental health are important aspects of general health. The knowledge that your teeth are straight and functional, having the ability to smile, chew, and talk, without pain, can all contribute greatly to feelings of well-being. Dentists are health professionals who specialize in the diagnosis and treatment of a range of problems that affect the mouth and teeth. Good oral health can contribute to good general health, dignity, self-esteem, social integration, and increased quality of life.

Education

The preparation of dentists is spread over 5yrs, and results in BDS or BChD. The training process consists of academic, theoretical, and practical training in all aspects of dental care. A wide range of postgraduate courses in specialist areas are also available. Dentists have to register with their professional body (in the UK this is the General Dental Council) before starting to practice.

Role of the dentist

A substantial focus of the dentist's role is in oral health promotion of the general public, in addition to dental treatment and surgery. A significant element of their role in dental care is preventing and treating dental and oral disease, correcting dental irregularities, and treating dental and facial injuries. People with ID are most likely to see dentists in NHS services, including family practices, community dental services, and hospital departments.

Oral health and people with intellectual disabilities

People with ID experience higher rates of dental disease than the general population. Good oral care is generally based on an individual's physical, mental, and cognitive ability to carry out effective oral hygiene, make informed choices about healthy eating, and to seek and comply with dental treatment. People with ID are seriously disadvantaged in some, or all of these areas, with multiple barriers in their access to oral care.

Potential barriers in access to good oral care for people with intellectual disabilities

- A lack of perceived need for good oral care or an inability to express the need for treatment
- A lack of awareness or ability in self-care
- An increased range of oral and facial development abnormalities
- Increased drooling, tooth grinding and dry mouth; dry mouth is sometimes linked to the side effects of medication
- An increased need for high-energy food supplements and sugar based liquid medication, leading to oral erosion
- Reduced access to oral health education and dietary advice
- Established fear and anxiety
- Reduced physical access to dental clinics
- Reduced choice in the range of dental services
- Lack of dental staff training in ID.

Recommendations for improving oral care for people with intellectual disabilities

A number of recommendations have been made in response to meeting the oral health needs of people with ID. These include the need for dentists and other dental team members, specialist health professionals, carers, and people with ID to share the responsibility for improving oral healthcare.

- Dentists need to identify and assess the needs of their patients with ID. Patients at high risk, or with active dental disease, should be seen at 3-monthly intervals. Persons with low risk should be seen 6-monthly.
- Education and behavioural interventions that ensure appropriate diet and daily routines of good oral hygiene, should be promoted and taught to people with ID, including carers, when necessary. Meeting oral healthcare needs should be considered for children within school medical assessments, and with adults in HAPs.
- Preventative therapies, including use of fluoride toothpaste or antimicrobiological agents, should be implemented, where indicated.
- NHS organizations, including dental commissioners, working with interdisciplinary ID staff teams, should facilitate training for all dental staff on working with people with ID. Placements for dental students within ID community settings should be developed.
- General oral advice sheets, covering a healthy diet, oral hygiene, and visiting the dentist, should be made available in an accessible format. A local strategy should be agreed across organizations on how these will be promoted actively and disseminated to all high-risk groups.

Further reading

The Royal College of Surgeons (2001). *Clinical Guidelines and Integrated Care Pathways for the Oral Health Care of People with Learning Disabilities.* Royal College of Surgeons: London.

Davies R, Raman B, Scully C (2000). Oral health care of people with special needs. *British Medical Journal* **321**, 495–498.

British Dental Health Foundation 🖳 www.dentalhealth.org.uk

British Dental Health Foundation. *Dental care for people with special needs.* 🖳 http://www.library. nhs.uk/oralhealth/ViewResource.aspx?resID=87622

Podiatrist

Registered podiatrists are also known in some services as chiropodists. Podiatrists are trained in the assessment, diagnosis, and treatment of the feet and lower limbs. They also offer advice on the prevention of foot problems and the management of sports injuries. They perform nail surgery and teach people how to care for feet. Podiatrists work from a number of different resource bases, including local health centres, general hospitals, health clubs, shops, and private hospitals. They also go out and visit patients in a range of different environments, including day centres, special schools, residential, nursing, and family homes, and sometimes work on their own, as members of interdisciplinary health teams or as members of skill-mixed foot care teams. Other team members include podiatry assistants and orthotic technicians. Podiatry chiropody services delivered through the NHS are free of charge, and are targeted at people with the perceived greatest risk of foot health problems. A high percentage of the general population pay for private chiropody treatment.

Education

Podiatrists become qualified after the completion of a Bachelors degree. As with all other health professionals allied to medicine in the UK, they have to be registered with the HPC before working in practice.

Key health priorities in foot care for podiatry services

- Treatment for older people with deteriorating health
- People with diabetes
- People with osteoarthritis
- People with rheumatoid arthritis
- Post surgical care
- Neurological conditions
- Immune deficiency
- Terminal illness
- Septic lesions and cellulitis
- Vascular conditions/heart disease
- Severe foot deformities
- Ingrowing toe nails
- People with severe physical or intellectual disabilities.

Podiatry and people with intellectual disabilities

Little research has been completed on foot health and people with ID. However, people with ID are known to experience greater health conditions that may require particular care of their feet. The number of people with ID with these conditions that receive chiropody support will be variable across the country. The fear of having a person work on one's feet and not fully understanding the rationale, particularly if discomfort is involved (even to reduce longer term pain) may be an additional challenge in providing foot care to people with ID, and may need to be actively addressed within HAPs.

There are a number of additional factors that may warrant additional monitoring in relation to foot care for people with ID, including:

- Limited ability in foot self care, including the cutting of toenails
- Limited ability of older family carers in providing foot care

- Difficulties in communicating foot pain, other foot abnormalities or infection
- Reduced detection rates of long-term health conditions, associated with a need for foot care
- Fear and anxiety related to medical appointments
- Non-attendance at medical appointments due to barriers to access
- Challenging behaviour or limited concordance with foot care or medical appointments
- The wearing of poorly fitting shoes
- Changes in mobility may relate to foot problems, rather than injury.

Nurses working with people with ID have a part to play in monitoring foot care. As a number of people have difficulties in self-reporting of foot problems, early signs may be seen to indicate a need for support. Regular preventative foot care should be promoted, where available with a chiropodist. Local protocols on the cutting of toenails, including the care of people with diabetes, should be developed and implemented at a local level.

Further reading

Mencap factsheets on foot care and people with a learning disability available from
🖳 http://www.mencap.org.uk/

Audiologist

National studies suggest that ~16% of the general population experience a significant hearing loss, with people with ID found to have over twice this amount. Much hearing loss in the ID population goes unrecognized. This may be masked by self-injurious and other problematic behaviours, which arise from pain in the ear or difficulties in hearing. The role of an audiologist is to identify and assess hearing and/or balance disorders, recommending and providing appropriate rehabilitation and management.

Education

There are currently 3 ways to become an audiologist. These are to complete a BSc, an MSc, or a postgraduate diploma. A BSc in audiology, the most common route into the profession, is 4yrs in length, with the time being shared between university learning and clinical placements. Once qualified audiologists are eligible to apply for registration to practice with the Registration Council for Clinical Physiologists.

Roles in practice

Audiologists work predominantly in hospital settings, with adults and children. They generally work as members of interdisciplinary audiology teams. Referrals for assessment are usually made by GPs, or speech and language therapists. Audiology services vary in role and distribution across the country.

Key roles of audiologists

- Newborn and school hearing programmes
- Screening for speech, cognitive communication or other related disorders that may impact on education or communication
- Identification and assessment of activities that identify hearing or balance problems
- Assessment and interpretation of auditory problems including non-medical management of tinnitus (noises, such as ringing in the ear)
- Assessment and provision of balance rehabilitation therapy
- Preventative strategies, including prevention of hearing loss and protection of hearing function
- Assessment, selection, fitting, dispensing of hearing assistive technology, including hearing aids
- Identification and work with populations of high risk of hearing loss or other auditory dysfunction e.g. people with ID
- Conducting clinical examinations of the ear, using an auroscope
- Assessment regarding potential surgery
- Partnership working with speech and language therapists, school staff, parents and carers
- Participation in noise measurements of the acoustic environment
- Evaluation and management of children and adults with auditory related processing disorders
- Development of culturally appropriate hearing programme based interventions, including hearing aids, counselling, and referral for speech and language therapy
- Advocacy for the communication needs of all individuals.

Audiologists and people with intellectual disabilities

The provision of audiology services for people with ID is gaining in importance, due to increasing evidence recognizing the unmet hearing needs of the population. Audiologists are often a limited resource, and some areas have difficulty in accessing their local service. Specific roles of an audiologist in working with people with ID may include:

- Early detection of hearing loss
- Developing approaches for the collection of baseline hearing measurements
- Supporting young children and adults in the introduction wearing, regular evaluation and maintenance of hearing appliances, based on individual need
- Supporting paid and family carers in the wearing of hearing appliances
- Working in partnership with hearing, speech and language therapists in relation to managing and responding to the hearing needs of individuals.
- Conducting otoscopys (clinical examination of the ear, using an auroscope) to detect impacted ear wax, or other conditions that may be contributing to the cause of hearing loss
- Educating staff on the specific factors that might indicate hearing loss in people with ID e.g. ear poking, head banging, behaviour change or discharge from the ear.

Further reading

Timehin C, Timehin E (2004). Prevalence of hearing impairment in a community population of adults with learning disabilities: access to audiology and impact on behaviour. *British Journal of Learning Disabilities* **32**(3), 128–132.

Dietitian

Eating and drinking well have an important role to play for our general health and quality of life. Dietitians are qualified professionals, having completed either a BSc in Dietetics, or a similar postgraduate qualification. Dietitians translate scientific information about food into dietary advice, to enable people to make informed and practical choices about managing food and lifestyle, in managing both health and disease.

Dietitians work in a variety of ways. Within the NHS, they work in both hospital and community settings, directly with the general public in health promotion, in public health, and in acute and chronic disease management. They influence food and health policy across the spectrum, from government to local communities and individuals. Within the UK, the title dietitian can only be used by those who have registered with the HPC.

Dietitians and people with intellectual disabilities

Dietetic provision varies across the country. In a few areas there are specialist dietitians. More commonly people with ID will meet a dietitian from within a wider community primary care or hospital service. Further information on what is available can be obtained from the local health care provider, GP, or dietetic department.

Recent documents (see 📖 Further reading) have highlighted the importance of good dietary support for this population and their carers. As a result of awareness of the nutritional problems found in people with ID, there has recently been a call for an increased number of dietitians working directly with this population. Nutrition related health problems are more common in people with ID than in the general population, and those people who require enteral feeding or adapted diets require the support of a dietitian.

> **Most common nutrition related causes of ill health in people with intellectual disabilities**
>
> - Underweight and overweight
> - Swallowing difficulties
> - Gastro-oesophageal reflux
> - Diabetes
> - Bowel disorders including constipation
> - Dental disease
> - Hypertension
> - Diabetes
> - Coronary heart disease
> - Mental health conditions
> - Other long-term conditions, e.g. dementia, epilepsy.

Dietitians working with people with ID focus their work in a number of different ways, including:

- Addressing the need for local availability of appropriate and accessible resources
- Training on specific medical conditions, as well as wider food and health issues e.g. food and health provision
- Completing nutritional assessments, and giving dietetic advice and support to people with ID.

> **Conditions that should trigger a referral to a dietitian working with people with intellectual disabilities**
>
> - Persistent underweight
> - Persistent overweight
> - Eating and drinking problems
> - Specific medical conditions requiring complex nutritional intervention e.g. phenylketonuria, coeliac disease, diabetes
> - Chronic constipation
> - Use of enternal feeding.

A significant focus of the role of all dietitians is to promote guidelines on healthy eating. Healthy eating, however, is not only the responsibility of dietitians. Everybody working with people with ID should promote the following key messages and tips for a healthy diet as advised by the Food Standards Agency. The two keys to a healthy diet are, eating the right amount of food for how active you are and eating a range of foods to make sure you are getting a balanced diet.

FSA (2008) 8 tips for eating well

- Base your meals on starchy foods
- Eat lots of fruit and vegetables
- Eat more fish
- Cut down on saturated fat and sugar
- Try to eat less salt
- Get active and try to be a healthy weight
- Drink plenty of water
- Don't skip breakfast.

Further reading

National Patient Safety Agency (NPSA) (2004). *Understanding the Patient Safety Issues for People with Learning Disabilities*. NPSA: London.

Crawley H (2007). *Eating Well: Children and Aults with Learning Disabilities*. The Caroline Walker Trust.

British Dietetic Association 🖳 www.bda.uk.com

Food Standards Agency 🖳 www.food.gov.uk

Food Standards Agency. *Eat well, be well* 🖳 www.eatwell.gov.uk

Physiotherapy

Physiotherapists work with people of all ages, helping them manage physical problems caused by illness, accident, impairment, and ageing. At the core of their work is the belief that body movement is central to the health and wellbeing of all. A physiotherapist's role is focused on preventing loss of movement and optimizing the functional potential of individuals.

Training

Physiotherapy is a popular healthcare profession. Training programmes are available at a number of different universities across the country. Physiotherapy is a science-based degree, leading to a BSc, which takes either 3yrs or 4yrs to complete. In order to practise as a physiotherapist, all qualified staff must register with the HPC.

Over the course of their training all physiotherapists will have gained experience in a wide and diverse range of adult hospital settings. These may include orthopaedics, general medicine and surgery, neurology, cardiology, and respiratory care. Other placements available include paediatrics, maternity and women's health, mental health, or a variety of community settings, including primary care. In many courses, during their training physiotherapists will seldom have had a placement focussed specifically on working with people with ID. Many will graduate having had little information and knowledge of the needs and skills of working with this population.

After qualification, physiotherapists may rotate through different hospital or community placements, until choosing to work in a specialist area. Further training will be available to them relevant to this specialism. In this role physiotherapists are likely to work as members of profession specific teams; this may include colleagues with different skills and levels of experience, including physiotherapy assistants. Physiotherapists also often work in wider multidisciplinary teams.

The core skills of a physiotherapist

- Holistic movement assessment, incorporating psychological, cultural, and social influences
- Analysis of movement and function
- Manual therapies e.g. movement, massage, manipulation, electrical stimulation
- Therapeutic exercise e.g. hydrotherapy, group activities
- Assessment for aids and appliances
- Educating carers and staff in the techniques of moving and handling.

Physiotherapists are increasingly found working in primary care settings. This is due to the current focus in the provision of care outside hospital, and the flexible role of the GP in the commissioning and provision of services to meet the needs of local communities.

How do physiotherapists work?

- Health promotion activities e.g. sports groups
- Preventative approaches e.g. postural care
- Individual treatment
- Rehabilitation.

There is no common national model as to how physiotherapists are employed. They may be employed by GPs, primary care trusts, acute trusts or charities, or may be independent contractors. They may be based in any range of primary health, acute hospital, and social care settings. These include:

- GP surgeries
- Private medical practice
- Community hospitals
- Special schools
- Leisure and sports
- Industry.

They may treat people in any of these environments or, where indicated, in the family home.

Physiotherapists in primary care and people with intellectual disabilities

People with ID experience many of the same conditions requiring physiotherapy as the general population. They use the same hospitals, hospital discharge teams, and health centres, and therefore may have access to the same hospital and community healthcare services. When physiotherapy is required, people with ID are frequently, and successfully, treated by the generic teams.

Specialist ID physiotherapists are a limited resource and may not always be available within specialist services, and they work closely with their physiotherapy colleagues in other services. They may refer people to generic services, helping the person access generic services and then help to support the staff in knowing the best ways to communicate and treat the person, in relation to their ID. Referral from the generic service to the ID service should be needed only where there are specific indications for a specialist service, such as communication difficulties, complex physical impairment, behaviour that challenges generic service delivery, specialist individual needs, in conjunction with an ID.

Further reading

Hodges C (2005). Getting to grips with learning disabilities. *Frontline* **June 15**, 21–23.

Occupational therapy

Occupational therapists (OTs) work with all age groups of people, in hospitals and across community settings. Their clinical role is based on the assessment and treatment of physical and psychiatric conditions. Through the use of specific purposeful activity they work to prevent disability and promote independent function, by addressing work and other aspects of daily life. Some occupational therapists may also undertake a close partnership with housing departments and social services in the provision of aids and adaptations to houses, where changes, such as a downstairs bathroom, are required, as a result of changes to a person's health and their ability to use household facilities.

In what areas do occupational therapists work?

- Mental health services
- Intellectual disability services
- Physical disability services
- Primary care
- Children's services
- Older peoples services
- Rheumatology
- Care management
- Environmental adaptation
- Equipment for daily living.

Education

OTs now undertake a 3yr (or 4yr in Scotland) degree. It can also be completed in 2yrs as a postgraduate qualification. All OTs must register with the HPC prior to practice. Throughout their education OTs complete a number of different placements, in a range of specialist areas. This might include ID; however, many OTs complete their education without having the opportunity to work in this area, and start to specialize after they qualify.

Role in practice

OTs in primary care often work as members of the primary care team. In some areas primary care OTs are an integral part of joint rehabilitation teams. These are joint teams set up to coordinate work between primary care trusts and social services. These teams, led by social services, are usually responsible for providing the equipment, or any adaptations required, to enable someone to live at home. They also increasingly work in teams that focus on community care, or care provision outside of hospital. OTs work with people that have injuries, illness, or disabilities on programmes of treatment based on an individual's lifestyle, environment and personal choices. An assessment of need may be done in the home, a community setting, or in hospital before discharge.

OTs may work with individuals for variable periods of time, depending on the need identified. Referrals to the service are usually made by other medical professionals. In some parts of the country OTs are increasing in number whereas in others they are becoming an extremely limited resource.

What is the role of an occupational therapist working in primary care?

- Rehabilitation after amputation injury or illness e.g. after a stroke or accident
- Rheumatology e.g. management of joint care in arthritis
- Falls prevention in vulnerable older people, promoting home safety
- Assessment and provision of aids and equipment, to facilitate independence or to support carers in their caring role
- Assessment of the home, developing designs for housing adaptation
- Provision of treatment e.g. in running limb rehabilitation clinics after injury, offering hand exercises, splinting, pain management
- Maintaining activities of daily living skills when living with a debilitating health condition e.g. multiple sclerosis
- Assessment of a person's work environment, to assess any aids required to facilitate a return to work
- Referrals for people who will need to use a wheelchair
- At times involvement in interventions related to behaviour management.

Occupational therapists and people with intellectual disabilities

OTs in primary care do not always have the communication skills or training in working with people with ID. Likewise OTs in ID services may not have the specialist skills required in primary care. Within adult services it is common practice for OTs in community ID teams to support primary care OTs in any rehabilitation work. This enables the sharing of skills to enable the individual to receive the best service. Where a person with ID has very limited communication or behaviour that challenges, the OTs in ID services may take a lead in the work. Children's disability teams based in either hospital or community settings usually have an OT working as a member of the team.

Further reading

(2008). The Occupational Therapy News **16**(9). This whole journal issue is focussed on OT services for people with learning disabilities.

Herge EA (2003) Beyond the basics to participation: occupational therapy for adults with developmental disabilities. *OT Practice*, **8**(21) CE-1-CE-8.

Lillywhite A, Alwal A (2003) Occupational therapists' perceptions of the role of community learning disability teams. *British Journal of Learning Disabilities*, **31**(3), 130–135.

Mountain G (1998) *Occupational Therapy for people with learning disabilities living in the community: a review of the literature.* London: Royal College of Occupational Therapists.

Optical care

Regular assessment of vision and good care of the eyes is essential for good health and well-being. Having a regular eye test does not just tell you how short or long sighted you are. It can also reveal eye conditions that might lead to loss of vision (e.g. glaucoma). In addition an eye test can detect evidence of general poor health or the existence of a previously undiagnosed health condition (e.g. diabetes).

The regularity of eye tests varies with age. Children are recommended to attend for an eye test 2-yearly, or more frequently as recommended by an optometrist. Adults are recommended to have regular eye tests from the age of 40yrs, the age when eyesight often starts to deteriorate, and the risk of cataracts and glaucoma is increased. Follow-up examinations should take place every 2yrs, or more frequently, as advised. People with ID should follow the same recommendations. If detected early the development of some eye diseases can be stopped or slowed down.

Eye tests are conducted by optometrists. Optometrists are also known as ophthalmic opticians, and have a different role to opticians. Optometrists work in private practice and for the NHS, in both hospital departments and primary care.

What is the role of optometrists?

- Conduct eye examinations to detect injury, disease, abnormality or defects
- Conduct eyesight tests
- Advise on eye care or visual problems
- Recognize abnormal eye conditions e.g. squints
- Prescribe corrective lenses
- Fit spectacles and contact lenses.

Education

A qualified optometrist has completed a 3yr training (4yrs in Scotland) and has obtained a university degree. On gaining the degree, an optometrist has to complete a year of salaried clinical experience with the NHS, and then pass a qualifying examination, before they can register with the General Optical Council. They are permitted to practice independently.

Role in practice

Optometrists work in private practice, or for the NHS, in both hospital departments and primary care. Optometrists work as members of eye care teams, other members include opticians, orthoptists, and ophthalmologists. Opticians are qualified to fit and adjust spectacles, some having an additional qualification to fit contact lenses and low vision appliances. Orthoptists are qualified to diagnose and work, nonsurgically, with people with eye problems. Based predominantly in hospital departments, orthoptists respond to GP, or other medical referrals, to carry out visual screening after stroke or head injury. Ophthalmologists provide services in hospitals and community settings and are specialists in diseases of the eye.

Optical care for people with intellectual disabilities

People with ID experience significant impairments of sight, much of it undetected, such as premature cataracts. In addition high levels of eye problems have been found in people with specific conditions, such as Down syndrome, progressive visual failure associated with Prader–Willi syndrome and people born prematurely, who may have received oxygen therapy, and in association with cerebral palsy.

In the planning and provision of optical care to people with ID, a proactive approach often needs to be taken. Only a small number of optometrists may have the knowledge and skills of working with the population.

What issues need to be considered in optical care for people with intellectual impairments?

- An inability to communicate eye pain or a change in visual function
- A range of behaviours, considered challenging e.g. eye poking, head banging, may indicate a visual problem
- Regular stumbling or falls may indicate a visual problem
- A lack of knowledge in the need for regular eye checks or where to go to get them carried out
- A fear of medical appointments and the use of unfamiliar optical procedures
- An inability to provide medical information, to support optical assessments
- Fear or behaviours that makes the wearing of glasses difficult for individuals.

Best practice suggests that people with intellectual disabilities should be well prepared when going for optical assessment or treatment. A list of accessible resources and a preparation assessment form called *Telling the optometrist about me* are available from ▣ www.lookup.org

Further reading

Royal National Institute for the Blind ▣ www.rnib.org.uk

Community nurses mental health

Community nurses mental health (CNMH), previously known as community psychiatric nurses (CPN), play a significant role in the delivery of services to people with mental health problems living in the community. Working as members of primary care, community mental health teams, and hospital outreach teams, they have a number of different skills in order to treat, to assess, and to provide specific intervention to support people living with mental health conditions, either at home or other community settings. They may also work as mental health liaison nurses in accident and emergency departments.

Education

CNMHs have widely differing areas of skill and qualification. Most qualified nurses hold a Registered Nurse qualification in mental health, taken at either diploma or degree level. In addition, some nurses hold other nursing qualifications, e.g. in ID or general nursing. After qualification, mental health nurses may work in hospital or residential settings where they gain a range of skills and experience, before moving into a community setting. Some undertake a post-basic qualification in community nursing. The skills of a CNMH may include:

- CBT
- substance misuse
- forensic psychiatry
- psychotherapy
- counselling
- family therapy
- nurse prescribing
- group therapy
- child and adolescent psychiatry
- mental health and learning disabilities.

What support does a CNMH offer primary care teams?

- Working with the team to help in the provision of care of people who are to the most seriously ill
- Helping the team to develop skills in working with people who are the less seriously ill
- Developing realistic health promotion approaches
- Facilitating link between the community mental health team and the primary care team.
- Updating the team on changes in mental health treatments and strategy.

CNMHs work across services, and are required to have a number of key skills that are essential for both clinical patient care and team working. Community orientated primary care, including the role of CNMH, is the main driver for improvement of mental health services.

Key organizational skills of CNMHs

- Communication
- Self-management
- Team working
- Leadership
- Professional support and clinical supervision
- Accountability, at professional, managerial, and clinical levels
- Referrals and caseload management
- Management of resources
- Evidence based practice
- Risk assessment.

Key clinical skills of CNMHs

- Assessment of physical and mental health
- Development of therapeutic relationships
- Treatment e.g. medication, psychological interventions
- Formulation of treatment plans
- Clinical monitoring of health status
- Carer support
- Research and audit
- Health promotion
- CPA
- Key worker responsibilities—case management and coordination.

CNMHs and people with intellectual disabilities

People with ID experience increased rates of long-term mental health conditions to that of the general population. Current UK policies promote the need for mental health services for the general population to be accessible to adults with ID. In some areas this approach is well supported, with good joint working between ID and mental health services, enabling this to happen. Best practice is considered to be where there is clear local agreement between mental health and ID services at a local level about the commissioning and provision of services.

Further reading

Sines D, Appleby F, Frost M (2005). *Community Healthcare Nursing*, 3rd edn. Blackwell Science: London.

Foundation for People with Learning Disabilities (2004). *Green Light for Mental Health*. Foundation for People with Learning Disabilities: London.

Secondary care

People with ID experience the same range of health needs, though their experience of ill health associated with both acute and chronic illness is greater than in the general population. Given that the health profile of the ID population is different to that of the general population, it is evident that they will be higher users of secondary healthcare services, with an estimated 26%/yr of people with ID being admitted to general hospitals, compared with 16% of the general population.[1]

Access to secondary health services

While most people avail of a comprehensive health service, people with ID continue to experience inequity accessing all aspects of healthcare, including secondary care. Evidence nationally and internationally identifies the barriers that people with ID encounter accessing secondary health care, being associated with their difficulties with learning and communicating, the lack of knowledge of healthcare professionals on the nature of ID and their health needs, and negative attitudes of staff.[1,2] Consequently, access to secondary care remains a concern for people with ID and their families. Although it is improving, there is growing evidence that the barriers identified above can in fact increase the risks to the safety within this environment. The NPSA suggests that 'people with learning disabilities may be at more risk of things going wrong than the general population, leading to various degrees of harm being caused while in general hospitals'.[3]

Ensuring equity of access

Health is a right for all, and people with ID have the same needs and rights to access health services as the general population. The Scottish Executive,[4] Department of Health,[5] Welsh Assembly,[6] and Department of Health, Social Services and Public Safety[7] clearly recognize and emphasize the need for secondary health services to be accessible and nondiscriminatory, through the provision of support to people with ID, so that they can understand and avail of the treatment required. In addition the Disability Discrimination Act[8] outlines the responsibilities of public services to ensure equity, and within secondary healthcare this means taking account of the needs of people with ID, and making reasonable adjustments to meet those needs.

Enhancing support

Supporting people with ID within secondary care is the responsibility of all staff, and though it may seem challenging at times, it is not without solutions. Effective communication is essential for equity of access to health, which can be facilitated by putting in place the foundations that support opportunities for accurate navigation through the hospital, and the receipt of appropriate assessment, investigations, and treatment, to meet the needs of this client group within an inclusive framework. This includes:

- Awareness by all staff of the distinct needs of this population
- Staff having a common understanding, that people with ID have the right to be treated as an individual
- The identification and removal of physical barriers to enhance access
- Flexibility with appointments to suit individual's needs

- The use of straightforward signs to direct people where to go
- The development of information in a format that is easily understood, with additions of pictures and signs, which would enhance understanding and reduce anxieties
- Staff needing to feel competent using various communication strategies to support patients to understand and express their needs and choices
- Respecting the right of the individual (adult) with ID to be involved in and adequately informed to support their healthcare decisions
- Having awareness that some people with ID may carry a statement of healthcare preferences, and that this needs to be respected
- An appreciation of the role of the families/carers in supporting the care of the patient while in hospital, so that they are not expected to be the principal care givers
- Introducing those concerned to the liaison nurse (if any)
- Having an awareness and record of support services that are available within or outside the hospital
- Ensuring frequent and timely communication occurs with the people with ID and their families/carers in a format that is understood, to plan appointments, admissions, support while in hospital, and safe discharge.

Further reading

Mencap (1998). *NHS. Health for All*. Mencap: London.

Michael J (2008). *Healthcare for All: Report of the independent inquiry into access to healthcare for people with learning disabilities*. Department of Health: London. 🖵 www.iahpld.org.uk/

1 Mencap (2007). *Death by Indifference*. Mencap: London.

2 Iacono T, Davis R (2003). The experiences of people with developmental disability in Emergency Departments and hospital wards. *Research In Developmental Disabilities* **24**(4): 247–64.

3 National Patient Safety Agency (2004). *Understanding the Patient Safety Issues for People with Learning Disabilities*. National Health Service: London.

4 Scottish Executive (2000). *The Same As You. A Review of Services for People with Learning Dsabilities*. The Stationary Office: Edinburgh.

5 Department of Health (2001). *Valuing People: A New Strategy for Learning Disability for the 21st Century*. HMSO: London.

6 Welsh Assembly (2002). *Reference Guide for Consent to Examination and Treatment*. Welsh Assembly: Cardiff.

7 Department of Health, Social Services and Public Safety (2005). *Equal Lives: Review of Policy and Services for People with Learning Disabilities in Northern Ireland*. Stormont: Belfast.

8 Disability Discrimination Act (2005). HMSO: London.

General hospital services

General hospitals are an integral part of the structure of health service for all members of the population, including people with ID. These hospitals are required to provide equity of access to people with ID. Contact with general hospitals can range from outpatient appointments and day procedures for investigations, review or minor procedures, through to contact with accident and emergency departments, the need for major surgical intervention, and repeated lengthy admissions because of complex health needs.

Unfortunately, despite some innovative services to promote access to acute general hospitals, the consistent findings of inquiries and research projects over the past 10yrs has been that people with ID experience major difficulties in accessing and receiving high quality services within many general hospitals, at times resulting in their unnecessarily premature death.[1] The failure of acute hospitals to make 'reasonable adjustment' to meet the needs of people with ID could of itself be seen as unlawful discrimination, and leaves a service open to legal challenge under the Disability Discrimination legislation.

Challenges in achieving equity of access and outcome

Challenges, although often presented as difficulties arising from the presence of ID in a patient, can arise from three major areas:

- the presence of ID and the associated difficulties that may result in communicating directly with the patient for staff who are unfamiliar with the person
- difficulties in providing information about procedures
- confirming consent and gaining cooperation.

However, difficulties in communication cannot solely relate to the presence of ID, and are also influenced by the lack of skills among staff in communicating non-verbally, lack of confidence in working with people with ID, and stereotypical attitudes which presuppose people with ID will not be able to understand, give consent, or will be difficult to manage. The risk of 'diagnostic overshadowing' has been highlighted as a potential major factor in failing to recognize the need to treat physical health conditions. This occurs when changes in physical (or mental) health are considered to be part of the presence of ID, even though the signs and symptoms are not associated with ID. As a result of this error in judgment, the necessary investigations are not undertaken, the appropriate diagnosis is not made, or the necessary treatment commenced. In addition, appointment systems, as well as inflexible policy-driven systems and procedures that are unable to adjust to meet individual needs, can result in difficulties when seeking to plan for or respond to the differing abilities and needs of a person with ID.

Promoting access to a quality service within acute hospitals (see 🕮 Secondary care, p.366)

A number of practical actions can increase the likelihood of an improved quality of care for people when in contact with general hospitals:

- Listen to people who know the person with ID, if they say something is wrong, investigate the possibility seriously.
- Ensure that all people with ID who have a planned contact with/admission to the acute general hospital should have the opportunity to have

an assessment of the additional support they may need to ensure their appointment/admission is a success.

- Clarify how the person with ID communicates, and ensure the necessary arrangements are in place to promote effective communication (including staff training).
- Provide information to people with ID and parents/carers about what they can expect when in contact with general hospital services. This should include contact details for key staff in both services that may be able to organize additional support, if required.
- In the first instance, information should be provided directly to people with ID in a format accessible to them, and they should be given the necessary time to comprehend as much of this as is possible for them to promote informed decision making.
- When information needs to be shared, the right of people with ID to confidentiality should be respected.
- Maintain frequent contact with the person with ID to monitor for any improvement or potential deterioration their health.
- At all times, see the person first (not the ID), remain alert to the possibility of physical health problems, and actively guard against diagnostic overshadowing. If you use the presence of ID to explain changes in behaviour, physical signs, symptoms, or overall health changes, you are probably making a mistake.

Further reading

Mencap (2007). *Death by Indifference.* Mencap: London.

NHS Networks. *Access to Acute: a network for staff working with people with learning disabilities to support access to acute medical treatment.* http://www.networks.nhs.uk/networks/page/592

Royal College of Nursing (2006). *Meeting the Health Needs of People with Learning Disabilities: Guidance for Staff.* Royal College of Nursing: London.

1 Michael J (2008). *Healthcare for All: Report of the independent inquiry into access to healthcare for people with learning disabilities.* Department of Health: London. www.iahpld.org.uk/

Practice nurses

NHS policy changes have encouraged a shift from hospital-based care to community-based care, with procedures that were once only undertaken as an admission into hospital now being undertaken within the PHCT. Practice nurses work in a GP surgery as part of a PHCT supporting the local people with their healthcare. The PHCT consists of a range of professionals, such as doctors, practice nurses, health visitors, dietitians, and counsellors.

What do practice nurses do?
- Offer health screening and health promotion
- Offer family planning advice
- Run nurse-led clinics
- Offer immunizations
- Offer smear tests
- Take bloods
- Treat minor injuries
- Help with minor operations under anaesthetic.

What does this mean for people with intellectual disabilities?

We know that the life expectancy of people with ID has increased significantly in recent years, which in part has been due to the reduction in preventable illnesses and an increase in health promotion. However, the health inequalities faced by people with ID has increased, and it is important that services and agencies work together to meet a person's healthcare needs. It is more likely that a person should be seen more regularly in primary care, this could mean seeing the practice nurse for a health check or to have a blood test.

As an ID nurse, you should work closely with the practice nurse to ensure that the person with ID is able to receive the same care and treatments, and/or advice, that is offered to the general population.

What does primary care have to offer people with intellectual disabilities?

People with ID should be able to access primary care services and receive the same care and treatment that would be offered to the general population.

The legal framework

The Disability Discrimination Act (2005) and the Disability Equality Duty is now law within the UK, and services need to be able to prove, not that they treat people in the same way, but that they are taking all reasonable adjustments to their services to ensure that people with ID are able to access their services. National policy drivers from across the UK, all advocate that people with ID should be able to access mainstream services, yet it is known that primary care services do not always get it right for people.[1]

Who is responsible for the health of people with intellectual disabilities?

It is everyone's responsibility. It is important that all services work together to address the person's healthcare needs. This should be written into a person's HAP. The ID nurse should work together with the practice nurse, supporting the person to access primary care and the practice nurse where possible; this may involve desensitization work, and working to make information accessible in order for the person to understand the information (see 🕮 Developing accessible information, p.68).

Developing collaborative working with practice nurses

- Exchanging contact details with the practice nurse
- Making regular visits to the health centre, perhaps for coffee
- Undertaking joint clinics
- Taking opportunities to shadow each other in roles
- Providing opportunities for practice nurses to visit people with ID in other settings
- Providing information to practice nurses on working with people with ID, and meeting their key health needs[2]
- Attending events held by practice nurses and inviting them to ID events.

Further reading

DRC (2007). *Closing the Gap: One Year On*. Disability Rights Commission: London.

British Medical Association (2006). *Focus on the quality and outcomes framework* 🖵 www.bma.org.uk/ap.nsf/content.focusqoffeb06

NHS Working in Partnership Programme. *Practice Nurse Tool Kit* 🖵 www.wipp.nhs.uk/99.php

---

1 Disability Rights Commission (2006). *Closing the Gap*. Disability Rights Commission: London.

2 Disability Rights Commission (2006). *Equal Treatment: Closing the Gap. Learning Pack for Health Professionals*. Disability Rights Commission: London.

Outpatient clinics

Outpatient clinics see more patients each year than any other hospital departments, and people with ID are high users of this service from childhood throughout their life due to their health profile. Evidence shows that people with ID are living longer and they experience greater health needs than the general population, and this is particularly so with chronic illness.[1,2]

For many people, including people with ID, the experience of the outpatient clinic is either the beginning of a period of investigations and treatment, or the end stage of healthcare at that time, for the specific problem. However, regardless of the outcome of the outpatient appointment, people need to have the perception that their needs were recognized, understood, and addressed.

Yet, people with ID continue to experience difficulties accessing healthcare service. Within the outpatient clinics, the barriers are associated with issues such as inflexible appointments, long waiting times, lack of communication, overcrowded waiting areas, lack of resources such as lifting equipment, lack of knowledge and understanding of ID, and poor staff attitudes. All of these can increase a patient's experience of distress, and contributes to the risk of harm.[3] Evidence highlights that regardless of the length of time or purpose of stay, hospitalization can be very distressing for people with ID; however, there are opportunities to support people with ID during their experience with the outpatient clinic.

Supporting people in outpatient clinics

A number of measures have been suggested by Barr[4] and Wharton et al.[5] to support people with ID in outpatient clinics.

- Work collaboratively with the acute liaison nurse (ID) if one is located in the hospital.
- Preparation for the experience should begin before the patient arrives at outpatients; the referral letter could indicate any special requirements, e.g. difficulties waiting in crowded areas, or lifting equipment required. In addition, the appointment letter could ask for confirmation of any requirements.
- Flexible appointments, either the first or last appointment of the individual clinic, or the day, when there may be fewer people around.
- If clinics are overrunning, there should be an opportunity for individuals and their families to leave the outpatient department for some time out, to seek refreshments, or to go to another area, in order to reduce anxieties associated with long waiting times. Staff should agree a new time to return to the outpatient department, without having to remain in the department if the appointment is delayed.
- Extra time should be given during the appointment to facilitate effective communication.
- Sufficient space should be provided to facilitate wheelchairs, and to maintain privacy and dignity.
- Where possible, there should be an option of alternative waiting arrangements, for people who may be distressed on the day.
- There needs to be ongoing education of healthcare professionals on ID, and on ways to enhance communication.

- Any journeys to another area of the hospital may need to be escorted, and access to the area facilitated.
- Special requirements should be communicated to other healthcare professionals e.g. by nurse in outpatients to the radiographer in X-ray department, so that they are ready for the patient's arrival.
- All communication to the individual needs to be in a format that is understood, and any further investigations, treatment, and care explained fully in order to support decision making.
- Consent to examination, treatment, and care must be sought from the adult patient with ID. If there is doubt that the person can give valid consent, then their capacity must be assessed accurately. If the individual is found to lack capacity, the healthcare that had been prescribed, still needs to be given, based on 'best interests'.
- Healthcare professionals need to have a clear understanding of the current legislation and guidelines on consent and capacity, to support decision making.
- There are many ongoing initiatives and good practice to improve access and streamline the patient pathways within outpatient clinics, and staff should seek understanding of these, to support their efforts.

1 Barr O, Gilgunn J, Kane T, Moore G (1999). Health screening for people with learning disabilities by a community learning disability service in Northern Ireland. *Journal of Advanced Nursing* **29**(6): 1482–91.

2 Disability Rights Commission (2006). *Equal Treatment: Closing the Gap.* Disability Rights Commission: London.

3 National Patient Safety Agency (2004). *Understanding the Patient Safety Issues for People with Learning disabilities.* NHS: London.

4 Barr O (2004). *Promoting Access. The experience of children and adults with learning disabilities and their families/carers who had contact with acute general hospitals in the WHSSB Area and the views of nurses in these hospitals.* A Report to the Western Health and Social Services Board: Londonderry.

5 Wharton S, Hames A, Milner H (2004). The accessibility of general NHS services for children with disabilities. *Child: Care, Health & Development* **31**(3), 275–282.

Radiology departments

Radiology departments are usually located within district and major secondary hospitals. These departments can vary considerably in size and the services they provide. While all offer X-ray investigations, and this equipment may also be seen within some dental surgeries and larger health centres, some radiology departments also provide more detailed scanning investigations in the screening, diagnosis, or interventions to treat health conditions.

Radiography departments use X-rays or other scanning equipment to check on bony injuries, soft tissues, the presence of thrombosis (clots), the condition of internal organs and new growths (tumours), and foreign bodies (e.g. pica, coins). It is also possible to use X-rays to view other body organs by introducing a medium that is visible on the X-ray. Radiology equipment may also be used to provide a 'picture' to guide and check the successful location of delicate internal procedures e.g. the insertion of central venous lines. Some treatments for cancer involve the use of radiotherapy, where the area of the body in which a tumour is present receives a targeted exposure to radiation.

Reason why people with intellectual disabilities may use radiology departments

People with ID may have contact with staff in a radiology department for any of the reasons outlined above in order to check for an injury, the functioning of body organs, or to receive treatment. This is often a key step within the processes of diagnosis, and therefore any difficulty in gaining cooperation for such procedures may delay diagnosis, often resulting in prolonged discomfort and reducing the chances of success in any treatments.

Some people with ID, including people with epilepsy, people with complex physical health needs, and older people, may be more likely to have contact with X-ray departments as a result of accidents, ill health (in particular chest infections), or as part of on-going monitoring of their health status.

Preparing for contact with radiology departments

In emergencies, it is not always possible to undertake detailed preparation for contact with a radiology department; however, patients with scheduled appointments known about in advance can be prepared. In seeking to support a person with ID who may have contact with a radiology department, the following actions may be helpful:

- With the agreement of the person with ID (or their parents, if a child) contact the radiology department to establish the reason for the visit and the nature of the procedure to be undertaken.
- Inform staff in the radiology department of any additional information they may need in relation to communication abilities, ability to wait, and additional physical mobility issues.
- Clarify with the person with ID what they understand about their forthcoming appointment/investigation.
- Provide information on the steps involved in using the department, including the possible need to change clothing, lying still, use of a scanner, using accessible information including photographs, and videos

if necessary. A preappointment visit to see the staff and equipment may be helpful if the department is nearby.

- Bear in mind that radiology departments are unfamiliar places for people not used to them. Investigations may include the use of equipment that is overhead or a large scanner, people are often required to lay still, staff may wear protective clothing, stand behind screens, lights may be dimmed, and sudden noises may come from the equipment. People may also be asked to move or allow a painful body part to be examined.
- At times practising to sit or lie still may be useful.
- Confirm if any pre-appointment preparation is required, such as increasing/restricting fluid/food intake, or taking premedication.

Support during contact with staff in radiology department

Arrival at department should be well planned, parents or carers accompanying a person should make available to radiology staff additional information using health passports, and confirm ongoing consent to investigation/treatment. Provide ongoing information during the appointment, particulary if the person is to be left alone, and involve acute liaison nurse if available. Give positive encouragement and feedback when things are going well.

Post appointment

It is important to clarify if there are any restrictions of contact with other people, and explain any alterations from normal, such as discoloured bowel motions. Before leaving confirm whether a review appointment is required, and the arrangements for this.

Children's health services

The number of children with complex physical healthcare needs has increased as paediatric and ID services have been able to support an increasing number of children with complex physical healthcare needs. Many of these children require intensive support throughout their childhood, at times being dependant on technology to receive adequate nutrition, and at times for breathing.[1]

Children's services should be characterized by effective interdisciplinary and interagency communication in community/hospital based provision, and integrated working that focuses on the needs of the child and family, rather than the needs of the service or professionals within the services.[2] 'Every child matters', which has been heralded as a 'new approach to the wellbeing of children and young people from birth to age 19', with the stated aim of 'every child, whatever their background or their circumstances, is to have the support they need to: be healthy, stay safe, enjoy and achieve, make a positive contribution and achieve economic wellbeing'(🖳 www.everychildmatters.gov.uk/aims/). In order to achieve the above vision of services, ID nurses need to consider their role in developing supporting services that recognize the abilities and needs of the child as an individual in a wider family context, and working across interdisciplinary service structures, including being employed in services other than ID services.

All children with ID and their carers may have contact with general children's health services in both primary and secondary care. Some children with complex physical healthcare needs may have more frequent contact with children's services, which are reviewing and monitoring their development, responding to acute episodes of ill health, or seeking to provide palliative care.

Promoting collaborative working with children's services

The development of more inclusive services promotes that children with ID should have equity of access to children's services, and that their general health needs should be met within children's services available to all children, rather than within a separate and possibly parallel ID service. While this may work for a large number of children, those children with complex physical healthcare needs will often require support from secondary specialist children's nursing teams in community and hospital settings. Many of these services have developed in the past 10yrs in a response to the growing number of children with complex healthcare needs. Such services have a valuable contribution to make, as do ID nursing services, particularly when children and teenagers also have difficulties arising from behaviour that presents challenges, or more time is required to teach new skills that can be provided by children's services. Collaborative working is also very important to facilitate a smooth transition of care from children's to adult services.

By working collaboratively it will be possible to provide the combined knowledge, skills, and commitment to support children and their families, which can be particularly valuable in the process of transition from child to adult services, and in child protection matters. It is accepted that collaborative working can bring its own challenges, and requires an investment in time and personal commitment if it is to be successful (see 📖 pp.282–285, and 📖 Community children's nurses, p.340). Nurses within ID services should develop contact with their nursing colleagues within children's hospital and community services, sharing information on the possible contributions to care of a child, expressing a willingness to work in partnership, exchanging knowledge, skills and contact details. There should be opportunities to meet regularly.

Many of these children are a 'new generation' of children with complex needs who would have been unlikely to survive into adulthood only 10yrs ago. Therefore, new service arrangements are required to effectively support children and their families. These should not be negatively impacted on by either ID or children's services claiming 'professional territory'. Such a position seeks to advantage one service, but little to enhance services for children.

Services for children with disabilities that appear to be most successful are characterized by:
- Listening to disabled children and young people
- Providing information and advice
- Positive attitudes and a coordinated approach
- Flexible support services, which are tailored to individual children's and families' needs
- Having more money—children and parents
- Measuring the actions of all statutory and voluntary agencies against the human rights of disabled children.

Further reading

Department of Health (2004). *National service framework for children, young people and maternity services: Executive summary.* Department of Health: London. ▣ www.dh.gov.uk/en/Publicationsandstatistics/Publications/PublicationsPolicyAndGuidance/DH_4089100

1 Elston S (2003). *Assessment of Children with Life Limiting Conditions and their Families: A Guide to Effective Care Planning.* ACT: Bristol.

2 Department of Health (2004). *National Service Framework for Children, Young people and Maternity Services.* Department of Health: London.

Accident and emergency departments

People with ID, because of their complex needs, may have more intense involvement with healthcare services, with a greater number of people being admitted to general hospitals (more so than the general population). Mencap suggests that ~26% of people with ID are admitted to general hospitals in comparison to 14% of the general population, yet their actual stays within hospitals are shorter.[1]

Barriers to support within the accident and emergency environment

Admission to hospital is predominantly through A&E, the area where primary and secondary care interface. Challenges are particularly associated with a lack of knowledge of ID, communication difficulties, and misunderstandings regarding the individual's right and ability to consent to healthcare. Consequently, this reduces the nurse's confidence to assess needs, plan, provide and evaluate care, and arrange discharge and referrals where appropriate.

Although nurses within A&E are expected to respond to all people who come into the service, few healthcare professionals have received education in the health needs of this population, or have clinical experience in assessing their needs, which increases the risk of needs not being identified, or met.[2] A&E is for many a fast-moving, noisy, bizarre, and unfamiliar environment, and for a person with ID, a lack of understanding of what is happening can increase their levels of anxiety and distress, which may be demonstrated in odd or challenging behaviours. There is the risk that these behaviours may be misinterpreted, being linked to the disability, and not seen as an indicator of distress.

Furthermore, Houghton suggests that conducting a safe assessment of an individual with ID may take up to 4 times longer than the rapid assessment nurses normally carry out.[3] This extra time may not be given to a person with ID, yet it is estimated that 40–50% of people with ID experience some difficulty with communication.

In addition, people with ID are often excluded from healthcare discussions and decisions. This is associated with many health professionals wrongly believing that adults with ID neither have the right to consent or withhold consent to healthcare, nor have the capacity to make such decisions (see 📖 Capacity and consent, p.98, and 📖 Consent to treatment, p.260).

Enhancing support

Some A&E services work closely with acute liaison nurses in their localities, and others have introduced procedures for giving priority to the needs of people with ID through the use of 'priority cards', which should be considered within the triage process. In order to enhance support, challenges need to be recognized and addressed, and nurses also need to be aware of the following:

- Any existing health passport that may be available for the individual—ask to see and make use of this document
- The need to identify their own areas for professional development, addressing any lack of knowledge of ID

- The high health needs of this population, and that these needs may be communicated and presented differently in them
- The need to reduce fears and anxieties by informing the patient of the journey and potential waiting times
- The difficulty that some people with ID have in communicating their needs, so must find out how they communicate, allowing extra time to inform decision making, assess, investigate, and provide treatment
- Individuals want to be autonomous, speak to the individual in the first instance, see the person first, before the disability
- Behaviour is a means of communicating, not a symptom of ID
- The need to seek support from family/carers to aid understanding
- Where possible, one nurse should remain with the patient throughout the patient's journey
- Adapting your communication style may significantly enhance communication. Use other communication tools to enhance effective communication e.g. The Hospital Communication Book
- All adults have the right to consent to healthcare, and if there are concerns regarding capacity to consent, this must be assessed
- The guidelines within their country on consent, and use the relevant guidance as a framework to aid decision making
- On discharge or referral, the information needs to be communicated in a format that is understood.

Further reading

Access to Acute (A2A) 🖳 www.networks.nhs.uk/networks/page/592

Sowney M, Barr O (2007). The challenges for nurses communicating with and gaining valid consent from adults with intellectual disabilities within the accident and emergency care service. *Journal of Clinical Nursing* **16**(9), 1678–1686.

1 Mencap (2004). *Treat Me Right*. Mencap: London.

2 Sowney M, Brown M (2007). People with learning disabilities: Issues for Accident and Emergency Practitioners. In: Dolan A and Holt L (eds.) *Accident and Emergency Theory into Practice*. Baillière Tindall: London.

3 Houghton BM (2001). Caring for people with Down syndrome. *Accident and Emergency Nurse* **9**(2), 24–27.

Dental services

Oral health, including dental health, is important in a number of ways e.g. the presence of well-developed teeth in making it possible for people to eat a well balanced diet, for clear speech, and confidence in one's appearance and smile. Good oral health is also important in preventing gum disease, halitosis (foul smelling breath), dental pain, and mouth ulcers.

Proactive steps to maintaining good dental and oral health include: the eating of a well balanced diet, an adequate intake of fluids, brushing teeth after meals, and regular check-ups by a dentist, in which they can examine the development and soundness of teeth and gums (see ☐ Dentists, p.350).

However, for many people with ID, achieving the above activities is difficult without practical support. The challenge to maintaining healthy teeth and gums can arise when some people with ID may find it difficult to brush their teeth effectively, are unable to eat orally, have irregularly placed teeth that need specific dental interventions, or find it difficult to cooperate with dental examination or treatment.

While most dental surgeries are based within community settings, it can be difficult to have people with ID who require dental treatment seen in a community based dentist, if they have any concerns about their own ability to manage, or other difficulties that may arise during examination or treatments. Although at times this can be accommodated by the community based dental practices, there may be mobile facilities that make the service more accessible for some people, in particular those with complex health needs. However, there can be long delays for people with ID in accessing dental services, and often these are provided within hospital dental departments and involve the use of a general anaesthetic. In order to reduce the need for such a service, it is important that carers for people with ID encourage effective dental and oral health from a young age.

Preparing for an appointment

It is helpful for people with ID to meet a dentist before intervention is required as an emergency when they are in pain. Pre-appointment visits to the dental surgery to meet the staff, sit in the dentist chair, experience some of the smells and noises of the dental surgery, letting the dentist look in their mouth, touch their gums (as well as applying a local anaesthetic), can be a worthwhile investment of time, and should provide an opportunity to develop cooperative relationships and to reinforce positive behaviour for the person with ID, their carers, and staff within the dental surgery.

If a visit to the surgery is not possible due to distance, time or other issues, then a 'photographic tour' of the dental surgery may be possible. This could involve using a series of photographs of staff or a video tour of waiting rooms, chairs, some equipment, e.g. overhead examination light, toothbrushes, as well as explaining that dentists may wear gloves and eye protectors, and nearby locations, to familiarize the person with staff and location before they attend.

Support during contact

The requirements for valid consent apply to examination and treatment, and therefore it is important that this has been obtained prior to attending the dental surgery and confirmed when there. While parents may give consent for children under 18yrs, (see ▢ Consent to treatment, p.260, and ▢ Vulnerability, p.266) good practice would seek to have all children involved in this process, because in reality parental consent will be of little practical use if the person will not cooperate with the dentist.

People with ID do not seek to be difficult patients; therefore, a lack of cooperation should be explored and actively responded to. Carers should explain to the dentist how the person receiving treatment shows signs of distress, and monitor carefully for these, responding promptly with ongoing encouragement, an explanation of what is required, break in treatment, and if necessary further anaesthesia/analgesia. Active cooperation while in the dentist chair will also increase the prospects of establishing a pattern of regular visits and opportunities for proactive treatment, and good dental and oral health.

Support after an appointment

Many visits to the dentist will not result in post-appointment pain, indeed it may relieve pain. However, care is needed in supporting people who have received anaesthesia, which will have numbed part of their mouth or cheek, to ensure they do not injure this. It is also important to assist the person with ID to follow the instructions they have received about eating and drinking hot and cold foods, care of teeth that have been treated, dental sockets after treatment, and the use of pain relief. Opportunities should also be used for reinforcing success with the person with ID and the dental surgery staff.

Further reading

The Royal College of Surgeons (2001). *Clinical Guidelines and Integrated Care Pathways for the Oral Health Care of People with Learning Disabilities.* The Royal College of Surgeons: London.

Davies R, Raman B, Scully C (2000). Oral health care of people with special needs. *British Medical Journal* **321**, 495–498.

British Society for Disability and Oral Health (2006). *A commissioning tool for special care dentistry.* BSDH: London.

Mental health services

People with ID have the right to use the same mental health services as any other citizen, and this is reflected in policy across the UK. This policy has not been met without apprehension, from professionals in both mainstream and ID services. Current policy also recognizes that some people will require specialist ID services for their mental health, though most people could and will use mainstream services with or without extra support. There is a changing role for ID services, moving towards a tertiary role, in that they will offer expertise, support and facilitate movement within and between services by providing advice and support to mainstream services. There are still issues in accessing mainstream services, and the main ones are discussed below, along with ideas on how they can be addressed.

Care pathways

Service boundaries and eligibility criteria have been problematic for people with ID and mental health problems, with them at times ending up with a limited or no service, until they reach crisis point. Many services are addressing this issue by developing joint protocols. This is where both mainstream and specialist services develop a care pathway for people with ID to access whatever service is best suited to meet their mental health needs, with both parties offering advice and support where needed.

Vulnerability

Like anyone else, people with ID may be vulnerable in mainstream mental health services, but vulnerability does not automatically indicate exclusion. For example are there separate services for people in catatonic states or those who are disinhibited? The answer is 'no', risk is assessed and managed. The risk to each person should be assessed individually, and it should be determined if plans can be put in place to minimize the risk. If this cannot be achieved, then specialist services should be accessed.

Developing knowledge and skills

Mainstream mental health staff often believe that they lack the skills or knowledge to support people with ID. This can be due to a lack of confidence and experience. It can also be because of a perceived fear of the unknown. Although the use of mainstream services is a relatively new concept, it is likely that mainstream staff have supported people with mild ID. It is probable that staff did not recognize them as having ID, as they may not have had a formal diagnosis or attended a special school. However, there are some particular issues where training and/or advice from a specialist service can help the transfer of skills:
- Rights and values
- Recognizing mental health problems e.g. atypical presentation
- Interviewing people e.g. reducing the risk of suggestibility and acquiescence
- Associated unmet health needs
- Adapting interventions e.g. simplification of cognitive behavioural techniques

- Unwanted effects of treatment e.g. side effects such as susceptibility to seizures
- ASD
- Range of specialist and support services available.

Communication

A significant number of people with ID will have specific communication needs, some of which are very apparent, and others that can be easily overlooked. Making sure that communication is pitched at the appropriate level is essential for ensuring an equal relationship between the person using the service and staff. Under the Disability Discrimination Act[1] service providers are required to make reasonable adjustments to enable people with disabilities to make use of that service. This can include making sure that any information provided about local services, the person's rights, and treatments are produced in an accessible format.

An example in practice

One example of how the inclusion agenda is being driven forward is the Green Light Toolkit in England.[2] It is primarily an audit tool that examines how well services are working together to meet the mental health needs of people with ID. It is based on a traffic light scoring system and offers examples of how services can be improved. It is a tool that should be used in partnership with those using services, their carers, and other local services.

Further reading

Hardy S, Chaplin E, Woodward P (2007). *Mental Health Nursing of Adults with Learning Disabilities*. Royal College of Nursing: London.

1 Department of Work and Pensions (1995). *Disability Discrimination Act.* HMSO: London.

2 Foundation for People with Learning Disabilities (2004). *Green Light for Mental Health.* Foundation for People with Learning Disabilities: London.

Planning for contact with health services

As noted in the earlier sections of this chapter, people with ID may seek access to a range of services from primary care, secondary care, and specialist services. As citizens of the country they should have equity of access to all health services (including mental health services, see 📖 Chapter 7, pp.213–248). There is a legal requirement on services to make 'reasonable adjustments' when people are unable to access services in the usual way. Failure to do so may result in a legal challenge of unlawful discrimination against health services.

Persistent challenges

A recent independent inquiry in access to healthcare for people with ID, concluded that people with ID continue to find it much harder than other people to access assessment and treatment for general health problems. A number of factors were noted as contributing to this situation including:

- Failure to make reasonable adjustments to support people with ID in accessing and using services
- The views of parents and carers of people with ID are often ignored by healthcare professionals
- Staff in general healthcare have limited knowledge about ID, and often hold negative stereotypical attitudes about the limited abilities of people with ID
- Staff in general healthcare services are not familiar with what help they should provide or from whom to get expert advice
- Limited collaborative working occurs between staff in ID services and general healthcare services.[1]

Planning for contact

Most contact between people with ID and general healthcare services is known about in advance by staff and family carers. This contact is often in the context of appointments within primary care services, outpatient appointments, planned day case admissions for minor procedures (e.g. dental treatment), or planned admission to a ward. In contrast, while people within ID may present specific challenges when admitted as an emergency,[2] such contact is less frequent.

Therefore, on most occasions, opportunities exist to plan more effectively for contact between people with ID and general healthcare services. Practical steps that can be taken to increase the likelihood of a successful outcome are as follows:

- Staff in health services should ask if a 'health passport' exists and make use of the information contained within it.
- Staff in ID services should exchange names, address, telephone, email details, and emergency contact arrangements with key colleagues in primary care, mental health, or general hospitals services.
- The person requesting the appointment/admission should identify that this individual may have additional needs and what these may include.

- Information should be provided to people with ID and parents/carers about what they can expect when in contact with general health services.
- The above information should be presented in accessible formats and provide contact details for key staff in both ID and general health services who may be able to organize support.
- The procedures for making appointments should take account of the extra time that may be needed to complete the necessary examination and treatment.
- Consideration should be given to the need to reduce the usual level of examination/treatment, and plan this over subsequent contacts, rather than trying to complete it all in one session.
- Appointments should be provided at the start of a clinic session, where this is convenient to people with ID, to increase the likelihood that the person is seen promptly.
- Staff in ID services should work collaboratively with their colleagues in general healthcare to assess additional support needed to ensure an appointment or admission is successful.
- Attention should be given to the practicalities of transport to and from the health service, parking, access to building/room, and toilet/changing facilities that may be required. Reasonable adjustments should be identified in advance and the necessary arrangements put in place.
- At the end of the contact, the success of the arrangements should be reviewed, and arrangements built upon for any subsequent contact.
- Feedback should be provided to staff, highlighting and reinforcing areas of good practice.

Further reading

Sowney M, Barr O (2004). Equity of access to healthcare for people with learning disabilities: a concept analysis. *Journal of Learning Disabilities* **8**(3), 247–265.

1 Michael J (2008). *Healthcare for All: Report of the independent inquiry into access to healthcare for people with learning disabilities*. Department of Health: London. ⌕ www.iahpld.org.uk/

2 Sowney M, Brown M, Barr O (2006). Caring for people with learning disabilities in emergency care. *Emergency Nurse* **14**(2), 23–30.

Discharge planning

People with ID have greater health needs in relation to both acute and chronic illness compared with the general population, and as such are higher users of healthcare. Although they are admitted to acute general hospitals more often than the general population, they actually spend less time within the hospitals, being discharged relatively quickly, though not necessarily appropriately.[1]

Discharge from hospital should be seen as a process and not an end in itself, where discharge planning is ongoing, involving the individual, their family, and multidisciplinary team. Although most people will be involved in their planned discharge, people with ID and their families/carers have often experienced problems with the discharge process.

Issues with discharge

The House of Commons Health Committee on Delayed Discharge have identified the following issues:[2]

- Discharge may occur too soon
- Discharge is often delayed
- Discharge is poorly managed from the patient/carer perspective
- Patients are often discharged to unsafe environments.

There is evidence that people with ID experience inequity when accessing healthcare, and that many health needs go undetected and are thus not met. If people are discharged too early in their care, there is a risk that needs may not have been identified or not appropriately addressed, which may have fatal consequences.[3] Conversely, if the individual's care is complete, then delaying discharge also poses a risk to the individual's safety. Evidence shows that the longer someone is within the hospital environment, the greater the risk of nosocomial infection and other untoward events.[4]

The key principle underpinning effective discharge is a partnership approach with patients and families, yet this is often not the case.[1] Carers report that people with ID are discharged too early, despite protests from families.[3]

In addition, many people with ID will be supported within the community by families or paid carers, so advanced warning is often needed to prepare for the discharge. If the environments into which the person with ID is transferred are not prepared, they may be unsafe.

Planning for discharge should be an integral aspect of planning care, and it is important for nurses within the clinical environment to ensure that good discharge plans are put in place. This can be facilitated through good working relations with the patient, carer, and multidisciplinary team to promote good clinical outcomes and a safe discharge.

Preparing for discharge

- A patient-centred approach must be taken prior to admission, or as soon after admission as possible to plan the individual's discharge.
- Working collaboratively with the acute liaison nurse if available in local services, and staff in local community ID team or residential services.

- The adult patient needs to be seen as an individual, with the right to be autonomous in decisions about his/her healthcare, and consent must be sought before any information is shared with family/carers.
- This approach should recognize the role of the family/carers. Information should be gained from them about the best way to support the patient through the hospital journey, including discharge.
- If the individual is in receipt of a care package, then the appropriate community support people need to be communicated regarding admission and discharge.
- Information regarding plans to discharge may be recorded within the individual's HAP.
- For people with communication difficulties, information should be provided in a timely fashion, and in a format that they understand. Sowney et al. suggest that people with ID and their families should have:[5]
  - information on their diagnosis and any treatment given in a format that is understood by them
  - clear advice on any treatment regimen to be followed at home
  - a contact number, should they require further advice or support
  - an evaluation of their understanding prior to discharge
  - an awareness of and links with the CLDT, and where possible liaise with the Liaison nurse.
- Consideration of the carers needs is crucial to effective discharge.
- Good communication with families/carers will facilitate a safe transfer from the hospital environment.

1 Department of Health (2003). *Discharge From Hospital: Pathways, Process and Practice*. Department of Health: London.

2 House of Commons Health Committee (2001). *Delayed Discharges (2001–02). Vol.1*. HMSO: London.

3 Mencap (2007). *Death by Indifference. Following up the Treat Me Right Report*. Mencap: London. 🖳 www.mencap.org.uk/html/campaigns/deathbyindifference/DBIreport.pdf [accessed March 2009]

4 National Patient Safety Agency (2004). *Understanding the Patient Safety Issues for People with Learning Disabilities*. National Health Service: London.

5 Sowney M, Brown M, Barr O (2006). Caring for people with learning disabilities within emergency care: Why emergency nurses need to sit up and take note. *Emergency Nurse* **14**(2), 23–30.

Tertiary care

Defining tertiary care

From a medical or nursing perspective, tertiary healthcare can be described as specialized consultative care provided by professionals who have the appropriate resources, facilities, and expertise to provide specialist investigations or treatment usually for long-term or chronic conditions. Specialist cancer care, incontinence advisors, epilepsy and dementia care specialists are common tertiary services required by people with ID. Referrals are usually made from primary or secondary care professionals.

Difficulties in accessing tertiary care

People with ID may have difficulties in accessing specialist care because:
- their health needs may be overlooked and thus remain unrecognized
- services do not talk to each other enough
- there is a lack of easy to read information
- there is little or no support for family carers
- there is a lack of awareness and understanding by hospital staff about ID
- hospital staff do not know about consent to treatment, the mental capacity legislation, and related consent policies.[1]

Additionally, physical, administration, communication, attitudinal, and knowledge barriers may make access to good healthcare difficult. Nurses supporting the individual with an ID need to address these issues in a proactive way to facilitate appropriate healthcare at all levels.

Facilitating tertiary healthcare

To support nurses in accessing appropriate tertiary healthcare, and to help support the person in preparation for hospital appointments, tests and investigations, roles such as health facilitator, and acute liaison nurses, have been developed in some places. The health facilitator role includes working alongside other professionals in the primary, secondary, and tertiary care teams to ensure that individuals with an ID gain full access to the healthcare they require when they require it. Their role is to facilitate, advocate, and support individuals (and their carers) to efficiently navigate their way around healthcare services.

Many people with an ID have a variety of tertiary health needs which, if remain untreated, may at best be uncomfortable, and at worse become life changing or indeed life threatening. Since some individuals may not be aware of their own health needs, or are not able to articulate personal concerns, nurses need to remain vigilant in spotting any changes in the person that may indicate changes in potential health status. Nurses who care for people with ID may be among those best placed to encourage healthier lifestyles, and key issues for the nurse around accessing tertiary care include working proactively to ensure the following.

Adequate preparation prior to hospital appointments—some individuals with an ID will not be familiar with (and/or may be fearful of) healthcare facilities e.g. outpatient departments or clinics. Familiar carers can plan for the visit—perhaps take photographs of any diagnostic instruments or equipment that is likely to be used, to explain to the patient beforehand, arrange a visit to the clinic prior to the appointment to promote familiarity. Contact the clinic to arrange extra appointment time for the person in case the person needs more time to be guided through the anticipated procedure, and provide time to have complex terms translated and explained in a language that they are more likely to understand.

Accurate assessment—communication can be the biggest barrier to accurate and appropriate assessment, and some health professionals may not be familiar with how to communicate effectively with people with ID. A familiar carer can support the individual by alleviating fears and anxieties during diagnostic consultations, by enhancing reciprocal communication, and in supplementing information with personal knowledge where appropriate. Assessments are crucial to establishing specific health need, and subsequently identifying appropriate treatment options.

Developing links with health professionals—collaborative working is the key to effective support, and includes establishing and maintaining up-to-date links with local health professionals, being aware of local and regional resources, and knowing when, where and how to refer for specialist care and intervention.

Health action plans—can also help to identify and monitor health needs from a holistic perspective, incorporating details of health needs and interventions, oral care, dental care, fitness and mobility, continence, vision, hearing, nutrition, and emotional needs, in addition to details of current medications, side effects, and screening tests records. Such a plan seeks to ensure that health needs are not overlooked and can be monitored.

Further reading

Department of Health (2001). *Valuing People: A New Strategy for Learning Disability for the 21st Century.* HMSO: London.

1 Michael J (2008). *Healthcare for All:* Report of the independent inquiry into access to healthcare for people with learning disabilities. Department of Health: London.
🖳 www.iahpld.org.uk/

Palliative, end of life nurses

Noticing that someone is ill

People with an ID may not recognize changes in their bodies that are indicators of potential palliative conditions. Additionally, some people may lack the verbal repertoire to explain any associated discomfort, identify changes in usual habits (such as eating, elimination and/or weight loss), and thus some conditions are likely to go unrecognized. Personal carers need to remain watchful in anticipation of such changes, which otherwise might go unrecognized in people with ID, to reduce late diagnosis and prevent poor prognosis.

End of life

When disease is deemed to be advanced, progressive and life limiting, the focus of care becomes that of comfort and quality of life. End-of-life care supports people with an advanced, progressive, incurable illness to live as well as possible until they die. It 'enables the supportive and palliative care needs of both patient and family to be identified and met throughout the last phase of life and into bereavement'.[1]

Palliative care

Palliative care is described as active, holistic care, in which the management of pain and other symptoms, and provision of psychological, social, and spiritual support is paramount. It aims to affirm life and regard dying as a normal process, offering a support system to help patients and their families live as actively as possible until death, and as such is an important part of the nursing role of all those involved with the patient who has been diagnosed with a life-limiting condition. Such care can be delivered to patients in their own homes, in hospitals, hospice settings, and also by those healthcare professionals who specialize in palliative care.

Specialist palliative care

Specialist palliative care nurses provide advice alongside the patient's own clinical team. They work in community, hospital, hospice, or care home settings, providing specialist advice in order to prevent or relieve suffering associated with a lifelimiting illness. This may include advice regarding pain and symptom control, or other problems relating to the patient's physical, psychosocial, or spiritual needs. However, studies indicate that healthcare professionals who specialize in palliative care may have little experience in caring for people with ID, and will require advice, education, and support from the ID nurse.[2]

Palliative care for people with intellectual disabilities

At the heart of good palliative care is a holistic assessment, which may prove difficult when the patient has an ID. The DisDat tool uses behavioural observations to assess distress in individuals who have limited verbal communication skills.[3] Similarly, the checklist 'Planning ahead to manage pain and distress confidently' helps carers to be proactive in identifying care strategies.[4] Nurses may be reliant on familiar carers to interpret symptoms and recognize indicators of distress, promote reciprocal communication thus enhancing high standard, individualized palliative care and support. Living with a life-limiting condition may bring a number of issues and problems, both for the patient and their family, which may change over time as the illness progresses and death approaches. It is important that the nurse identifies and anticipates any inherent changes and is able to:

• recognize and assess the holistic needs of the patient and the family in relation to their physical, psychological, social, spiritual, and informational needs
• provide the care and support in order to meet those needs within the limits of their own knowledge, skills, and competence in palliative care
• understand when they need to seek advice or refer to the specialist palliative care service
• collaborate with specialist palliative care services, families, and other health and social care professionals, in order to meet all of the needs of the patient with ID who has a lifelimiting condition.

End of life care must be relevant to the patient's normal way of life, with an emphasis on quality of life. For the patient with an ID, this will require a careful and collaborative approach by those healthcare professionals involved in the patient's care. See also 📖 Support associated with loss and bereavement, p.326

Further reading

NHS End of Life Care Programme 🖥 www.endoflifecareforadults.nhs.uk/eolc/

1 National Council for Palliative Care (2007). *Palliative Care Explained* 🖥 www.ncpc.org.uk

2 Tuffrey-Wijne I, McEnhill L, Curfs L *et al.* (2007). Palliative care provision for people with intellectual disabilities: interviews with specialist palliative care professionals in London. *Journal of Palliative Medicine* **21**, 493–499.

3 Regnard C, Mathews D, Gibson L (2003). Difficulties in identifying ditsress and its causes in people with severe communication problems. *J Palliative Nursing* **9**(3), 173–176.

4 Brown H, Burns S, Flynn M (2005). *Dying Matters: A Workbook on Caring for People with Learning Disabilities who are Dying.* The Mental Health Foundation: London.

Continence advisors

Continence advisors are experienced qualified nurses who have undertaken specialist training. Their primary role is to support people with bladder and bowel problems, promoting continence and the management of incontinence. The continence advisor works together with the person with continence problems, their carers and other health professionals, providing education and specialist advice and equipment to enable the person and relevant others to effectively manage the problem.

Working in partnership

The ID nurse will often have an in-depth knowledge of continence, with many undergoing further training in this area. It is important that the ID nurse works in partnership with the continence advisor to ensure the person with ID and/or their family members are able to benefit from the wide range of knowledge, skills, and services available within the primary care, ensuring the person has access to the people with the right skills at the time they are needed most. This partnership could be facilitated by the development of joint care plans and/or HAPs.

Continence

Acquiring continence is a complex process; everyone is born without bladder and bowel control and needs to learn the necessary control and the socially acceptable places to go.

To achieve continence a person needs to:
- recognize the need to urinate or defecate
- identify the right place to go
- be able to reach the place
- hold on until the place can be reached
- pass the urine or faeces once there.

Incontinence is a major problem for some people with ID, and while manageable when the child is small, becomes a major difficulty for parents as the child grows. However, it is important to recognize that incontinence is a symptom, and not a disease, affecting all age groups, but is not an inevitable part of disability or illness. It is important, however, that incontinence is not accepted as inevitable just because the person has an ID. It is clear that becoming continent will be difficult for many people, but it is important that every person is supported, using the usual 'toilet training' techniques where possible. This should be discussed with the child, the parents, the nursery nurse, the schoolteacher as part of the child's development, and should be made fun.

Communication

It is important to think about the language you use when talking to people and/or their carers about their continence problems; remember this can be embarrassing, and people may not use or know the correct terms. The correct terms should be introduced to parents and/or carers, but ask them what terms they use and try to use a mixture of these (if appropriate) when talking about their problems. Language can be a real barrier; this could be due to the sensitive nature of the work, language difficulties, or different cultural backgrounds. It is important when working with families and carers to communicate clearly, sensitivity, and in a culturally appropriate manner in order to be effective. It is important to support the person and/or their families to feel at ease as far as possible to gain an understanding of the issues.

Aids, adaptations, and equipment

- The continence advisor will have a wide knowledge of the range of aids and equipment that is available from specialist companies, and will be able to advise people on the most appropriate type to help to effectively manage their problem. These are often available for trial from the local services to aid independent living.
- All-in-one continence aids are available for children and adults with ID, and can be accessed following an assessment from either a health visitor/continence advisor, or ID nurse.
- Specialist seating or toileting aids are available following an assessment from an occupational therapist.

Further reading

Bladder and Bowel Foundation http://www.bladderandbowelfoundation.org/

Epilepsy specialist nurse

The main aim of epilepsy management is to maintain the person's functional capacity to its maximum potential through the control of seizures. To achieve this it is essential that the management of their care involves a multidisciplinary approach, incorporating the individual, medical/social service professionals, parents, relatives, friends, and carers. Although they are few in number, specialist epilepsy ID nurses provide an important role supporting the person with epilepsy and carers in the community.

Qualifications and skills

Epilepsy nurse specialists are usually registered nurses with experience in neurology/ID. The range of qualifications held can vary considerably, ranging from postregistration certificates to diploma, degree or Masters in epilepsy. Some may also hold qualifications in independent and supplementary prescribing. Research has shown that epilepsy nurse specialists can lead to improvements in epilepsy care. This is illustrated by the development of the therapeutic relationship between nurse and client. A reason for this is often that the nurse will see the individual more frequently than the doctor, and have more time to spend in the consultation.[1]

Key principles in supporting people with epilepsy

- Using a person-centred approach[2]
- Improving quality and continuity of healthcare
- Monitoring AED medication
- Facilitating access to specialist and generic services
- Advocating, educating, and communicating for and on behalf of individuals
- Promoting independence by helping to reduce overprotection while maintaining safety and balancing risks.

See ☐ Epilepsy, p.156, and ☐ Supporting people with epilepsy, p.158.

Role of the nurse for people with epilepsy

The nurse is a clinician and acts as an educator, advocate, and liaison for the person with epilepsy and other parties i.e. health, social, education, and voluntary sector. In seeking to promote and maintain self-management by the person with epilepsy, the nurse will:

- Provide accurate information and advice to people with epilepsy and their families in the management of their condition at different stages of their life
- Support the doctor with the newly diagnosed person, using counselling skills to help the person adapt to the changes this may create
- Coordinate the interdisciplinary service needs of people with epilepsy
- Co-ordinate care between primary and secondary levels i.e. acute hospital/GP/community
- Provide a nurse-led epilepsy clinic
- Seek to achieve concordance with AED therapy
- Identify possible barriers to concordance i.e. lifestyle, work
- Give basic information about prescribed medication.

- Give advice about medication systems that promote self-administration of drugs i.e. monitored dosage system/pill box, drug wallets
- Advise when trips abroad are planned e.g. prophylactic AED, vaccinations
- Advise about daily life, such as recreation, alcohol
- Give information on epilepsy aids i.e. helmets, alarms etc
- Provide epilepsy training to clients, carers, relatives
- Establish/undertake epilepsy assessments/individual epilepsy guidelines, and risk management plans.

Outcomes of the epilepsy nurses' interventions[3]

- Improved communication about epilepsy between healthcare providers and individuals with epilepsy
- Increased access to healthcare
- People obtain better control of their seizures
- Improvement of independence
- Individuals with epilepsy and their carers were more informed about their condition, particularly as the nurse has good knowledge and understanding of epilepsy
- Through training of carers in the management and administration of e.g. rectal diazepam and buccal midazolam, fewer admissions to A&E may occur.[4]

Further reading

Epilepsy Action ▣ www.epilepsy.org.uk

National Society for Epilepsy ▣ www.epilepsynse.org.uk

1 Mills N, Campbell R, Bachmann MO (2002). What do patients want and get from a primary care epilepsy specialist nurse service? *Seizure* **11**, 176–183.

2 Department of Health (2001). *Valuing People: A Strategy for People with Learning Disabilities for the 21st Century.* Department of Health: London.

3 Goodwin M, Higgins S, Lanfear JH, Lewis S, Winterbottom J (2004). The role of the clinical nurse specialist in epilepsy. A national survey. *Seizure* **13**, 87–94.

4 Cole C, Pointu A (2007) Epilepsy awareness and the administration of rectal diazepam. *Learning Disability Practice* **10**(1), 10–15.

Dementia nurse specialists

Dementia is one of the richest areas of human work, and staff supporting people with dementia require specific knowledge, training, creativity, and insight. The dementia care field has been criticized for an over reliance on a 'medical model of care', and a failure to adopt a bio-psychosocial approach focused on the holistic needs of the person.[1] Using Kitwood's and other person-centred models, nurses have the potential to move care to a new culture, acknowledging that people with dementia require support emotionally, socially, psychologically, and physically, to maintain their quality of life.

Due to the increased evidence of dementia in people with ID, and unique, complex issues around screening, assessment, diagnosis, care, and end of life, the development of advanced level nursing posts within the field of ID nursing is also critical. Such developments also build on the unique personcentred ID nursing perspective, and apply it to caring for persons with dementia, recognizing that each person is unique, and will experience and respond differently to the challenges inherent in dementia (see 📖 Dementia, p.236).

Previous and ongoing work by McCarron[2] contends that addressing the care needs of people with ID and dementia requires leadership, a multidimensional approach, and the development of a strategic plan, which incorporates:

* routine baseline screening, comprehensive diagnostic workup, and consensus diagnosis, operationalized through a memory clinic model
* the development of a continuum of residential options to support the changing needs of the person and their carer at different stages of dementia
* appropriate dementia-specific day programmes
* training and education for staff, family and peers
* evidence-based research to guide practice and policy.

Developing appropriate educational pathways and working closely with academic institutions to equip ID nurses to respond to this advanced role will continue to be critical. Specialized nurse training to support these initiatives is required; there are examples including the 'Higher Diploma in Specialist Nursing in Ageing and Dementia in Persons with Intellectual Disability' at Trinity College Dublin. A cadre of nurse specialists is now beginning to emerge within ID services able to respond to dementia care challenges and develop the needed services with providers, and to address problems highlighted nationally and internationally, including:

* Addressing the lack of screening and the tendency for late diagnosis
* Understanding and implementing effective supportive interventions to address and minimize common behaviours, which challenge in dementia
* Addressing and diagnosing health comorbidities in order to maximize health and well being
* Addressing end of life and palliative care needs of persons with endstage terminal dementia, including support of peers, staff, and family members.

Nurses who have completed such courses may have the following roles.

Clinical—screenings, operation of memory clinics, work with multidisciplinary teams, and support of primary care teams and families in the diagnosis and management of symptoms of dementia.

Education and training—direct delivery and support for training for professional carers, families, peers and multidisciplinary team members on all aspects of dementia and dementia care, and supporting clinical sites for nursing students.

Advocacy—negotiating the full range of support for persons with dementia and their families, including grief and bereavement support.

Audit and research—participation and leadership in clinical audits, giving people with ID access to evidence-based interventions emerging from the dementia field, and contributing to the development of effective interventions.

Consultancy—acting as a specialist resource on dementia care.

ID nurses are in a prime position to advocate for and coordinate interdisciplinary approaches that maximize the capability of the person and their quality of life through a seamless person-centred model of care delivery.

Further reading

Alzheimer's Society ▪ www.alzheimers.org.uk

Cooper RA (2001). Health care workforce for the twenty-first century: The impact of nonphysician clinicians. *Ann Rev Med* **52**, 51–61.

1 Kitwood T (1997). *Dementia Reconsidered: The Person Comes First.* Open University Press: Buckingham, UK.

2 McCarron M (2005). *A Strategic Plan on Dementia, Daughters of Charity Service.* Trinity College: Dublin (unpublished).

Forensic nursing

Risk assessment and management

Context

The ID nurse has a key role working within forensic services, which will importantly focus on risk assessment management strategies in order to inform person-centred care and treatment approaches. Inglis *et al.* have identified that the ID nurse is at the centre of care and treatment of ID people in secure settings.[1] It is imperative, therefore, that ID nurses working within these settings receive *additional* education and training in addition to their pre-registration nurse education programmes. This should be linked to their KSF and personal development planning.

Inglis *et al.* have stated that the ID nurse may work with people in the context of *forensic nursing* for a number of reasons, including people who:[1]

- have not committed an offence but whose behaviour has brought them to the attention of the police
- have not committed an offence but whose illness or behaviour leads them to being held under the Mental Health Act
- have committed a minor offence but their primary need is for treatment, and whom it is not in the public interest to detain
- have committed an offence and who will be prosecuted
- have committed an offence and may enter the prison population with a mental health problem
- develop a mental health problem in prison
- are considered unfit to plead.

Assessment of risk

Johnston has identified that a review of literature on risk assessment and management revealed little direct evidence for this specific population.[2] Good risk assessment and management is a particularly important aspect of care and treatment for this group of people, as it will help to identify current presenting issues, and the required care and management interventions. The process of assessment should aim to be a structured and supportive process.

While there are a number of tools which may be used, the *Best Practice in Risk Management* guide[3] has recommended that risk assessment tools should be seen as part of the overall clinical assessment process, and choosing the right tool for the job is a complex job (see Fig. 11.1).

The process of risk assessment should be person centred, involving the individual concerned and significant others, be multiprofessional and multiagency, and enhance the therapeutic relationship between the nurse and client. This is often demonstrated through the implementation of the CPA.

The consequences of poor risk assessment and management planning can be serious, not only for the individual but for others.

Forensic risk assessment should be about taking a dynamic appreciation of risk and risk management as opposed to risk elimination. This development, according to Johnston, is more in line with the normalization of risk taking in ID.[2] The ID nurse working in these specialist settings may encounter people detained under mental health legislation. *Best Practice in Risk Management*[3] has identified a number of different assessment tools when working with people with forensic needs, which are applicable to working with a person with ID.

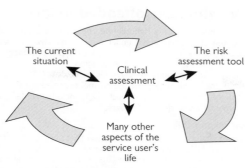

Fig. 11.1 The clinical assessment process. Reproduced from *Best practice in managing risk: principles and guidance for best practice in the assessment and management of risk to self and others in mental health services*, Department of Health, 2007.

Scenario

Bill attends a local day service. He is a 48yr gentleman who lives with his parents. He likes visiting shops and eating out, but does not like crowds and noisy places. Bill has a history of physical attacks on young children. He arrives from home to the day centre in a highly agitated state. Staff supporting Bill decided to go out for lunch, as this was something that Bill liked. It was half-term holiday from the local schools, and the height of lunchtime in the restaurant. The food was delayed, which resulted in Bill becoming increasingly agitated. While being escorted from the restaurant Bill attacked a young child.

Following this event the police were called and an investigation was conducted. This highlighted that no risk assessment or management plan were conducted prior to or during the outing.

When working with people with a forensic history, it is important to remember that risk plans are not static, and ongoing risk assessment and risk management planning is essential, and takes account of previous and present factors.

Conclusion

Risk assessment and management with people in ID with a forensic history requires systematic assessment, clear documentation, partnership working, and effective communication with all those involved with the person's care. It is imperative that consideration is also given to the different levels of security that the nurse and client might be working in e.g. high, medium, and low secure services. Inadequate or non-existent risk assessment and management can have serious consequences, not only for the person with ID, but also for others.

1 Inglis PA, Robinson MA, Thornton P, English G (2003). *Partnerships in Nursing & Education: Enhancing the Role of the Specialist RNLD in Forensic Settings.*

2 Johnston S (2002). Risk assessment in offenders with ID, the evidence base. *Journal of Intellectual Disability Research* **46**(1), 47–56.

3 Department of Health (2006). *Best Practice in Risk Management.* HMSO: London.

People who have offended in law

The term 'offender' can only rightfully be applied to a person who has been convicted of an unlawful act under the criminal law. In order to be convicted of an offence there must be evidence 'beyond reasonable doubt' that the person did the unlawful act/s in question.

A range of factors including ID can affect decisions about whether or not a person should be subject to the normal processes of the criminal law. Within the criminal justice domain ID is included under guidance relating to mentally disordered offenders.

Criminal responsibility

It is a fundamental assumption within the law that people who are prosecuted for unlawful acts will be held criminally responsible and liable to legal punishment. Factors that may negate or diminish criminal responsibility include considerations regarding the alleged unlawful act and about the person, including ID and other mental disorders. In practice the application of the criminal law would not be considered appropriate for most people with more severe ID. A very small minority of people with ID will be prosecuted for more serious offences and found unfit to plead under the Criminal Procedure (Insanity and Unfitness to Plead) Act 1991.

Considerations

- The alleged act (offence) must be **voluntary** (*actus reus*) and **intentional** (*mens rea*).
- Potential mitigating factors include mistake, accident, duress, and provocation.
- Personal factors/characteristics that may result in exemption or diminish criminal responsibility include mental disorders—ID, mental illness, personality disorder, and ASD.

The journey to a conviction

Pre-arrest and arrest

The police have a duty to investigate any criminal offence that is reported to them. The police investigation can lead to the arrest of the person who is suspected of having committed the offence. The police have a substantial degree of discretion and must balance a range of considerations when they make decisions regarding the appropriateness of arrest, and the nature and seriousness of the alleged offence including:

- The context of the alleged offence, including the setting in which the offence occurred, the ability and willingness of any victims to make a complaint and provide a reliable statement
- The mental capacity of any offender—this may be affected by the presence of ID and other mental disorders.

Post-arrest

All people who have been arrested have certain rights that are laid down in the Police and Criminal Evidence Act (PACE) 1984 (revised 2008):

- Right to remain silent
- Right to see a solicitor in private at any time
- Right to have someone told you are at the police station
- Right to look at the PACE Codes of Practice.

There are additional safeguards for people who are identified as being mentally vulnerable (PACE Code C), including people with ID (See 📖 Rights of person offending, p.408).

Prosecution

The CPS is the principal public prosecuting authority for England and Wales. In most cases the CPS, in consultation with the police, are responsible for deciding whether a person should be charged with a criminal offence, and if so what the offence should be. The CPS applies a threshold test to these decisions:

- Is there is a realistic prospect of conviction?
- Is prosecution in the public interest?
- Will conviction result in a significant sentence?

Disposal

Disposal is the term that is used for the outcome of a successful prosecution. There are strict guidelines for the judiciary to follow regarding the sentencing options that are available depending on the severity and circumstances of the offence and other factors (Crime Sentences Act 1997). Sentencing options include community sentences (e.g. community supervision orders, fines, community service etc.) and custodial (prison) sentences. In practice, community sentences are less likely to be considered for people with ID unless specialist learning disabilities are involved, and advice and support is provided to the criminal justice agencies dealing with the case (see 📖 Working with criminal justice agencies, p.432).

Diversion

In 1990 in the UK, the government of the day recommended that mentally disordered offenders, including people with ID, should be diverted from the criminal justice system and receive care and support from health and welfare services (Home Office Circular 66/90). In practice people who engage in offending behaviour are diverted away from the normal criminal justice process at various stages. see 📖 Rights of person offending, p.408; 📖 Admission for assessment, p.414; 📖 Admission for treatment, p.416.

Further reading

Stone N (2003). *A Companion Guide to Mentally Disordered Offenders.* Shaw & Sons: Kent.

Department of Health (2008). *Revised Mental Health Act Code of Practice.* Department of Health: London.

People in mainstream prison

In 2008 there were over 80,000 people in prison and the numbers are rising. As the number of people in prison has grown, there are increasing concerns regarding mentally disordered people in the prison population.

Research shows that the prevalence of people with ID in the prison population is higher (~7%) than in the general population (2.3%). While some of these people will cope adequately with a term of imprisonment, many will be very vulnerable, having difficulty coping, and struggle to access the range of services within the prison to meet their support, offence related, and healthcare needs.

About prisons

There are over 130 prisons in England and Wales, including Youth Offenders Institutes for 15–21yr-olds, adult male prisons, women's prisons (17), and 10 independently provided prisons. Prisons vary in size, with the largest (HMP Liverpool) accommodating almost 1500 men, to much smaller establishments. Some prisons cater only for sentenced prisoners, and others also accommodate prisoners on remand. Prisons are categorized in terms of security levels:

- Category A—prisoners whose escape would be considered highly dangerous to the public.
- Category B—prisoners who do not need the highest level of security but for whom escape must be made difficult
- Category C—prisoners who cannot be accommodated in open conditions but who are deemed not to have the ability or resources to make a determined attempt to escape
- Category D—prisoners who are deemed safe to serve their sentence in open conditions

Specialist prisons

Some prisons specialize in dealing with specific groups of offenders particularly those convicted of sexual offences. These prisons are sometimes referred to as treatment prisons.

Allocation

Prisoners may be allocated to any prison in England and Wales according to their offence, security needs, and individual circumstances. There is no right to be located close to home. Information regarding particular vulnerabilities, such as those associated with ID, may be taken into account when a decision is made regarding allocation; however, this may not be possible if prison vacancies are severely limited.

Purpose of prisons

- Hold prisoners securely
- Reduce the risk of prisoners reoffending
- Provide a safe and well-ordered establishment in which prisoners are treated humanely, decently, and lawfully.

Prison healthcare

Healthcare services in prison should include the same range of services available in the community, including primary health services, dental services, and specialist mental health, drug, and alcohol services. Many prisons have a healthcare wing to which prisoners can be admitted if their healthcare needs cannot be met on an outpatient basis. The prison service will also support prisoners who need treatment for physical health needs to access acute hospital services.

Few prisons have specific services to meet the needs of people with ID. People with ID may need additional support to enable them to access the services that are available.

Vulnerability

Mental health, self-harm, and suicide

Questions about mental health needs, self-harm, and suicide should be asked as part of the routine screening on reception into prison, in order that safeguards can be put in place by the prison service where required. People with ID may have difficulty providing accurate information regarding their own needs (see 📖 Risk of suicide, p.548).

Programmes/rehabilitation

Prisons provide a range of activities aimed at reducing the risk of future reoffending including offence specific programmes, e.g. sex offender treatment, anger management, enhanced thinking skills courses. Educational provision is also available in most establishments. While specific programmes are available in adapted form, people with ID may have serious difficulties accessing or benefiting from the available provisions, and will be considered ineligible for some programmes. This may cause significant problems, particularly in cases where eligibility for parole/release is contingent on completion of a specific sentence plan (i.e. indeterminate public protection sentences).

Role of specialist intellectual disability services

- Establish links with prisons in their area and alert prisons to the presence of prisoners with ID
- Raise awareness of the needs of people with ID and provide advice on how these can be met in the prison setting, including access to healthcare services, education, and offence related programmes, and links with other services where appropriate
- Provide information regarding specific needs and risks to inform the care of the person during remand or when serving a sentence
- Provide information on how people with ID who cannot be adequately supported in the prison setting can be referred to specialist secure services i.e. access to assessment for admission to secure hospital services (see 📖 pp.414–417)
- Maintain contact with the prison and contribute to release planning by attending pre-release meetings, providing information, and agreeing input if the person is returning to their local area on release.

Rights of victims

All victims of crime have a range of rights. These rights apply regardless of the status of the offender. People with ID who have offended against another person may therefore be subject to arrangements aimed at protecting any victims.

People with ID are also at increased risk of being the victims of crime. When this is the case, they should be afforded the same rights as anyone else who is a victim of crime (see 📖 People with intellectual disabilities as witnesses, p.412).

Police

When a crime is reported to the police the alleged victim should be given an opportunity when interviewed by the police to describe all the effects on them. This will include physical and material harm, and may also include any emotional and psychological effects/harm that have resulted from an alleged offence. This information may be taken into account in any subsequent court proceedings e.g. may have a bearing on the sentence if the offender is convicted. This information may also have a bearing on whether the court agrees to special measures if the victim is required to act as a witness (see 📖 People with intellectual disabilities as witnesses, p.412).

Domestic Violence, Crime and Victims Act 2004

The Domestic Violence, Crime and Victims Act includes a Victim's Code regarding the services to be provided to victims of criminal conduct. Under specified circumstances these services may also be available to others acting for the victim i.e. where the victim has died or is unable/incapable of exercising their rights as a victim.

Victims' rights

These rights will only be afforded if the local probation board is satisfied that the person requesting them has been the victim of an offender who has been detained or imprisoned for a sexual or violent offence.

The victim has the right to receive information about the offender, including:

- information regarding plans for release/discharge
- whether or not they will be subject to license conditions or supervision requirements
- whether or not they will be subject to conditions on their discharge
- what the conditions/requirements of discharge are, including any restrictions specific to the victim
- information regarding any variations/changes made following release/discharge
- other information considered relevant to the victim.

Offenders detained under the Mental Health Act 1983 (revised 2007)

The Victims' Code covers victims of offences committed by offenders who have been detained under Part III of the Mental Health Act, which deals with patients who are concerned with criminal proceedings or under sentence (see 📖 Admission for treatment, p.416).

Multiagency public protections arrangements

Disclosure

MAPPA are the statutory arrangements for managing sexual and violent offenders. The police, probation, and prison services are the responsible authorities for MAPPA. Other public bodies, including the National Health Service and social services have a duty to cooperate with the MAPPA. Under the MAPPA the responsible authorities can disclose information about an offender and the plans for their management in the community to third parties, including victims and others who may be at risk.

Offenders detained under the Mental Health Act 1983 (revised 2007)

Hospitals where offenders are detained have a duty to notify the owning MAPPA area when an offender is admitted to hospital, and when there is a prospect of discharge/return to the community. The relevant MAPPA area will consider victim issues, including plans for the protection of any previous and potential future victims, and disclosure of information to others (including victims) (see 📖 Management in the community, p.430).

People with intellectual disabilities as victims of crime

People with ID are often vulnerable in their local communities, and may be at increased risk of being the victims of crime; this may include hate crime.

Victim support schemes

Victim support schemes are available in all areas to provide help to people to cope with crime. The police will routinely provide information about local schemes when a crime is reported.

Role of specialist intellectual disability services

Specialist ID services should raise awareness of the needs of people with ID, and assist people to access, and make use of, support when they are the victims of crime. In a forensic context staff have a role to inform offenders with ID about the rights of victims, including their right to information about future plans for the offender.

Further reading

Ministry of Justice National MAPPA Team (2009). *MAPPA Guidance 2009*. Ministry of Justice: London.

Mencap (1999). *Living in Fear*. Mencap: London.

Victim Support website: 🖵 www.victimsupport.org.uk

Rights of person offending

People with ID who come into contact with the criminal justice system because of offending behaviour have the same rights as others. They may face particular problems, however, including a range of vulnerabilities, an increased potential for wrongful conviction, and limited access to the range of services available to non-disabled offenders (see 📖 People who have offended in law, p.402).

Police

The Police and Criminal Evidence Act 1984 (revised 2008) sets out the procedures for the detention, treatment, and questioning of people by the police.

Pre-arrest

When a crime is reported, police have a duty to investigate but also have a substantial degree of discretion regarding the decision to arrest. In practice the police will often decide that a person with ID lacks capacity to form intent and cannot be held fully accountable for their conduct, and conclude that arrest is therefore inappropriate.

Arrest

If a person with ID is arrested, they have the same rights as anyone else:
- Right to remain silent
- Right to see a solicitor in private at any time
- Right to have someone told you are at the police station
- Right to look at the PACE Codes of Practice (see 📖 Rights to a solicitor, p.410).

Additional safeguards for 'mentally vulnerable' suspects

- Clinical assessment regarding fitness for detention and fitness for interview
- Simplified explanation of the right to remain silent
- Presence of an appropriate adult to support, advise, and assist the detained person, particularly when they are being questioned
- Guidance/training for police for interviewing vulnerable suspects, including adaptations in normal police interviewing style
- Request for a psychiatric assessment/assessment under the MHA.

If these safeguards are not provided, where appropriate the reliability of the investigation may be questioned, and evidence gathered from the suspect may be ruled inadmissible in court.

Detention

The rights of all suspects who are detained by the police are laid down in PACE Code C (1984), including time limits, level of care, and medical attention. The appropriate adult role includes ensuring these requirements are met.

Disposal—Police

After the police have arrested a suspect and undertaken an initial investigation they can decide between various possible courses of action. In practice these decisions will often be made in consultation with the CPS. The decision made at this stage will depend on the severity and circumstances of the offence, and whether or not the suspect has admitted to the offence. If the suspect has ID (or another mental disorder) this may also affect the decision. People with ID should be afforded the same range of options as other suspects.

- **No further action or discontinuance**—due to lack of evidence or because prosecution is not deemed to be in the public interest
- **Informal warning** issued by the police
- **Non-judicial criminal punishment**—e.g. fixed penalty notice
- **Civil enforcement**—e.g. application for antisocial behaviour order, sexual offences prevention order (see 📖 Management in the community, p.430)
- **Formal caution**—if the suspect admits to the offence and consents to being cautioned. It is important that the suspect understands the implications of admitting to the offence and the caution
- **Police bail**—if it is considered safe, the suspect is released with conditions pending further investigation
- **Charge**—if the suspect is charged, a decision must be made regarding the need to detain the person or release him until he appears in court.

Courts

All cases in Court are dealt with under strict rules governing court proceedings. The burden of responsibility for proving 'beyond reasonable doubt' that an offence has taken place rests with the prosecution, and all suspects have a right to defend themselves. The defence lawyer's role is critically important in protecting the rights of vulnerable defendants, as it provides the means by which information about the person, the need for psychiatric reports, evidence that the person is unfit to plead, and other mitigating factors are taken into consideration. During the course of proceedings the court may seek psychiatric advice and remand an accused person to hospital for reports on his mental state under Section 35 of the MHA (see 📖 Admission for assessment, p.414).

Sentencing/disposal

Sentencing is subject to strict guidelines (Crime Sentences Act 1997). A pre-sentence report will normally be prepared by the probation service to inform decisions about sentencing. The court may sentence a person with ID to any sentence available for the offence for which they have been convicted, including custodial and community sentences. The court may also consider expert reports (including psychiatric reports) and make a disposal under the MHA (see 📖 Admission for treatment, p.416).

Further reading

Stone NA (2003). *Companion Guide to Mentally Disordered Offenders*. Shaw & Sons: Kent.

Jacobson J (2008). *No One Knows*. Prison Reform Trust: London.
🖥 www.prisonreformtrust.org.uk

Rights to a solicitor

Code C of PACE 1984 (revised 2008) sets out the procedures for the detention, treatment, and questioning of people by the police. PACE Code C includes the right to legal advice.

Research suggests that the legal rights of mentally disordered suspects, including those with ID, are best ensured by the presence of a legal advisor at the police station, and when the suspect is interviewed by the police.[1]

PACE Section 58

A person who is detained in police custody:
- has the right to consult a solicitor, in private, at any time
- is entitled on request to have a solicitor present when they are interviewed.

Police responsibilities

The police custody officer is responsible for ensuring that suspects know their legal rights. All suspects should be verbally informed of their right to legal advice. The words that are used are:
"You have the right to an independent solicitor free of charge."

Further information about the right to legal advice is normally given in writing in the form of a Notice to Detained Person, as follows:
- You can speak to a solicitor at the police station at any time, day or night. It will cost you nothing.
- Access to legal advice can only be delayed in exceptional circumstances.
- If you do not know a solicitor, or you cannot contact your own solicitor, ask for the duty solicitor. He or she is nothing to do with the police. Or you can see a list of local solicitors.
- You can talk to a solicitor in private on the telephone, and the solicitor may come and see you at the police station.
- If the police want to question you, you can ask for the solicitor to be there. If there is a delay, ask the police to contact the solicitor again. Normally the police must not question you until you have spoken to a solicitor. However, there are certain circumstances in which the police may question you without a solicitor being present.
- If you want to see a solicitor, tell the custody officer at once. You can ask for legal advice at any time during your detention. Even if you tell the police you do not want a solicitor at first, you can change your mind at any time.
- Your right to legal advice does not entitle you to delay procedures under the Road Traffic Act 1988, which require the provisions of breath, blood, and urine specimens.

Role of the intellectual disability nurse

Suspects with ID can be at greater risk when they are accused of offences if they do not understand and exercise their right to legal advice. ID nurses in forensic and criminal justice liaison roles can assist the police to support suspects with ID through a period of detention and interviews by the police:
- Explain the information contained in the Notice to Detained Person in simple language.

- Ensure that suspects with ID know that they are entitled to have a solicitor to support them and give them legal advice.
- Encourage people with ID who are suspected of an offence, arrested and held in police custody to exercise their right to legal advice.
- Work with the police and other agencies to raise awareness of the needs and vulnerabilities of people with ID in the criminal justice system. (see 📖 Rights of person offending, p.408, and 📖 Working with criminal justice agencies, p.432)

Further reading

Jacobson J (2008). *No One Knows*. Prison Reform Trust: London.
🖥 www.prisonreformtrust.org.uk

1 Robertson G, Pearson R, Gibb R (1996). Police interviewing and the use of appropriate adults. *Journal of Forensic Psychiatry* **7**(2), 297–309.

People with intellectual disabilities as witnesses

People with ID are at least as likely to witness crime as others in the general population, and may be at increased risk of being victims of crime. The presence of an ID may, however, be taken as an indication that a person is unable to provide reliable information in order to make a statement to the police, and be unable to act as a witness in criminal proceedings. A range of provisions are available to enhance the evidence provided by vulnerable and intimidated witnesses, including people with ID.

Special measures

The Youth Justice Act 1999 introduced a range of 'special measures' that can be used to facilitate the gathering and giving of evidence by vulnerable and intimidated witnesses.

The police

- Detailed guidance for the police regarding how to plan and conduct interviews with vulnerable and intimidated witnesses (including children)
- Video recorded interview in the presence of a responsible adult who will ensure that the witness understands questions asked and provides reliable information.

Court proceedings

If a person with ID is required to act as a witness in court, their capacity to give reliable evidence may be called into question as part of the defence case. With the agreement of the court, special measures can be made available to assist a person with ID to participate in court proceedings as a witness:

- Screens to shield the witness from the defendant
- Live link to enable the witness to give evidence and be cross-examined from outside the court room via a video link
- Exclusion from the court of members of the public and the press
- Removal of wigs and gowns by judges and barristers
- A video recorded interview may be admitted to the court as the witness's evidence in chief. If a video recorded interview has been agreed, video recorded cross-examination may also be admissible
- Examination of the witness via an 'intermediary' (see 📖 Intermediaries)
- Aids to communication—provided that the communication can be verified and understood by the court
- Protection of the witness from cross-examination by the accused person
- Restrictions on evidence and questions about the witness's sexual behaviour.

Intermediaries

All witnesses who are considered vulnerable can get help from an intermediary. Intermediaries come from a range of professional backgrounds (speech and language therapist, psychologists, social workers) and are specially trained for the role, and registered with the Intermediary

Registration Board. Vulnerable witnesses are matched to a suitably skilled intermediary on the basis of individual need. The role of the intermediary is to help witnesses at each stage of the criminal justice process to understand questions, and to communicate on behalf of the witness where required.

Witness support schemes

Witness support schemes are not able to advise on specific cases but do provide emotional and social support for vulnerable witnesses at all stages of the criminal justice process, including police interview, and prior to and during court proceedings/trial.

Roles for specialists in intellectual disabilities

- Witnesses who are known to have ID are generally interviewed by police officers, with additional training in the case of alleged sexual offences, but less often in the case of non-sexual offences—Specialists in ID should raise awareness of the need for appropriately trained officers to interview people with ID when non-sexual offences are reported.
- It is rare for the police and CPS to consult specialists/experts in ID about witnesses' disabilities or their implications—Specialist services for people with ID should raise awareness of available expertise, and engage with criminal justice agencies to provide expert advice on the effects of ID for those who are victims or witnesses.
- The availability of special measures to adult ID witnesses is still limited—Specialists in ID, particularly those in criminal justice liaison roles, should raise awareness/advocate for the wider use of special measures where these could assist ID witnesses to give evidence.
- Many witnesses with ID would benefit from specialist support and preparation prior to appearing in court, but it is not always clear which agency is responsible for providing this—Specialists in ID should raise awareness of their services and work jointly with witness support schemes to facilitate access to preparation and support for ID witnesses who are required to attend court.

Further reading

Home Office (1998). *Speaking Up For Justice. Report of the Interdepartmental Working Group on the Treatment of Vulnerable or Intimidated Witnesses in the Criminal Justice System.* Home Office: London.

Victim Support website 🖳 www.victimsupport.org.uk

Admission for assessment

Many ID nurses in forensic roles work in inpatient and secure services, and their day-to-day work involves working with people who have been detained in hospital for assessment and/or treatment. In England and Wales[†] the involuntary admission of people to hospital for assessment and treatment of mental disorder is governed by the MHA 1983.

Involuntary admission

Involuntary admission to hospital can take place only if a person is suffering from mental disorder within the meaning of the MHA, and detention in hospital is necessary for their own health and safety and/or the protection of other people. Mental disorder means any disorder or disability of the mind. A person with ID cannot be considered to be suffering from mental disorder within the meaning of the MHA unless their disability is associated with abnormally aggressive or seriously irresponsible conduct.

Part II Mental Health Act

Part II of the MHA provides civil arrangements for compulsory admission to hospital and guardianship. The vast majority of people who are involuntarily admitted to hospital for assessment and/or treatment of mental disorder are admitted under Part II of the Act.

Part III Mental Health Act

Part III of the MHA provides arrangements for patients who are concerned with criminal proceedings or under sentence to be detained to hospital for assessment and/or treatment of mental disorder.

Assessment or treatment

It can be unclear whether a patient who needs to be detained should be admitted for assessment or treatment. Patients who are admitted for assessment will often need and receive treatment, and patients who are admitted for treatment will often need to be assessed as part of the treatment process. The core focus of assessment for most people with ID will be to gain an understanding of problematic and offending behaviour, and any association between their ID and behaviour that could result in harm to self and/or others.

Indications for assessment

- The patient has never previously been admitted to hospital and/or has not been in regular contact with specialist services.
- The diagnosis/cause of the patients' problems is unclear. Previously established treatment/interventions require reformulation, including assessment of the potential for informal treatment.
- The presenting needs/condition of the patient are judged to have changed since an earlier involuntary admission.

Table 11.1 The Mental Health Act 1983. Admission for assessment

Admission for assessment

Section No	Purpose	Duration	Requirements
Part II: Compulsory admission to hospital and guardianship			
Section 2	Admission for assessment	Up to 28d	Evidence of mental disorder/cannot be assessed without detention
Section 4	Admission for assessment in an emergency	Up to 72hrs	Urgent necessity with a view to admission for assessment under S.2
Section 5 (2)	Doctor holding power	Up to 72hrs	Patient already receiving treatment of mental disorder as in-patient—with a view to admission for assessment under S.2
Section 5(4)	Nurses holding power	Up to 6hrs	Evidence of immediate risk of harm—need to secure attendance of responsible/approved clinician
Section 135	Warrant for the police to search for and remove a patient to place of safety for a mental health assessment	Up to 72hrs	Evidence to suggest mental disorder and need for a mental health assessment
Section 136	Police power to remove a person from a public place to a place of safety for a mental health assessment	Up to 72hrs	Evidence to suggest mental disorder and need for a mental health assessment
Part III: Patients concerned in criminal proceedings or under sentence			
Section 35	Remand to hospital for report on accused's mental condition	Up to 3 periods of 28d—not to exceed 12 weeks in total	Evidence to suggest that an accused person who is to be remanded awaiting trial or sentence is suffering from mental disorder that requires assessment in hospital

Further reading

Stone N (2008). *A Companion Guide to Mentally Disordered Offenders*. Shaw & Sons: Kent.

Department of Health (2008). *Revised Mental Health Act Code of Practice*. Department of Health: London.

† Readers from Northern Ireland and Scotland should refer to their own specific legislation.

Admission for treatment

Many ID nurses in forensic roles work in inpatient services, some of which are secure services. Their day-to-day work involves working with people who have been involuntarily admitted to hospital for treatment. The involuntary admission of people to hospital for treatment of mental disorder is governed by the MHA 1983 (revised 2007).

Involuntary admission

Involuntary admission to hospital can take place only if a person is suffering from mental disorder within the meaning of the MHA, and detention in hospital is necessary for their own health and safety, and/or the protection of other people (see 🕮 Admission for assessment, p.414).

Part II Mental Health Act

Part II of the MHA provides civil arrangements for compulsory admission to hospital and guardianship. The vast majority of people who are involuntarily admitted to hospital for assessment and/or treatment of a mental disorder are admitted under Part II of the Act.

Part III Mental Health Act

Part III of the MHA provides arrangements for patients who are concerned with criminal proceedings or under sentence to be involuntarily admitted to hospital for assessment and/or treatment of mental disorder.

Treatment

Treatment for many people with ID who are involuntarily admitted to hospital will be focused on addressing the 'abnormally aggressive' and 'seriously irresponsible conduct' that resulted in their detention. In the context of forensic nursing, treatment may include:
- **Behavioural interventions**—i.e. development or implementation of effective behavioural support and management plans that can be generalized to other settings/risk management plans
- **Offence specific treatment**—i.e. sex offender treatment programmes, treatment of fire setting behaviour, and treatment of violent offending
- **Related treatment**—e.g. anger management, anxiety management, problem solving, cognitive skills programmes
- **Interventions to improve day-to-day functioning**—social skills programmes, activities for daily living skills programmes, and interpersonal skills training.

Some people who are admitted involuntarily for treatment will also require treatment for mental illness (e.g. schizophrenia, bipolar affective disorder).

Appropriate treatment test

The availability of appropriate treatment is a requirement of detention to hospital for treatment of mental disorder. Treatment must be appropriate, taking into account the nature and degree of the person's mental disorder, and all the other circumstances of the person's case. The MHA Revised Code of Practice provides extensive guidance regarding this appropriate treatment test.

Further reading

Department of Health (2008). *Revised Mental Health Act Code of Practice*. Department of Health: London.

Table 11.2 The Mental Health Act 1983. Admission for treatment

Admission for treatment

Section No	Purpose	Duration	Requirements
Part II: Compulsory admission to hospital and guardianship			
Section 3	Admission for treatment	2 periods of 6 months and then renewable annually	Suffering from mental disorder which needs treatment in hospital and cannot be treated without detention
Part III: Patients concerned in criminal proceedings or under sentence			
Section 36	Remand of accused person to hospital for treatment	Up to 3 periods of 28 days—not to exceed 12 weeks in total	Evidence an accused person who is to be remanded awaiting trial or sentence is suffering from mental disorder which requires treatment in hospital
Section 37— with or without restriction order (S.41)	Hospital order— power of courts to order hospital admission for treatment May include Ministry of Justice restrictions in discharge (section 41MHA)	2 periods of 6 months and then renewable annually	Conviction for an imprisonment offence—requires treatment in hospital for mental disorder. Hospital order replaces sentence.
Section 38	Interim hospital order	Periods of 28 days renewable by the court for a total period not exceeding 1 year	Conviction for an imprisonment offence. Requires period of treatment in hospital to allow assessment regarding appropriateness of section 37
Section 47—with or without restriction order (S.49)	Transfer to hospital of a person serving a prison sentence. May include Ministry of Justice restrictions in discharge (section 49MHA)	S49 restriction order expires	Person serving a sentence of imprisonment requires treatment for mental disorder in hospital

Emergency holding powers

The detention of people for assessment and treatment of mental disorder is governed by the MHA 1983 (revised 2007). Section 5(4) and 5(2) of the MHA 1983 makes provision for patients who are already in hospital informally to be detained for a short period in order for a MHA assessment to be undertaken.

Use of Section 5(2)

The provisions under Section 5(2) can be used by a doctor or approved clinician to detain a patient who is already in hospital informally for treatment of mental disorder for up to 72hrs. Once Section 5(2) is invoked, the patient must be assessed for detention for assessment treatment under the MHA 1983 within 72hrs.

Indications for use

- The doctor or approved clinician in charge of the treatment of the patient (or their nominated deputy) has concluded that an application for admission under the MHA should be made.
- Detention of the patient under Section 5(2) is necessary in order for an application for admission to be made.

Considerations and safeguards

- Section 5(2) can be invoked only by the doctor or approved clinician (or their nominated deputy) in charge of the treatment of the patient's mental disorder.
- Detention commences at the moment the doctor or approved clinician's report has been delivered to the hospital managers.
- Section 5(2) can be used only for people who are already being treated for mental disorder as inpatients, and cannot be used for anyone attending hospital as an outpatient.
- When Section 5(2) is invoked, hospital staff may use the minimum reasonable force to prevent the patient leaving the hospital (see 📖 Use of restraint, p.426).

Other settings

Emergency holding powers in the MHA can be used only in hospital settings, including NHS hospitals and registered independent hospitals. For predictable emergencies and crisis situations in other settings, contingency plans can be agreed as part of a community care package. If a person is prevented from leaving, this may constitute restraint. Any use of restraint may have to be justified under common law doctrine of necessity, which provides a general power to take the steps that are reasonably necessary and proportionate to protect others from immediate risk of significant harm. If it is considered necessary to regularly prevent a person leaving, consideration should be given regarding the need for a legal framework.

Guardianship Section 7 and Section 37 MHA 1983—this is a framework for working with a patient in a community setting, where this cannot be provided without compulsory powers. This may include a condition of residence to which the person can be returned if required.

Deprivation of liberty safeguards MHA 2005—An application for deprivation of liberty can be made for a person who lacks capacity, if this is necessary and justifiable in their best interests, and there is no less restrictive alternative. This protects staff who are responsible for the person's care and safety, and provides legal safeguards to the person whose liberty is curtailed (see 📖 Use of restraint, p.426).

Other agencies—police/criminal justice system

The police have a range of powers to detain people where this is necessary to protect against harm and/or in order to investigate alleged crimes:

- Powers to remove a person suspected of being mentally disordered to a place of safety under sections 135 and 136 of the MHA 1983
- Powers to arrest and detain people suspected of committing an unlawful act (see 📖 People who have offended in law, p.402)
- Powers to restrain a person to protect life and property
- Conditions of residence as part of bail arrangements, community (probation) orders.

Further reading

Department of Health (2008). *Revised Mental Health Act Code of Practice.* Department of Health: London.

Department of Health (2008). *The Mental Capacity Act 2005 Deprivation of Liberty Safeguards Addendum to the Mental Capacity Act Code of Practice.* Department of Health: London.

Nurses holding power

The detention of people for assessment and treatment of mental disorder in England and Wales is governed by the MHA 1983 (revised 2007). Section 5(4) of the MHA 1983 makes provision for patients who are already in hospital informally to be detained for a short period by a registered nurse in order for a MHA assessment to be undertaken.

Use of Section 5 (4)

The provisions under Section 5(4) can be used by a registered nurse (mental health or ID) to detain a patient who is already in hospital for treatment of mental disorder for up to 6hrs. Once Section 5(4) is invoked the patient must be assessed within 6hrs by a doctor or approved clinician who has the power to use Section 5(2) of the MHA 1983 (see 📖 Emergency holding powers, p.418).

Indications for use

- Immediate necessity to prevent the patient leaving the hospital for the sake of their own safety and/or the protection of others
- Not practicable to secure the attendance of a practitioner who can complete a report under Section 5(2) MHA 1983 (see 📖 Emergency holding powers, p.418).

Considerations and safeguards

- A nurse cannot be instructed by anyone else to use Section 5(4) to detain a patient.
- In reaching a decision to use Section 5(4) the nurse should fully assess the circumstances and presenting needs of the patient including:
  - how soon arrangements can be made for the patient to be assessed by a doctor or approved clinician
  - whether the patient can be persuaded to remain until they can be assessed by a doctor or approved clinician
  - the harm that might occur if the patient leaves hospital before the doctor or approved clinician.
- The registered nurse who is responsible for invoking Section 5(4) must record the decision, the reasons for it, and the time it was invoked in the patient's records. This record must then be sent to the hospital managers.
- When Section 5(4) is invoked, hospital staff may use the minimum reasonable force to prevent the patient leaving the hospital (see 📖 Use of restraint, p.426).
- If a doctor or approved clinician has not attended within 6hrs, the patient must be released from detention.

Further reading

Department of Health (2008). *Revised Mental Health Act Code of Practice*. Department of Health: London.

Mental Health Review Tribunal

The detention of people for assessment and treatment of mental disorder in England and Wales is governed by the MHA 1983 (revised 2007). The MHA provides several safeguards for patients who have had their liberty curtailed under the Act, including the MHRT (Section 65 MHA).

Purpose

* An independent judicial body for detained patients to appeal against detention
* To review the cases of detained and conditionally discharged patients (Section 41 MHA)
* To review the cases of patients subject to Community Treatment Orders (section 17A MHA) and Guardianship Orders (sections 7 and 37 MHA).

Mental Health Review Tribunal rules

MHRTs must be arranged and conducted in accordance with the rules laid down in the MHA 1983.

Applying for a MHRT

Applications must be made in writing. Hospital managers have a duty to ensure that patients and their nearest relative (unless the patient requests otherwise) are informed of their right to apply for a MHRT. Applications can be made when:

* the patient is first detained in hospital for assessment or treatment, or made subject to a Guardianship Order (Section 7 or 37 MHA)
* a patient is transferred from guardianship (Section 7 or 37 MHA) to hospital or discharged from hospital subject to a Supervised Community Treatment Order (section 17A MHA)
* when detention in hospital is renewed
* when a Supervised Community Treatment Order is extended or revoked
* when the patient's status under the MHA changes e.g. from Section 2 to Section 3. (see 📖 Admission for assessment, p. 414; 📖 Admission for treatment, p.416; 📖 Management in the community, p.430)

Under specified circumstances when the patient has not exercised the right to apply for a MHRT, the managers of the hospital must make an application on behalf of the patient.

Composition

* The MHRT must comprise at least 3 members, including a legal member, medical member, and a non-medical member
* The legal member will be the chair
* Non-legal members are required to have some relevant specialist expertise.

Powers (Section 72 MHA)

The powers of the MHRT are:

* to direct the discharge of a detained patient if they are not satisfied the patient is suffering from mental disorder (within the meaning of the MHA) to a nature or degree that warrants detention in hospital

- to direct the discharge of a detained patient if detention is not justified in the interests of the health and safety of the patient and/or for the protection of others
- to specify that the patient must be discharged on a date in future.

Considerations

In reaching a decision whether to direct discharge, the MHRT must consider all the relevant circumstances of the case including the:
- availability of appropriate treatment (Section 145 MHA) and the likelihood of treatment alleviating or preventing deterioration in the patient's condition
- the likelihood of the patients being able to care for himself, to be able to obtain the care he needs, or to guard against serious exploitation.

Other safeguards
- Hospital manager's hearings
- Independent mental health advocates (Revised MHA Code of Practice 2008)
- MHAC (Section 121 MHA)
- PALS

Role of the intellectual disability nurse

- Ensure that patients are aware of their rights to apply for a MHRT
- Take all possible steps to provide information about MHRTs in a form that is accessible and understandable to the patient. Provide this information as frequently as necessary
- Assist patients who are physically unable to do so (e.g. unable to read or write) to apply for MHRT. This may include making a written application on their behalf or enabling access to advocacy services
- Ensure detained patients are aware of their entitlement to free legal advice and representation
- Assist detained patients to request the services of an appropriate legal representative
- Provide the necessary support and assistance to enable detained patients to have contact with their legal representative
- Contribute as part of the multidisciplinary team to assessments that will inform reports for consideration by the MHRT.

Further reading

Department of Health (2008). *Revised Mental Health Act Code of Practice*. Department of Health: London.

Mental Health Act Commission

The detention of people for assessment and treatment of mental disorder in England and Wales is governed by the MHA 1983 (revised 2007). The MHA provides several safeguards for patients who have had their liberty curtailed under the Act, including the MHAC (Section 121 MHA). The MHAC is empowered to review care and treatment provided to detained patients in NHS and independent hospitals, and care homes.

Purpose

The purpose of the MHAC is to safeguard the interests of all people detained under the MHA.

Functions

- To review the operation of the MHA in respect of patients liable to be detained under the MHA
- To visit and interview in private, patients detained under the MHA in NHS and registered independent hospitals (including mental health nursing homes)
- Investigate complaints that fall within the remit of the MHAC
- To appoint medical practitioners and others to give second opinions where this is required under the MHA
- To monitor the implementation of the MHA Code of Practice (revised 2008)
- To provide regular reports to Parliament relating to the operation of the MHA.

Structure and roles

The MHAC is comprised of lay people, lawyers, doctors, nurses, social workers, psychologists, and other specialists. Commissioners work at local and area levels to keep the operation of the MHA under review.

Local commissioners

- Visit detained patients
- Examine patients records
- Take up immediate issues on behalf of detained patients
- Identify issues for action and decide how they can be resolved
- Maintain supportive but objective relationships with local services who provide care and treatment to detained patients.

Area commissioners

- Coordinate the work of the MHAC
- Develop and maintain working relationships with providers, social services departments, user groups, and other relevant agencies
- Provide annual reports to the Boards of all providers who deal with detained patients.

Second opinion doctors

When a detained patient is incapable of giving consent or refusing to consent to treatment, the responsible clinician or approved clinician has a duty to obtain a second opinion. The MHAC are responsible for the appointment of second opinion doctors for this purpose. A second opinion is required for *detained patients* who lack capacity to consent:
- when medication is continued beyond the first 3mths of treatment
- if ECT is to be used.

Other safeguards

- Hospital managers hearings
- Independent mental health advocates (Revised MHA Code of Practice 2008)
- MHRT (Section 65 MHA)
- PALS.

Further reading

Jones R (2008). *The Mental Health Act Manual*, 10th edn. Sweet and Maxwell: London.

The Mental Health Act Commission website— 🖳 www.mhac.org.uk

Use of restraint

Restraint can be described as the intentional restriction of a person's movement or behaviour.[1] Restraint, which is also referred to as physical intervention, may be a required and justifiable component of patient care to prevent harm to the patient and to other people.[2] Restraint may also be used by other agencies, including the police and prison service, to manage people who pose a risk of harm to themselves, others, and property. There is a range of interventions that can constitute restraint.[3]

Types of restraint

- *Mechanical restraint*—in a forensic context, physical security, including locked doors, baffle locks, keypads, fences, and the use of seclusion, can be described under the heading of mechanical restraint.
- *Physical restraint*—one or more members of staff holding the person, moving the person, or blocking their movement
- *Technological surveillance*—includes tagging, pressure pads, closed-circuit television, and door alarms.
- *Chemical restraint*—the use of medication to restrain movement, including regular and as-required medication
- *Psychological restraint*—can include telling someone that what they want to do is not allowed and depriving people of their lifestyle choices (see 🕮 Behavioural interventions, p.302).

When can restraint be used?

Restraint may be necessary in these situations:

- Where the patient's behaviour has the potential to cause harm or is causing harm to themselves e.g. deliberate self-harm, attempted suicide, other dangerous actions
- Where the patient's behaviour has the potential to cause harm or is causing harm to other people e.g. violence
- To prevent a person leaving who is subject to legal orders e.g. detained under the MHA.

Principles

- Complete assessments to identify and address underlying reasons for violence, aggression and self-harm (see 🕮 Risk assessment, p.100, and 🕮 Risk assessment and management, p.400)
- Respect for privacy and dignity
- Use restraint (physical intervention) only as a last resort
- Use the least restrictive option available to manage risk
- Proportionate—use only that force necessary to respond to the risk
- Use restraint only for as long as necessary to manage the risk of harm
- Use only those techniques for which you are trained.

Considerations

Legal and ethical issues

All interventions that constitute restraint must be justifiable under the common law doctrine of necessity, which provides a general power to take the steps that are reasonably necessary and proportionate to protect others from immediate risk of significant harm. Nurses should be aware that restraining another person without their consent may constitute a criminal offence. The need to protect staff must always be properly balanced with the duty to provide care and protection.

Professional issues

All nurses who are involved in the use of restraint are accountable for their own practice, and must abide by current professional standards and the policy of their employing organization relating to the use of restraint.[3]

Individual responsibilities

- Understand what restraint is and the circumstances in which it may be legally and ethically used
- Minimize the need to use restraint
- Understand the relevant legal and ethical frameworks
- Take action when inappropriate or abusive use of restraint is suspected or observed
- Understand how to minimize the risks if restraint is used.

Negotiated care plans or advanced directives

Wherever possible the views of clients/patients should be taken into account when care/management plans are developed. This can include negotiated plans, where specific approaches can be agreed in advance in the event of restraint being necessary.

Training

Training should cover prevention and management of aggressive and violent behaviour, including recognition, prevention and de-escalation, in addition to techniques used in restraint.

Safety

It must be recognized that there is always a risk of harm when restraint is used. There is clear evidence that death can occur during restraint of a highly resistant person in a face-down position. This is called positional asphyxia. Organizational policies and training should include safeguards against this risk.

Other agencies

Other agencies will abide by their own professional standards, codes, and policies when using restraint.

1 Counsel & Care UK (2002). *Showing Restraint: challenging the use of restraint in care homes.* Counsel & Care UK: London.

2 National Institute for Clinical Excellence (2005). *The Short-term Management of Disturbed/Violent Behaviour in Psychiatric In-patient Settings and A&E Departments.* NICE: London.

3 Royal College of Nursing (2008). *Let's talk about restraint. Rights, risks and responsibilities.* Royal College of Nursing: London.

Keeping yourself safe

Forensic nursing involves working directly with people who may engage in a range of behaviours that have the potential to cause harm to others. Personal safety is an important consideration for all nurses who undertake forensic roles. All registered nurses have a responsibility for their own safety. In addition, organizations that employ nurses to work with people who have the propensity to harm others have a duty to ensure that staff are appropriately trained and supported to undertake their work safely.

Types of harm

Forensic nurses are likely to encounter a range of potentially harmful behaviour in the course of their practice. This places them at risk of various types of harm:

- Physical injury as a result of being a victim of violence and/or as a result of involvement in the management of violent incidents or physical interventions and restraint (see 📖 Use of restraint, p.426).
- Emotional and psychological harm as a result of the demands of the role, and associated with working in direct care roles with people who have significant difficulties in relationships with others.
- Risk of harm as a result of indirect actions e.g. allegations made by patient/clients.
- Risk of sexual harm as a result of sexual assault and/or abusive behaviour.
- Risks associated with the nature of this area of practice including those arising from involvement in decision making about risk and the potential for things to go wrong.

Risk assessment and management

A thorough and objective understanding of the needs and risks of patients is a key component for safe practice.

- Take all available information into account and avoid unnecessary risks.
- Do not compromise your own safety—take time to familiarize yourself with information about the person and avoid short cuts. Tell senior colleagues if you are concerned that you lack the necessary knowledge and understanding to keep yourself safe.
- Ensure all activities that could give rise to risk are discussed and agreed with the person's care team and others involved in the person's care and management.
- All nurses strive to develop positive therapeutic relationships with their patients; never conclude that a special relationship with the person will protect you from harm. Always balance factual information regarding previous behaviour and risks with other opinions, including impressions gained from your personal relationship with the person.
- Always abide by agreed risk management plans regardless of whether you consider these overly cautious or restrictive.

Physical danger

Some nursing roles involve working with people who engage in violent behaviour, and pose a risk of injury or harm to others, including staff:

- Staff should receive training in the management of disturbed and violent behaviour (see 📖 Use of restraint, p.426).

- Clear policies and guidance should be in place regarding the management of violence covering all types of interventions used to manage potentially dangerous behaviour, including restraint, observations, seclusion, training. Always familiarize yourself with these policies, and report any issues that affect your ability to abide by them.
- Additional safeguards should be provided for staff where they are deemed necessary. These may include personal and environmental alarm systems, use of mobile phones, seclusion facilities, debriefing, and other staff support arrangements, and policy on lone working.

Recording and reporting

- Always share any concerns with colleagues and use formal reporting procedures to record and report any and all concerns that could affect your own safety and/or the safety of others. This may include statements and opinions expressed by patients as well as threats and statements of intent to harm other people.
- Report all incidents, including those which could have resulted in harm (near misses), and less serious incidents that are indicative of risk.
- If you are a victim of violence you may report this to the police. Even though the police response may be affected because the incident involves a person with ID, you have the same rights as any other victim (see 📖 Rights of victims, p.406).

Code of conduct

All nurses must abide by the NMC code of conduct, performance, and ethics. The code includes important requirements for safe practice:

- Respect people's confidentiality—you must disclose information if you believe someone may be at risk
- Share information with colleagues
- Work effectively as part of a team and manage risk
- Keep clear and accurate records
- Maintain clear professional boundaries.

In the interests of clients, patients, and registrants, the NMC recommends that registered nurses have professional indemnity insurance in the event of claims of professional negligence.

The forensic process is adversarial, and nurses may experience serious conflicts between their caring and custodial/public protection roles. Role clarity is absolutely essential for safe practice and you must ensure that you always work strictly within the boundaries of your role and competence.

Further reading

Nursing and Midwifery Council (2008). *The Code: Standards of Conduct, Performance and Ethics For Nurses and Midwives.* Nursing and Midwifery Council: London.

Management in the community

Offenders should always be managed using the least restrictive option available that is sufficient to protect other people and prevent further offending. For many offenders a community disposal will be sufficient, and will enable the offender to receive ongoing input and supervision without recourse to a custodial sentence. Offenders with ID should have access to the same range of community options as other offenders. This can be problematic unless additional support is available to help the person understand what is required of them and to assist them to abide by any conditions that may be imposed to manage the risk of harm. For many offenders with ID, a shared approach that involves joint working between the criminal justice system, specialist ID services, and social services, will provide the most effective means of reducing reoffending and managing the risk of harm.

Options for community management

Community sentences

Community sentences are a combination of punishment and interventions to change the offender's behaviour. Community sentences can also include a condition that the offender participates in treatment, and can be used to encourage an offender to deal with problems that might be contributing to their offending i.e. drinks and drugs, mental disorder. A range of different orders have recently been replaced with a single generic community order (previously called a probation order), which can be personalized to a specific offender with a range of possible conditions and requirements:

- Compulsory/unpaid work
- Participation in specified activities, including offending behaviour programmes, and attendance for treatment of associated problems e.g. mental health problems, drug or alcohol problems
- Prohibition from certain activities
- Curfew
- Exclusion from specified areas
- Residence requirement
- Supervision by the probation service
- Technological restrictions, including tagging.

A community sentence is not available unless the offender is able to give an informed indication that they are willing and able to comply with the order itself, and any requirements. It should not be assumed that people with ID cannot benefit from a community sentence. Specialist ID services can advise the probation service and the courts regarding the use of community sentences, and advise on how ID offenders can be supported to understand and comply with any requirements, and to benefit from the order.

Civil enforcement

These orders are intended to manage harmful behaviour in the community. The orders can be made by lower courts (in their civil capacity) or a county court. The police can apply for an order.

Antisocial behaviour orders (ASBOs)

- The police and other agencies can apply for an ASBO
- Application must be supported by evidence of antisocial behaviour

- Order includes specified conditions to prevent antisocial behaviour
- Breach of the order is a criminal offence.

Sex offender prevention orders (SOPOs)
- The police can apply for a SOPO
- Application must be supported by evidence of behaviour that is sexually risky or indicative of the risk of sexual harm
- May include general and specific prohibitions e.g. to remain at a specified distance from a local school, not to enter parks
- Breach of the order is a criminal offence.

Appropriate behaviour contracts (ABCs)
An ABC is an informal agreement with the police in the form of a written contract agreed and signed at a meeting involving the individual. The potential for legal action to be taken can be stated in the contract. People with ID can benefit from these arrangements but care should be taken to ensure that the person concerned has the capacity to understand what is expected of them, and the consequences if they fail to abide by the requirements of civil enforcement order. Specialist ID staff can help people to understand these orders and provide advice to the police regarding appropriate requirements.

Multiagency public protection arrangements (MAPPA)
MAPPA are the statutory arrangements for managing sexual and violent offenders. The police, probation and prison services are the responsible authorities for MAPPA. The MAPPA provides structures and mechanisms for agencies to come together to agree risk management plans for offenders, including plans for people being released from prison.

Mental Health Act 1983
The MHA includes options that can support a package of care and treatment in the community:
- Guardianship Order—Section 7 & 37 MHA
- Supervised Community Treatment Order—Section 17A
- Section 17 leave—including trial leave prior to discharge
- Section 117 aftercare

Joint working
The most effective means of community management is through joint and collaborative working between the various agencies that have a responsibility for public safety. This shared approach should provide shared decision making about risk. Wherever possible the responsibility for risk should also be shared with the individual concerned. ID services should engage with partners in other agencies to ensure that all reasonable steps have been taken to support people in their communities.

Working with criminal justice agencies

There is a great deal of guidance for professionals in the criminal justice system and staff in health and welfare organisations which focuses upon inter-agency and joint working with mentally disordered offenders. Decisions on law enforcement, diversion from the normal process of criminal law, and disposal options for people with ID who are alleged to have committed offences and/or who are convicted, are inconsistent and at times seem arbitrary.

The criminal justice system

The National Offender Management Service (NOMS) has overall respon-sibility for correctional services, and provides a bridge between custodial and community services. The criminal justice system is made up of several agencies that have general responsibilities in terms of crime prevention and reduction, and specific responsibilities to address the needs and risks of offenders and alleged offenders. These agencies work closely together to fulfill their responsibilities, and provide a range of custodial and community services. The main services that make up the criminal justice system are:
- Police
- Probation service
- Prison service
- Courts.

Multiagency public protections arrangements

MAPPA are the statutory arrangements for managing sexual and violent offenders. The police, probation, and prison services are the responsible authorities for MAPPA. Other public bodies, including the NHS and social services, have a duty to cooperate with the MAPPA. The MAPPA approach to collaborative working can be applied to specialist health roles that involve joint working with criminal justice agencies.

Criminal justice liaison

People with ID who get into trouble with the law constitute a small minority group who are not a high priority for the criminal justice system. Criminal justice agencies need specialist advice and input to adequately address the particular needs of this group, and improve access to the responses, services, and interventions available to all offenders, where these are appropriate and could manage and reduce the risk of offending.

Staff in ID teams, including nurses, can provide valuable support in the form of criminal justice liaison roles:
- Support people with ID who get into trouble with the law to understand their own situations and the decisions that are made as part of the criminal justice process
- Develop working relationships with local criminal justice agencies, including police, probation service, prisons, and courts
- Develop a knowledge base regarding the operation of the criminal justice system, and identify points at which practical help, specialist advice, input, and support could be beneficial
- Provide advice to inform decisions about people with ID who get into trouble with the law

- Provide advice/information regarding other services, including contact details.

Role clarity is absolutely essential when working at the interface between health services and the law:

- At all times be aware that you may be called upon to justify/defend your opinions in a legal arena.
- Work strictly within the boundaries of your role and competence.
- Get full support from your line manager/employer for all aspects of your practice.
- Communicate and discuss the details of your involvement with your team and through clinical supervision.
- Seek advice and support from others in similar roles, including practitioners in other areas if required.
- Undertake training that equips you for the role, including training specific to mentally disordered offenders, and the law as it applies to people with mental disorder.

Joint working

The most effective means of supporting ID offenders is through joint and collaborative working between the various agencies that have a responsibility for public safety. This shared approach should provide shared decision making about risk. Wherever possible the responsibility for risks should be shared with the individual concerned. ID services should engage with partners in other agencies to ensure that all reasonable steps have been taken to support people in their communities.

Further reading

Riding T, Swann C, Swann B (Eds) (2005). *The Handbook of Forensic Learning Disabilities*. Radcliffe Publishing: Oxford.

Care Services Improvement Partnership & Valuing People Support Team (2007). *Positive Practices Positive Outcomes: A Handbook for Professionals in the Criminal Justice System Working with Offenders with Learning Disabilities*. CSIP & VPST: London.

Lifestyles

Citizenship

The idea of citizenship is based on the relationship between the individual and the state. It embraces the notion of reciprocal rights and responsibilities between citizen and state. If we believe in the existence of rights, it follows that we also believe in corresponding duties. We have a notion of a 'good citizen' who lives up to his responsibilities in society, and believe that the state has an obligation to meet the welfare needs of its citizens. The principle of representation is fundamental in society. It is connected closely with the concept of citizenship, which centres on the relationship between the individual and the state. Marshall has referred to citizenship as a status bestowed on those who are full members of a community.[1] He described three elements of citizenship:

- Civil
- Political
- Social.

The civil element comprises the rights that are necessary for individual freedom. These include personal liberty, freedom of speech, thought and faith, the right to own property, and to conclude valid contracts. The right to justice, a significant civil right, is the legal right to defend all of one's rights on an equal basis by means of the legal process. The political element concerns participation in the exercise of political power at local or national level. It may involve participation either as an elector or as a member of an elected body (local government, parliament) that is invested with political authority. Marshall's social element refers to the whole range, from the right to a modicum of economic welfare and security to the right to a full share in the social heritage, and the right to live the life of a civilized being according to the standards prevailing in the society. Citizens require access to social resources, including health, education, and social services, in order to further their own and other people's civil and political rights. Community care legislation in the UK[2] has emphasized the importance of representation of service users. A central aim of the policy was to give people more say in the services they use. Local authorities, which provide social services, are required to consult with service users and user organizations. The consumer's voice is important, and particularly significant for members of vulnerable groups. Recent years have seen developments in policy and practice in the UK relating to the welfare and interests of disadvantaged groups. The implementation of the Human Rights 1998 sends a clear egalitarian message. Article 14 states that *'the rights and freedoms set forth in this Convention shall be secured without discrimination on any ground'.*[3] While these rights had existed previously, the advantage of the Human Rights Act is that challenges can now be made in UK courts.

Further reading

Walmsley J (1993). Talking to top people: some issues relating to the citizenship of people with learning difficulties. In: Swain J, Finkelstein V, French S, Oliver M, Eds. *Disabling Barriers, Enabling Environments*. Open University and SAGE Publications: London.

1 Marshall TH (1991). *Citizenship and Social Class and Other Essays*. Pluto Press: London.

2 HMSO (1990). *National Health Service and Community Care Act*. HMSO: London.

3 The Human Rights Act 1998. HMSO: London.

Residential alternatives

In most Western countries residential care for people with ID has been influenced by political, ideological, and economic factors. Given that people with ID have been, and still are, often misunderstood this has sometimes resulted in inappropriate residential care being offered to them and their families. In this section a range of residential alternatives for people with ID are outlined. This range currently includes group homes, residential units, hospital type accommodation, intentional communities, tenancy agreements, supported living, home ownership, and family placements.

Hospital type accommodation

Despite the closure of most of the long-stay ID hospitals, some residential care provisions, known as 'residential campuses', have remained. Generally speaking these types of provisions retain therapists, nursing and medical staff, and provide a specialist focus of care.

Some ID hospitals remain in England; ~1500 people with ID still live in hospitals,[1] and in Wales, Scotland, Northern Ireland, and the Republic of Ireland there is long-term hospital care provision.

Across the UK the planned closure dates were: England by 2004, Scotland by 2005, and Wales by 2006. The date set for Northern Ireland is 2010 through a planned programme of reduction in beds.

In the UK and elsewhere there remains some resistance to the final closure of these facilities, and in some countries this kind of residential provision has now moved into the private sector.

This type of residential provision, when compared with others such as village communities and dispersed housing schemes, has failed to uniformly demonstrate quality service, and there appears to be no easy answer to explain why.[2]

Hostels

Hostels emerged during the 1960s and 1970s. Typically they catered for ~12–30 people, were often referred to as 'half-way houses', and were usually run by social service departments.

Many of these establishments remained institutional in nature and continued to perpetuate systems of block treatment and depersonalized forms of care.[3]

A development of the provision of hostel accommodation was that of 'core and cluster' arrangements, where a number of smaller, 'ordinary' houses were clustered around a larger residential unit.

Family placements for adults

Adult placements evolved from the fostering of children with special needs from the 1970s. There are many adult family placement schemes to be found across the countries of the UK and the Republic of Ireland.

People with ID are placed in families other than their own, as an alternative to residential care. The families are approved and trained by an official agency.

Because of the vulnerability of some people with ID, they are highly regulated, with extensive procedures and policies.

Further reading

Grant G, Goward P, Richardson M, Ramcharan P (2005). *Learning Disability: a Life Cycle Approach to Valuing People*. Open University Press: Milton Keynes.

Emerson E, Matton C (1996). *Residential Provision for People with Learning Disabilities: A Research Review*. Hester Adrian Research Centre: Manchester. ⊞ http://www.lancs.ac.uk/fass/ihr/publications/res_review.pdf

1 Department of Health (2001). *Valuing People: A New Strategy For Learning Disability For the 21st Century*. CM 5086. HMSO: London.

2 Emerson E, Robertson J, Gregory N *et al.* (1999). *A Comparative Analysis of Quality and Costs in Group Homes and Supported Living Schemes*. Hester Adrian Research Centre: University of Manchester.

3 Heron A (1982). *Better Services for the Mentally Handicapped? Lessons from the Sheffield Evaluation Studies*. King's Fund: London.

Supported living and home ownership

The preferred residential alternatives for people with ID, at least in Western countries, would appear to be supported living that incorporates homeownership.

Supported living

Supported living might best be thought of not as a single model, but as a range of residential alternatives for people with ID; however, central to all alternatives are living in one's own home, participating in one's own community, this is what has become known of as inclusion, and with all planning centred on the individual.

The Scottish Executive has described supported living as 'a form of intensive domiciliary service (support provided to people in their own home)'.

Supported living was developed in the USA and was born from frustration of the then dominant residential alternatives for people with ID.

Supported living represents a way of constructing services that takes services to people's own homes, and then develops around them the kinds of support that they need to live as independently as possible.

Typically this type of service will include staffing and agency management costs, and may also include a support tenant.

The costs are met from a combination of housing benefits and any other grants from central government and local social services (or in Northern Ireland—Health and Social Care Boards).

Within this type of residential alternative a range of options should be available, including rented or leased accommodation, or ownership of one's own property.[1] Barr et al. reported on the use of focus groups to collect data from people with ID to review accommodation and support preferences.[2] They pointed to a number of important themes to emerge, and these related to the importance of social networks, inclusion, reciprocal relationships, privacy, and security. They concluded that maintaining contact with their families and their local community was important in commissioning the location of new accommodation.

As this is a developing and relatively new approach it is likely that further evaluation will be needed to demonstrate the longer-term success of this approach.[1]

Further reading

Simons K, Ward L (1997). *A Foot in the Door: the Early Years of Supported Living for People with Learning Difficulties in the UK.* Joseph Rowntree Foundation: York

Joseph Rowntree Foundation ▦ http://www.jrf.org.uk/

Paradigm ▦ http://www.paradigm-uk.org

1 Simmons K, Watson D (1999). *The View from Arthur's Seat: a Literature Review of Housing and Support Options 'Beyond Scotland'.* The Scottish Office Central Research Unit, The Stationery Office: Edinburgh.

2 Barr O, McConkey R, McConaghie J (2003). Views of people with learning difficulties about current and future accommodation: the use of focus groups to promote discussion. *Disability & Society* **18**(5), 577–597.

Village and intentional communities

In 2001, the Department of Health in England defined village communities as '[a] service operated by [an] independent organization comprising houses clustered on one site together that share facilities'. An intentional community was defined as 'services operated by [an] independent sector organization comprising houses and some shared facilities on one or more sites based on philosophical or religious belief'.[1]

Village communities

The origins of such communities lie in the Camphill Village movement, established by Dr Karl König in Scotland during the 1940s.

This movement is based on the educational theories of Rudolf Steiner (1861–1925), and it was from his philosophy that the idea of therapeutic communities was developed.[2]

Therapies are supported by anthroposophical ideas and homoeopathic medicines, which, alongside the community experience, are designed to: '*foster the harmonious development of the whole human being—body, soul and spirit—to create a healthy balance between thinking, feeling, and with activity, and to engender morality, social cooperation and responsibility*'.[3]

In such communities, residents contribute what they can to the well-being of other members, according to their abilities. The idea is to foster mutual help and understanding in an environment that seeks to counter some of the supposed 'harmful' ways of modern life.

Non-disabled members of the community are not referred to as carers, rather as coworkers. They do not receive financial remuneration for their efforts and the nature of the relationship between other village members is based on equality.

Intentional communities

A problem with the description '*village communities*' is that not all such communities can properly be described as villages, and so an alternative term, '*intentional communities*', has emerged, which perhaps describes them more accurately.

Other types of residential community include L'Arche, a federation of communities in the UK, France, Denmark, Belgium, Norway, USA, and India, and Cottage and Rural Enterprise, and the Home Farm Trust.

Conclusion

There are numerous configurations for different types of residential care provision that can be made available for people with ID. However, where and how people with ID live should ultimately be a matter of their choice.

Further reading

Grant G, Goward P, Richardson M, Ramcharan P (2005). *Learning Disability: A Life Cycle Approach to Valuing People*. Open University Press: Milton Keynes.

The Orchard Trust 🖬 www.orchard-trust.org.uk

L'Arche 🖬 www.larche.org.uk

The Home Farm Trust 🖬 http://www.hft.org.uk/p/27/About_Us.html

1 Department of Health (2001). *Valuing People: A New Strategy for Learning Disability for the 21st Century*. CM 5086. HMSO: London.

2 Jackson R (1999). The case for village communities for adults with learning disabilities: an exploration of the concept. *Journal of Learning Disabilities for Nursing, Health and Social Care* **3**(2), 110–117.

3 Fulgosi L (1990). Camphill communities. In: Segal S (Ed). *The Place of Special Villages and Residential Communities*. AB Academic Publishers: Oxford, 39–48.

Risk management

Definition

Whereas 📖 Risk assessment and management (p.400) looked at the topic in the context of forensic nursing, this section looks more broadly at risk in the context of lifestyles. There are many definitions of risk management currently available, but broadly risk management in healthcare may be broken down into two aspects:

Strategic risk management, in which the emphasis is on doing 'the right thing', this should be stated clearly within an organization's business plans, operational policies, and procedures and risk registers. A risk register provides an assurance framework for the organization, and should be supported by an action plan, created to each of the risks identified. It is important that all staff make themselves aware of their role and responsibilities in relation to an organization's risk management processes.

Operational risk management, where the emphasis is on ensuring that all staff are 'doing things right'. This has clear links to the NMC professional code of conduct, clinical competency and governance, and general management of services.[1] The care programme approach provides a systematic framework for managing risks in clinical settings. This area is addressed in more detail in 📖 Risk assessment and management, p.400. As operational risk management is an ongoing process, there is a clear need that this is linked with practitioners' ongoing development, and should be linked for all staff to the knowledge and skills framework, and clinical and management supervision processes.

Policy

Within the NHS, there are clear policies and procedures for the management of risk within organizations. There are many organizations that are relevant to healthcare delivery and risk management, including: Health and Safety Executive, National Institute for Health and Clinical Excellence, NHS Litigation Authority, National Patient Safety Agency, Mental Health Act Commission, Healthcare Commission, Commission for Social Care Inspection.

All individuals are accountable for maintaining their knowledge around risk management policies and strategies, within their organization and in other agencies. ID nurses should know how this impinges on their day-to-day practice and be able to communicate risk issues.

Litigation

The NHS Litigation authority administers the Clinical Negligence schemes for NHS trusts,[2] and thereby provides a means for organizations to fund the cost of clinical negligence claims.

Person-centred risk management

Good person-centred risk management (see Fig. 12.1) is needed for services and for people with ID. Risk management principles must support people, and must not restrict the provision of good quality person-centred outcomes. Saunders has identified that strategies should signify (person-centred) values rather than be controlling, and they should not be seen as a way of protecting organizations from litigation.[3]

When supporting an individual to manage risks associated with their lifestyle, it is crucial to determine that the person has the capacity to make decisions specific to that particular risk. When someone makes an unwise decision this does not imply incapacity. It is essential that when addressing issues of capacity that ID nurses are fully compliant with the Mental Capacity Act 2005. Guidance may vary across the 4 countries of the UK and Ireland, but the key principles remain important.

Conclusion

The NMC has clearly stated in relation to risk management that all reg-istrants have a responsibility to deliver safe and effective care based on current evidence, best practice, and where applicable, validated research.[4] Registrants have a duty to their patients and clients to ensure they receive safe and competent care as well as being responsible for minimizing risk to patients or clients. The relevant clauses in the NMC Code to support issues concerning risk and risk management are 1.4, 8.1, 8.2 and 8.3.[4]

Steps must be taken to ensure that the patient's autonomy is respected and their consent always obtained. There may be times where there is conflict between professional accountability and patient autonomy. When facing professional dilemmas, the first consideration of the ID nurse must be the interests and safety of patients.

The role and dilemma facing ID nursing is to balance the rights and choices of the people they are supporting to lead an independent life and to experience new opportunities, while not exposing people to unneces-sary dangers or being too restrictive. The recent Healthcare Commission Report: *A Life Like No Other* (2007) has highlighted the needs for good risk management strategies.[5]

Further reading

Bowden D (1995). Is clinical practice improved by risk management? *Journal of Evaluation in Clinical Practice* **1**(1), 77–79.

1 Nursing and Midwifery Council (2004). *Code of Professional Conduct.* Nursing and Midwifery Council: London.

2 NHS Litigation Authority (2007). *Pilot Risk Management Standards for Mental Health and Learning Disability Trusts.* 🖳 http://www.nhsla.com/RiskManagement/ [accessed April 2009]

3 Saunders M (1999). *Managing Risk in Service for People with Learning Disabilities.* York Association of Practitioners in Learning Disability (APLD).

4 Nursing and Midwifery Council (2006). *A-Z advice sheet, Risk Management.* Nursing and Midwifery Council: London.

5 Healthcare Commission Report (2007). *A Life Like No Other.* Healthcare Commission: London.

Productive work

Many people with ID want to work. They can become productive workers if given the opportunity. Indeed it is vital that this happens. Being a worker:

- increases their status within the family and society, and they are seen as having talents and abilities
- reduces their dependency on others; it takes away some of the strain of care-giving within families and services
- enhances their self-esteem and self-confidence; being trusted with responsibilities brings other personal gains, in physical well-being and mental health
- provides opportunities for socializing; relationships can be formed and a greater range of social supports accessed.

Opportunities for work

As Fig. 12.1 shows, there are many opportunities for people to become productive workers. These can be grouped into three strands.

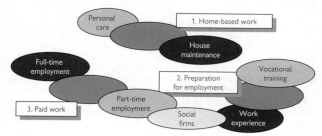

Fig. 12.1 Opportunities for productive work.

Home-based work—this can start at an early age as children and teenagers learn to care for themselves e.g. eating, washing, and dressing. These family-based experiences can be extended into household chores such as cooking and cleaning. As their competence grows, a variety of house main-tenance tasks become possible e.g. window cleaning, painting, gardening. These skills can be used in their own homes, but this type of work can also be done for neighbours and friends on a voluntary basis. Indeed, these skills may form the basis for obtaining paid work. Families and schools are key to promoting these forms of work opportunities.

Preparation for employment—this strand provides opportunities for acquiring the general skills required to hold down a job e.g. time keeping, communication, and cooperation, as well as the specific competences needed to undertake certain jobs. These skills can be acquired as part of training courses undertaken in schools and colleges alongside work expe-rience opportunities in realistic settings. Voluntary work also offers many opportunities to acquire and develop work-related skills, e.g. assisting in a charity shop, helping in old people's homes or care-taking duties in a community centre. Increasingly schools promote these options as well as colleges and specialist employment services.

Options for paid work—growing numbers of people are attaining their ambition to be in paid employment. In the past this type of work has been mainly around 'sheltered' employment, specifically for persons with disabilities. However fears of exploitation have seen these options replaced by 'social firms' in which workers with disabilities are treated more as employees or as trainees. Part-time paid employment with one or more employees can be especially suited to people with disabilities and avoids some of the problems around reduction in benefits, although full-time employment has been possible for some and reduces greatly their dependency on services. Self-employment opportunities are also developing, e.g. baking specialty products. The advent of specialist employment services for people with disabilities has increased these options.

Creating productive workers

Start young—children can learn self-help skills from an early age and should be encouraged to take responsibility for certain tasks around the house. These skills can be further developed in the teenage years and into adulthood. However, it is never too late for people to learn.

Common expectations—person-centred planning is the forum in which the young person, the family, schools and support staff can identify 'work' goals across the spectrum shown in Fig. 12.1, and plan together on how they will support the person's learning. These expectations include completing work to a high standard. Shoddy performance should be discouraged.

Opportunities to work—the experience of work is vital to help young people to test out their talents and appreciate what particular jobs entail. This will also help them to acquire the discipline needed to ensure the job is completed efficiently.

Building intrinsic motivation—work should be personally satisfying, and ways of making it so should be incorporated into any training strategy, e.g. by identifying their preferences and ensuring they feature in the work.

Social skills—among the reasons for people failing in paid employment is a lack of social skills needed to work as part of a team, and acting immaturely. Hence attention needs to be paid to the wider employability skills as well as the specific skills required by particular jobs.

Forward planning—progress reviews will help to identify potential difficulties before they become major problems, and revised plans drawn up to overcome them. Career development plans will provide a context for any further training and help to chart job progression.

Further reading

McConkey R (2007). Leisure and work. In: Gates B (Ed). *Learning Disabilities: Towards Inclusion (5th edn)*. Elsevier: London.

in Control ▣ www.in-control.org.uk

Supported employment

Supported employment is founded on the principle of 'place and train' rather than the idea of 'train then place', which had dominated work opportunities within ID services in the past.

The goal of supported employment is to find paid employment for the person in line with their talents and interests. He or she is trained 'on-the-job' by a 'job coach' who also adjusts the working environment if necessary and enlists the assistance of coworkers to provide additional monitoring and support. The job coach gradually fades out but remains in contact with employers and coworkers to give further advice and support should any problems arise.

Specialist supported employment services have been established in many locations. In the main, these have served clients with mild and moderate disabilities, although there are examples of people with severe disabilities and challenging behaviours also benefiting. They take referrals from various sources, such as school-leavers, FE colleges and career advisers, as well as from individuals and their families.

These services approach employers and undertake an analysis of jobs available in each setting. A profile will be completed of each job seeker, including their present competences, interests, and past experiences. Arrangements will be made for clients to have 'work tasters' by placing them with local businesses for a defined period of time. Also further training courses may be arranged, notably those that lead to an accredited award, such as NVQ.

Clients will be assisted in drawing up a CV, and coached in interview skills. When they are successful in gaining a position, a 'job coach' will be allocated who will teach the skills required for the job to the client in the workplace. The job coach will attend alongside the person until such time as the client can competently complete the work—this may extend from days to weeks.

During the training phase the salary of the new worker may be reduced to reflect the level of their productivity. However, the goal is for the client to be paid at least the national minimum wage or the going rate for that particular post.

The job coach maintains contact with the client, the coworkers and employer to offer advice and support should any difficulties arise. Regular job reviews will be undertaken in line with the client's career development plans.

There is growing evidence for the cost-benefits of these services in getting people into paid work alongside high levels of user satisfaction. To date only a minority of people have been able to access these services, and issues around long-term support have not been resolved. One solution is to engage a wider range of staff in seeking and supporting people in work settings; e.g. staff in supported living schemes could be allocated this function, and personal assistants paid through Direct Payments.

Six key steps in structured teaching

1. Set learning targets—these should be tasks of interest to the person and for which he or she has some of the necessary competences. In other words, it is not going to prove too difficult for them to learn.

2. Graded steps—the task is broken down into discrete steps so that the person can practice doing one step at a time. When they have accomplished one, they can move to doing two steps, then three and so on.

3. Examples—the person needs to be shown what they are expected to do. Telling them is not enough: e.g. digital photographs of the different stages can be used as 'prompts' or verbal cues given to remind them of key steps.

4. Praise—learners' achievements need to be recognized with praise. This serves the dual purpose of letting learners know they are correct while making them more willing to persevere. Equally any mistakes should be quickly pointed need out and an example given of the correct action.

5. Practice—it takes practice for any new skill to be done fluently across different settings and to a consistent standard. 'Over-learning' is recommended for people with ID to minimize mistakes.

6. Realistic settings—the learning and practice is best done in the actual setting where the task is to be performed. Although some practice can be done in 'pretend' settings, the person still has to transfer their skills to the real world. People with learning disabilities can find this difficult to do.

Structured teaching

Job coaches use structured techniques to teach people work skills. These strategies have a long history of success with people with ID e.g. in teaching self-care and household skills. These techniques are based around careful observation and ongoing assessment of each person's competences in one-to-one teaching sessions. Although it may take people longer to learn, they can achieve levels of competence on a par with non-disabled peers. Various training manuals are available to guide front-line staff in how they can implement these and other training strategies.

Benefits

One of the main disincentives to entering into paid employment is the impact of earnings on social security benefits paid to people with ID and their families. Advice should be sought from benefit specialists about the best way of structuring earnings from employment and the.

Further reading

Information on supported employment is available from:

British Association for Supported Employment. — 🖳 http://www.afse.org.uk

European Association for Supported Employment. — 🖳 http://www.euse.org

Networks of support and friends

Everyone needs the support of other people throughout their lives. Often this comes from family and friends rather than formal services. For people with ID, it is the reverse. They overly rely on services and the staff in them, hence many lead lonely and isolated lives. Most people with ID have few friends, irrespective of where they live, and this is often unnoticed.

Of all the assessments carried out by nurses on people with ID, the one least likely to be done is an examination of their friendships and social relationships!

The benefits of friendship are well known. It means having the company of others, times of laughter and adventure, people to give you advice and guidance, practical help, emotional support and protection, and above all, friends to whom you can show love and affection and who will do the same for you. Quality of life studies constantly stress the importance of friendships, and this is no less so for people with ID. Nurses need to promote friendships if they are to promote the health and well-being of people they support. Promoting friendships has its risks. Might they choose the wrong kind of person? Could they be taken advantage of? Will they get hurt if the friendship is not reciprocated? These risks can be managed and they are not an excuse for inaction.

Friendships are founded on three fundamentals:
• Friendships cannot be made for other people; friends choose one another. At best we can build up a network of acquaintances out of which friendships may develop.
• Friendships usually grow out of shared interests and activities, and from among people already known to the person. This is the starting point.
• Friends choose one another. You need to constantly consult and listen to the people you are trying to help. We must not impose our values and desires on to another.

In this section and in 🕮 Encouraging friendships (p.452), three inter-linked strategies are described for promoting friendships and building networks of support.

Expanding social networks

A social network is composed of people who interact socially. We belong to many different networks. We can make this happen for people with ID by getting them involved in leisure, work, and family networks. Often their closest friends will be among other people with a disability—certainly that's how many experience an intimate relationship.

Creating shared interests

Discover the person's interests by talking with them and giving them opportunities to try new things. Photographs will prompt them to remember. Build their self-confidence and encourage a spirit of adventure in trying new things. There are literally hundreds of indoor and outdoor pursuits in which people can get involved.

Respecting self-determination

People are looking for and get different things from friendships. We need to support their informed choices. Avoid being judgemental, but equally explain the risks and safeguards that are sensible. Discretely observe the interactions if you have concerns.

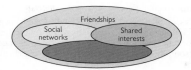

Fig. 12.2 Strategies for promoting friendships.

Getting acquainted

There are three approaches nurses can use to help people become better acquainted with people from their local community.

Supporting community involvement

People need to be supported to be involved in community activities. Doing some form of work in social settings can provide regular contact with other people (see 📖 Productive work, p.446). This can be voluntary or part-time paid work. The volunteer bureau is a good source of information. Citizen's Advice Bureaus will let you know about clubs and societies that meet locally. Support staff may be needed to support people initially in joining these groups.

Supporting friendships through invitations

We can support people with ID to invite their family, friends, neighbours, and workmates and so on, to their home or their centre. Celebrations are a good excuse. Make sure people spend time in activities together. Likewise they need to be supported in accepting invitations to meet other people.

Planning and recording relationships

Each person's individual plan must document the significant friendships in their lives—with photos and contact details listed—and the range of interests and activities they participate in. All staff should receive training on the importance of social relationships in the lives of people they support. This rarely happens at present, as it is not seen as a priority. The high turnover rates among support staff makes it essential to record the valued relationships in people's lives so that continuity of support is provided.

Encouraging friendships

In this section two approaches are described that have proved somewhat successful in developing friendships. There are other ways that can be more effective—through the promotion of advocacy and employment opportunities—when friendships are a bonus from other intended outcomes.

Circles of support

The idea of 'circles of support' or a 'circles of friends' began in Canada as a means of supporting people to belong to their local community.[1] In essence the concept is very simple—a group of people meet regularly to support a person who needs extra assistance to enrich their social and community life.

The circle might include family members, such as siblings, cousins, aunts and uncles, alongside neighbours and acquaintances, the co-workers of people in work settings, and members of clubs, churches etc. who know the person. The size of the circle does not matter, a few interested people can make a start. However, it does not have paid professional workers as members, although they can have a key role in facilitating the formation of the circle or acting as 'go-betweens' for the supported person.

The circle meets from time-to-time to explore with the person and each other the contributions they are making to each other's lives. Activity plans might develop as to how the circle supports the person in the coming weeks and months.

"In all circles of support people are encouraged to dream."[2]

Without a vision of what might be possible, the old routines and disappointments persist for the person with ID. Fulfilling their dreams often involves taking risks, but:

"the circle itself is a safety-net and each time a new risk is safely negotiated greater encouragement is generated to renew the risk-taking effort".[2]

The idea of circles of support can find expression in different ways. For example Key Ring is a housing provider for people with ID that works by building up mutually supportive networks among the tenants living within a geographical area as well as linking them into the communities where they live.[3]

Likewise new forms of day provision often operate on the basis of creating social networks for their clients by slotting them into educational, employment and recreational opportunities in the community.[4]

There is no prescription for the form and format circles of support take as they will be guided very much by the wishes and needs of the person with ID, as identified in their person-centred plan. Indeed the richest plans often develop when a circle of support is recruited to assist in developing the person-centred plan, rather than leaving this to paid support staff.

Befrienders

People can be recruited to act as 'buddies' or 'befrienders' for a person with a disability on either a paid or voluntary basis. They are best thought of as another form of support staff, such as a personal assistant, although a genuine, mutual friendship may develop. Often their role is to accompany the person to leisure activities they both enjoy. Unlike paid staff, they are linked with one person and their times are flexible.

Variations of this idea are found in recruiting host families who are prepared to take a child or an adult into their homes for short breaks, or acting as job coaches in introducing people to work settings (see 📖 Supported employment, p.448).

With the advent of individualized (direct) payments, people with ID or their family carers may recruit their own befrienders.

Befriending schemes need to be planned and implemented carefully to be successful. In particular, a lot of effort has to go into the recruitment and selection of befrienders. Similarly payments of expenses or fees need to take account of implications for tax and social security payments. Increasingly these schemes are provided by agencies who specialize in this form of service provision—usually voluntary organizations.

- Find out if such schemes operate in your area—the local volunteer bureau is a good starting point.
- Identify the particular needs that a befriender might meet for the person with ID. This will help you to arrive at a 'person-specification' for the befriender.
- Explore a range of options for linking the person with other people in addition to seeking a single befriender. Remember too that people with ID can make very good befrienders of each other.
- Introduce yourself to the befrienders and give them your contact details. From time-to-time contact them to find out how things are going, as well as doing it for the person with ID.
- In life, friendships come and go. The loss of a friendship is more noticeable the fewer friends one has. Hence the need to develop circles of support alongside befrienders.

Further reading

McConkey R (2005). Promoting friendships and developing social networks. In: Grant G, Goward P, Richardson M and Ramcharan P (Eds.) *Learning Disability: A Life Cycle Approach to Valuing People*. Open University Press: Milton Keynes.

Circles Network 🖳 http://www.circlesnetwork.org.uk/

The Buddy Scheme 🖳 http://www.kvc.org.uk/buddyscheme

Shared Care Network 🖳 http://www.sharedcarenetwork.org.uk

1 Neville M, Baylis L, Boldison SJ, et al (1995). *Circles of Support: Building Inclusive Communities*. Rugby: Circles Network.

2 Neville M and McIver B (2000). Circles of support. In Kelly B and McGinley P (eds). *Intellectual Disability: The response of the church*. Lisieux Hall Publications: Chorley.

3 Simons K (1998). *Living support networks: An evaluation of the services provided by KeyRing*. Pavilion Publishing: Brighton.

4 Towell D (2000). Achieving positive change in people's lives through the national learning disabilities strategies: Lessons from an American experience. *Tizard Learning Disability Review*, **5**(3), 30–36.

Retirement

Our knowledge is developing about the needs and characteristics of older service users with lifelong disability, which has been documented in recent texts.[1] Planning for retirement has proved to be significantly related to greater life satisfaction and better adjustment to the retirement process.[2] Person-centred later life planning for service users with ID places the person at the centre of the decision making process. One important principle is that 'successful' transition into new life phases are largely a product of informed and active planning.

The limited research that has been conducted suggests that older service users with ID are often constrained by a lack of understanding of concepts such as retirement, and a lack of awareness of choices.[3] When older people with ID are faced with the option of retirement, many may lack an understanding of the concept and may not be aware of the consequences of their retirement or of the alternatives. Research has shown that older people with ID may find that retirement from paid employment brings the cessation of a socially valued role, as well as disruption to daily activities, social supports, and income.[4,5] Researchers into transition in the lives of older people with ID have explored the impact of role loss and change,[6] in particular retirement,[4] housing relocation,[7] disability and loss of independence.[8,9] The loss or change of friends when moving to a new work environment can pose a significant barrier, and many are reluctant to retire to alternative employment because of fear of losing their workshop or job income, and close network of friends made in the workplace.[10,11]

Research indicates that pre-retirement attitudes about retirement and leisure activity participation can be two of the strongest contributors to retirement and life satisfaction for older service users.[12] Later life planning has been suggested as one means of facilitating an enhanced awareness of later life options for older people with ID.[2,13] Heller *et al.* have suggested that a later life planning training programme can be an effective means of teaching older people with ID about later life issues.[2]

In Ireland a survey was conducted to provide a picture as to the extent to which service providers were addressing the needs of the older people with ID in relation to retirement.[14] This research indicated that in recent years, an increasing number of services have been recognizing the importance of making strategic plans to cater for the changing age structure of their ID populations. In general the findings indicated that there was recognition of the need for retirement options, although little attention had been directed towards formalizing these services through policy making. When people with ID are approaching retirement years they are yearning for a slower pace of life, less structured days, and a balance between activities and time to rest. Services now need to be aware of the ageing process—what to expect and how they can adapt the service to meet these needs. Older service users want more flexibility around shorter days in day programme activities. Little attention has been given to the transition of older service users with an ID from work to retirement. Older people with ID can lead productive healthy, sociable lives following retirement.

1 Bigby C (2002). Ageing service-users with a lifelong disability: Challenges for the aged care and disability sectors. *Journal of Intellectual & Developmental Disability* **27**(4), 231–241.

2 Heller T, Factor A, Sterns H *et al.* (1996). Impact of person centred later life planning training program for older adults with mental retardation. *Journal of Rehabilitation* **62**(1), 77–84.

3 Mahon MJ, Goatcher S (1999). Later life planning for older adults with mental retardation: a field experiment. *Mental Retardation* **37**(5), 371–382.

4 Jonsson H, Borell L, Sadlo G (2000). Retirement. An occupational transition with consequences for temporality, balance and meaning of occupations. *Journal of Occupational Science* **7**, 29–37.

5 Rosenkoetter MM, Garris JM, Engdahl RA (2001). Postretirement use of time: Implications for preretirement planning and postretirement management. *Activities, Adaptations and Ageing* **25**, 1–18.

6 Moen P, Dempster-McCain D, Erickson MA (2000). *RoleTransitions, Project 2015: The Future of Aging in New York State*. Office for the Aging: New York State, 129–133.

7 Lutgendorf SK, Reimer TT, Harvey JH *et al.* (2001). Effects of housing relocation on immuno-competence and psycholosocial functioning in older adults. *Journal of Gerontology Medical Sciences* **56**, 97–105.

8 Ward MC, Higgs P (1998). Psychosocial aspects of adjusting to disability in older people. *Review in Clinical Gerontology* **8**, 251–256.

9 Wilmouth JM (2000). Unbalanced social exchanges and living arrangements transitions among older adults. *The Geriatrics*, **51**, 36–45.

10 Janicki M (1990). Growing old with dignity: On quality of life for older persons with lifelong disability. In: Schalock R (Ed). *Quality of Life: Perspectives and Issues*. American Association on Mental Retardation: Washington DC, 114–126.

11 Janicki M (1994). Policies and supports for older persons with mental retardation. In: Seltzer M, Krauss M, Janicki M (Eds). *Life Course Perspectives on Adulthood and Oldage*. American Association on Mental Retardation: Washington DC.

12 Heller T, Miller AB, Hsieh K *et al.* (2000). Later life planning: promoting knowledge of options and choice making. *Mental Retardation* **38**(5), 395–406.

13 Hogg J, Lambe L (1999). *Older People with Intellectual Disabilities: A Review of the Literature on Residential Services and Family Care Giving*. Foundation for People with Learning Disabilities: London.

14 Lawrence S (2008). Examining pre-retirement and related services offered to service users with an intellectual disability in Ireland. *Journal of Intellectual Disabilities* **12**(3), 239–252.

Retirement options

The 21st century will see growing numbers of people with ID living into old age. This reflects the improved medical care that they will have received compared with past generations. However, this new client group will pose major challenges to services as they may present with a different sets of needs.

Guiding principles

Don't be age fixated!

People with certain conditions, such as Down syndrome, may show signs of ageing at an earlier chronological age than others. Hence services designed for older persons may need to use functional entry criteria rather than ages.

Maintain friendships

Ensure that older people have opportunities to maintain contact with their younger friends and acquaintances, through visits and social celebrations.

An active lifestyle using person-centred planning

Although people may not be as *physically* active as they once were, they will still benefit from a range of stimulating educational and leisure activities beyond watching television. In some ways this becomes even more important with older persons as the effects of ageing are often quite varied. Individually tailored supports will become increasingly necessary. 'Futures plans' can also be drawn up to cover anticipated life changes (see 📖 Planning for the fourth age, p.457).

Ageing in place

Although it will not always be possible, people often prefer to maintain contact with familiar routines, people and places.

Options for the third age

An active retirement is the 'third age' for most European citizens and can be too for older persons with ID. Their options can include:

Availing of mainstream services for older persons

In all localities there are various activities organized for older persons e.g. luncheon clubs, tea dances, and bingo. People with ID can be supported to join by having a staff member or volunteer to accompany them.

Retirement clubs and home-based pursuits

Groups of retired persons may wish to meet for a programme of activities designed to suit their interests and capacities. These groups could be located in a leisure or community centre, with the members taking responsibility for a programme, which can include outings and visits, as well as centre-based events. Friendship circles can invite one another to their homes for coffee mornings or afternoon tea, or to take part in organized activities such as craft circles or to sing songs. A visiting 'tutor' may be recruited to provide activities such as yoga or aromatherapy.

All-age pursuits and befrienders
In most localities there are opportunities that include all ages of people, e.g. faith communities, spectator sports and clubs. Older persons can be encouraged to join, and perhaps this is best done when they are younger, as this will provide continuity for them. Volunteer helpers of a similar age can be recruited to visit the person at home, to transport them to activities, and to befriend them at social events or activities.

Family placement
Similarly, families could be recruited to offer short-breaks in their home to older persons, on either a daytime or overnight basis. These schemes have proved particularly suitable for persons with ID who have taken on caring roles with their ageing parents. Organizations such as Help the Aged and Age Concern should be able to provide information and advice, particularly when age discrimination is suspected.

Planning for the fourth age
An active retirement gives way to a fourth age that is typified by increased dependency on others through loss of functions such as mobility and self-care. However, in planning ahead for the fourth age, the principles noted in 📖 Options for the third age still apply, although it can be even more challenging to fulfill them.

- A plan for the future will set out the preferred options of the person (as far as they can be ascertained) and those of the nearest relatives, regarding their living and support arrangements.
- Most older persons want to continue living in their own home, and it is likely that people with ID are no different. Any necessary housing adaptations can be planned and undertaken in advance.
- The availability of mainstream services to provide additional and perhaps specialist support, e.g. palliative care, should be explored and referrals made as appropriate.
- Regular assessments of care needs should be undertaken to avoid delays in accessing additional support. Whenever possible, the same team of support staff should continue to provide the bulk of the care.
- Support staff should be trained in advance in caring for persons at the end-of-life and in the procedures to be followed on the death of the person they have supported.

Further reading
Help The Aged 🖥 http://www.helptheaged.org.uk/en-gb

Age Concern 🖥 http://www.ageconcern.org.uk/

The law

Mental Health Act 1983

Purpose

The scope and purpose of the MHA 1983 is outlined in Section 1 of the Act. It states that the Act makes provision for the compulsory detention and treatment in hospital of those with mental disorder.

The Act is in 10 parts:

- The scope of the Act
- Compulsory admission to hospital and guardianship
- Patients concerned with criminal proceedings or under sentence
- Consent to treatment
- MHRTs
- Removal and return of patients within the UK
- Management of property and affairs of patients
- Miscellaneous functions of local authorities and The Secretary of State
- Offences
- Miscellaneous and supplementary.

Implementation

Admissions to hospital under Part II of the Act (compulsory admission) can be made only where there is a formal application either from an ASW, or the nearest relative. An application is founded on two medical recommendations from two qualified medical practitioners, one of which must be approved for this purpose under the Act. It should be noted that Section 4 of the Act (see 🕮 Emergency holding powers, p.418) allows for emergency admission that requires the recommendation of only one medical recommendation in the first instance.

Definitions

The Act attempts to define the types of mental disorder that the Act is intended to cover by using the following definitions:

Mental disorder

Mental disorder includes mental illness, arrested or incomplete development of mind, psychopathic disorder and any other disorder or disability of mind.

The Act then offers 3 sub-categories of mental disorder:

Severe mental impairment—a state of arrested or incomplete development of mind, which includes severe impairment of intelligence and social functioning and is associated with abnormally aggressive or seriously irresponsible conduct on the part of the person concerned.

Mental impairment—a state of arrested or incomplete development of mind (not amounting to severe impairment), which includes significant impairment of intelligence and social functioning, and is associated with abnormally aggressive or seriously irresponsible conduct on the part of the person concerned.

Psychopathic disorder—a persistent disorder or disability of mind (whether or not including significant impairment of intelligence), which results in abnormally aggressive or seriously irresponsible conduct on the part of the person concerned.

The definitions of 'severe mental impairment' and 'mental impairment' are the ones most pertinent to the field of ID nursing. It should be noted that ID alone is not a reason for detention under the Act. It should be the case that these definitions become applicable under the Act when 'associated' with 'abnormally aggressive' or 'seriously irresponsible conduct'.

Mental illness is not defined in the Act. Irrespective of this it has been necessary for a working definition to be used when a diagnosis of mental disorder has been disputed. The DHSS Memorandum offered guidelines relating to the symptomology of mental illness, and stated that those having a mental illness will display one or more of the following characteristics:[1]

- More than temporary impairment of intellectual functions shown by failure of memory, orientation, comprehension, and learning capacity
- More than temporary alteration of mood of such a degree as to give rise to the patient having delusional appraisal of his situation, his past or his future, or that of others, or to the lack of any appraisal
- Delusional beliefs, persecutory, jealous, or grandiose
- Abnormal perceptions associated with delusional misinterpretation of events
- Thinking so disordered as to prevent the patient making a reasonable appraisal of his situation or having reasonable communication with others.

The nature of the disorder should be of such a degree that it warrants the detention of the person in their own best interests and that of others. It should be noted that these definitions will be abolished under The MHA 2007, and replaced by a single definition (see 📖 Mental Health Act 2007, p.462):

Statutory exclusions—the Act states that a person cannot be deemed to have a mental disorder based only on the following criteria:

- Promiscuity
- Other immoral conduct
- Sexual deviancy
- Alcohol or drug dependency.

1 DHSS Memorandum (1983). *The Mental Health Act*. HMSO: London.

Mental Health Act 2007

Readers should note that the MHA 1983 has been amended by the MHA 2007. This new Act became law in July 2007, and its main amendments are scheduled to come into force in October 2008. For the purposes of the sections within this book, most issues discussed in relation to the MHA 1983 will remain the same, or be very similar to how they have been out-lined. Some will have minor amendments, and therefore readers should check with the new Act for these. There is one major issue relating to definitions (discussed below). The major changes to the MHA 1983 that will influence practice are:

Criteria for detention—this includes a new appropriate medical treatment test.

Professional roles—a broadening of the range of practitioners who can take on the roles currently performed by approved social workers and responsible medical officers.

Nearest relative—this gives patients the right to apply to have the nearest relative displaced if there are reasonable grounds for doing so.

Supervised community treatment will allow for some people with mental disorder to receive compulsory treatment in the community.

MHRT—there will be a reduction in the time before cases are referred to the tribunal.

Age appropriate service—those under 18yrs who are admitted to hospital for a mental disorder must be accommodated in suitable environments.

Advocacy—there will be a duty by a national authority to make arrangements for the provision of independent advocates.

ECT—there will be new safeguards for patients.

The change that applies most directly to people with ID relates to Section 1 of the MHA 1983 (see 📖 Mental Health Act 1983, p.460). The new Act will have only one definition of mental disorder, which will apply throughout the Act. The categories of severe mental impairment, mental impairment, and psychopathic disorder will be abolished. The single definition will be:

'Mental disorder means any disorder or disability of the mind; and mentally disordered shall be construed accordingly.'[1]

---

1 Department of Health (2007). *Mental Health Act 2007*. HMSO: London.

Compulsory admission to hospital for assessment and treatment

Compulsory admission to hospital under the MHA 1983 for assessment and treatment is largely covered by 3 sections of the MHA outlined below.

Section 2—Admission for assessment

This allows for a person to be detained in hospital for assessment for up to 28d. This period should allow for an assessment to be made. If it is believed that the person needs to be detained further, it is customary to implement Section 3 for this purpose. An application can be made by the nearest relative or an ASW who has seen the person within the 14 days leading up to the signing of the application. Two medical representations are required for this section to be used.

Circumstances

An application can be made if it is felt that:
- an individual is suffering from a mental disorder of a degree that warrants detention in hospital for assessment, or for assessment followed by treatment for at least a limited period
- the individual should be detained in the interests of their own health and safety, or to protect others.

This section may be appropriate if:
- the person has not been detained before and diagnosis/prognosis is currently unclear
- significant time has elapsed between admissions
- the effectiveness of compulsory treatment under the MHA is not currently known.

Section 3—Admission for treatment

This section allows for the detention of a person for treatment for a maximum period of 6mths after which it can be renewed for a further 6mths, and then for 12mths at a time. It requires the recommendation of two doctors who must confirm that:
- the person is suffering from one of the 4 categories of mental disorder defined by Section 1(2) of the Act (see 📖 Mental Health Act 1983, p.460)
- if the person has a psychopathic disorder or a mental impairment, treatment is likely to alleviate or prevent deterioration
- the treatment is necessary for the health and safety or protection of others, and it cannot be provided unless he is detained under this section.

Section 4—Emergency admission for assessment

The provisions of this section are as for Section 2; however, it is intended to be used for emergency admissions. Section 2 would be used if it were not for the urgency of the situation. Unlike Section 2, only one medical representation is required.

Duration is for up to 72hrs. During this period a second medical representation can be obtained, and this converts the Section 4 to a Section 2.

Circumstances are as for Section 2, and additionally:
- It is an urgent necessity that the person be admitted and detained under Section 2
- The Section 2 requirement of obtaining a second medical representation would involve an undesirable delay.

It should be noted that Sections 5(2) and 5(4) (outlined in 📖 Emergency holding powers, p.418) are also used for compulsory detention under the Act.

Emergency holding powers

The detention of people in mental health and ID services is currently governed by the MHA (England and Wales). This chapter outlines the main provisions of Section 5(2): Detention of an inpatient, and Section 5(4): Nurses' holding powers.

Section 5(2)—Detention of an inpatient

This section allows for an approved doctor to detain an informal patient for up to 72hrs by reporting to hospital managers. Before this period of time elapses an application can be made for a Section 2 or 3 to be applied, or the individual can revert to informal status. Although this section can be used only by doctors, nurses need to be aware of it as it will affect the care and management of the client.

Section 5(4)—Nurses' holding powers

This section allows for the registered ID nurse or registered mental nurse to prevent a person from leaving an inpatient environment if it is considered to be in their best interest or that of others. This holding power can last for up to 6hrs. As soon as it starts, a doctor with authority to detain the individual must be alerted, and when the doctor arrives, the nurse's holding power ceases. Should further detention be required then the doctor must complete an assessment of the detained person.

Clinical considerations that may lead to the nurse applying Section 5(4):
• The person's stated intent
• The likelihood of suicide
• The person's current behaviour, particularly any changes from the usual
• The likelihood of violence
• Any recently received news from relatives or friends
• Any recent disturbances within the ward/hospital environment
• The person's known unpredictability.

Legal/procedural considerations when applying Section 5(4)

Section 5(4) can only be applied to a person who is an inpatient being treated for a mental disorder. It cannot be applied to a person being treated in a general hospital for a physical illness and who becomes mentally unwell.

Section 5(5) of the MHA dictates that the nurse must make a report to management as soon as possible after applying Section 5(4). The person detained under Section 5(4) must be informed of their rights as soon as possible after the section has been applied. Persons detained under Section 5(4) cannot have medication administered against their will, as this section is not governed by Part 4 of the Act (consent for treatment).

If the RMO detains the person under Section 5(2), then the 72hr period of detention allowed by this section starts from the time the nurse made the report of detention under Section 5(4).

Although it is not encouraged as it is not 'in the spirit' of the Act, a nurse can apply Section 5(4) for a further 6hrs if the RMO has not arrived before the initial 6hrs has elapsed. As outlined above, the nurse must make a report to the managers of the service setting as soon as possible under Section 5(5).

Section 5(4) allows a nurse to use the minimal restraint to prevent the person from leaving the hospital.

The decision to use Section 5(4) is the responsibility of the nurse applying it. No one can instruct a nurse to implement this section.

Mental Health Review Tribunals

In essence, the role of MHRTs is to review the situation of persons detained under the MHA 1983 who appeal against their detention, and to direct the discharge of those who meet statutory criteria. MHRTs are independent judicial bodies composed of the following members:

- Legal representatives
- Medical practitioners
- Lay members.

MHRTs are not public meetings but could be so if the patient requests it. The process of appeal might vary, and this is dependent on which section of the Act a person is being detained under. These variations pertain to issues such as when a person can appeal, who can appeal on a person's behalf, and the interim period between appeals. Readers should therefore read further to clarify the stipulations relating to specific sections; however, in broad terms, Sections 66 and 69 of the Act allow for appeals to the MHRT where an individual has been:

- admitted for assessment under Section 2
- admitted for treatment under Section 3
- received into guardianship under Section 7
- made subject of a hospital order or guardianship order by the courts under Section 37
- detained (or made subject to guardianship) for a further period under Section 20
- deemed to have a different form of mental disorder from that originally cited
- transferred from guardianship to hospital
- made subject to either a restriction order or restriction direction
- conditionally discharged
- made subject to supervised discharge.

Appeals can also be made to the MHRT if the nearest relative has been:
- barred by the responsible medical officer from discharging the individual detained in hospital
- replaced by acting nearest relative as the result of a court order.

Applications

Most tribunal hearings are the result of applications made by or on behalf of the patient, in some cases by the nearest relative. The Act also requires hospital managers to refer to the MHRT any patient admitted under Part II of the Act, who on renewal of the section has not had a tribunal hearing within the previous 6mths.

The powers of the MHRT

The MHRT can discharge individuals from certain sections of the Act. Individuals detained under Section 2 must be discharged if:

- they are not suffering from a mental disorder (as defined in Section 1 of the Act—see 📖 Mental Health Act 1983, p.460) that requires detention for assessment, or that section cannot be justified in the best interests of the detained person or others.

The MHRT can also discharge individuals from other sections other than Section 2 if it is satisfied that:

- the person is not suffering from a mental disorder that needs detention for treatment, or detention cannot be justified in the interests of the health and safety of the person or others, or if discharged the patient would not be a danger to themselves or others.

The role of the nurse

- To provide reports for the MHRT if required
- To give evidence to the MHRT if required
- To ensure the patient has the required information about the appeal
- To assist in finding legal representation
- To manage the process of appeal.

Procedures before MHRT hearing

- Applications must be made in writing
- Assistance should be offered and given to patients in completing the application form and to seek legal advice
- Patients should be informed of their rights—particularly to legal representation
- The nearest relative should be informed of their right to attend the hearing, and of their right to provide information before the hearing.

The Mental Health Act Commission

The MHAC was established under Section 121 of the MHA 1983. The Secretary of State is required to direct the MHAC to act on his behalf as a Special Health Authority. It comprises around 170 members (commissioners) and these include:
- Doctors
- Nurses
- Lay persons
- Social workers
- Psychologists
- Other specialists.

Functions of the MHAC

The MHAC provides a safeguard for those detained in hospital under the MHA. Its functions are to:
- keep under review the operation of the MHA 1983, in respect of patients liable to be detained under the Act
- visit and interview, in private patients detained under the Act in hospitals and mental nursing homes
- investigate complaints that fall within the remit of the commission
- review decisions to withhold the mail of patients, detained in high security hospitals
- appoint medical practitioners and others to give second opinions in cases where this is required by the Act
- publish and lay before Parliament a report biennially
- monitor the implementation of the Code of Practice and propose amendments to ministers.

The role of the commissioners—there are two types of commissioners. Area commissioners have a largely coordinating role. Local commissioners have the following roles:
- Visit detained patients
- Examine patient records
- Immediately take action on behalf of patients
- Prioritize issues for action and decide how to resolve them
- Maintain constructive and objective relationships with care providers at a local level
- Take part in national visits on specific topics.

The commissioners make frequent short notice and unannounced visits to all NHS properties and care homes in England and Wales, where people may be detained under the MHA.

The MHAC and people with intellectual disabilities

A key role of the MHAC is to appoint medical practitioners to give second opinions in situations where the detained person is incapable or refuses to give consent. This is a common issue relating to people with ID. In such instances the RMO has a statutory obligation to seek a second opinion from an independent second doctor appointed by the MHAC.

The MHAC and the role of the nurse

The nurse who is likely to work within settings where people may be detained under the MHA 1983 should ensure their practice is in accord with the Mental Health Code of Practice (COP). The COP is monitored by the MHAC and it influences their roles and functions. The COP is not legally binding but it does offer guidance on good practice, and should be adhered to. Nurses should consult this, as it is helpful for:

• Clarification of responsibilities
• Recognizing the individual needs of patients
• Setting objectives
• Raising standards
• Gaining resources
• Drawing up procedures, protocols and practices
• Evaluating practice
• Raising and maintaining human rights
• Encouraging multidisciplinary working
• Identification of poor practice
• Preparing people for discharge as soon as it is clear that detention is no longer necessary.

Once again readers should note that the MHA 1983 has been amended by the MHA 2007. The major provisions of the 2007 Act came into force in October 2008. As part of the new Act, the COP will be revised. It would appear that the revision will be in essence similar to that of the 1983. Interested readers should consult further reading to examine the proposed revisions.

Further reading

Jones R (2004). *The Mental Health Act Manual*, 9th edn. Sweet and Maxwell: London.

The Mental Health Act Commission ▣ www.mhac.org.uk

Department of Health (2003). *The Mental Health Act Code of Practice*. HMSO: London.

Department of Health (2007). *Mental Health Act 1983: Consultation on the Draft Revised Mental Health Act 1983 Code of Practice*. HMSO: London.

Sexual Offences Act

Summary

The Sexual Offences Act 2003 is an Act of Parliament that became law on 1 May 2004. It updates and makes many changes from the Sexual Offences Act of 1956 (which had been amended in 1976 and 1994). The major purpose of the Act is to govern non-consensual sexual behaviour. It is an extensive piece of legislation and therefore readers requiring more extensive detail should consult further reading. The Act is divided into a number of sections. The sections most relevant to people with ID, their carers, and nurses are Sections 30–41. For the purposes of the Act, ID falls under the umbrella term 'mental disorder'. This is the same definition used in the MHA 1983 and is:

'Mental illness, arrested or incomplete development of mind, psychopathic disorder, and any other disorder or disability of mind.'

Most relevant sections:

Sections 30–33 relate to offences against people who cannot legally consent to sexual activity because of a mental disorder impeding choice.

Sections 34–37 relate to offences against people who may or may not be able to consent to sexual activity but who are vulnerable to inducements, threats, or deceptions because of mental disorder.

Sections 38–41 relate to specific offences committed by care workers who engage in sexual activity with a person with a mental disorder receiving care in the setting they work at.

Role of the nurse

Nurses are referred to within Sections 38–41 of the Act. Their role should involve working within the provisions of the Act, monitoring for potential infringements covered by it, and acting accordingly. Under the Act any sexual activity between care worker and a person with a mental disorder is prohibited while that relationship continues. A relationship of care is one in which a person with a mental disorder (ID) is regularly or likely to be involved face-to-face with another person where their care needs arise from a mental disorder. This applies to both paid and voluntary people and includes:

- Doctors, nurses, advocates, cleaners, medical receptionists
- Care home and agency workers
- People who provide care within the individual's home
- People involved in face-to-face care who escort those with a mental disorder on regular outings
- Friends or family members if they provide care, assistance, or services relating to the individual's mental disorder.

The Act covers the following areas that relate to care worker offences.

Sexual activity with a person with a mental disorder—this covers all intercourse and sexual touching of any part of the body, clothed or unclothed, with the body or an object.

Causing or inciting sexual activity—this relates to causing or persuading a person with a mental disorder to engage in any sexual activity with someone else, or making them strip or masturbate. This offence applies even if the intended sexual activity does not take place.

Sexual activity in the presence of a person with a mental disorder—it is an offence to engage in sexual activity when you know you can be seen by a person with a mental disorder who is in your care, or that you intend/believe that they can see you, and where you gain sexual gratification from them watching you.

Causing a person with a mental disorder to watch a sexual act—it is an offence to intentionally cause someone with a mental disorder to watch someone else engaging in sexual activity. This includes looking at pornography, photos and webcams, and where it is for your own sexual gratification. This is not intended to prevent sex education.

Exceptions—there are situations in which care workers' offences apply. These are where a care worker is legally married to the person with a mental disorder or it can be proved that the sexual relationship predated the relationship of care, and as long as the sexual activity was lawful.

Further reading

Guide to the Sexual Offences Act 2003 ▣ http://www.homeoffice.gov.uk/documents/adults-safe-fr-sex-harm-leaflet

Disability Discrimination Act 2005

The DDA 2005 is an Act of Parliament that extends the scope of the 1995 DDA. The main purposes of the Act are to protect disabled people from discrimination in the following areas:
- Employment
- Education
- Access to goods and services
- Transport.

Definition

The DDA defines a disabled person as someone who has or has had a physical or mental impairment that has substantial and long-term adverse effect on their ability to carry out normal day-to-day activities. The effects of this have already or are expected to last for at least 12mths. The Act offers further explanation of this as follows:

Impairment—the Act does not give a specific definition of impairment; however, it is intended to cover sensory impairments, physical impairments, mental impairments, and ID.

Substantial adverse effect—the disability must substantially affect a person's ability to carry out normal activities. Even where a disability can be successfully treated, for the purposes of the Act the disability is assessed according to the effect it would have without treatment.

Long-term adverse effect—impairment is regarded as long term if it has or is expected to last for at least 12mths. For conditions such as epilepsy and rheumatoid arthritis that can be expected to recur then the person remains protected under the Act.

Normal day-to-day activities—under the Act, impairment can be judged to affect a person's ability to carry out day-to-day activities if one of the following areas are affected: mobility, manual dexterity, physical coordination, continence, ability to lift, carry or move everyday objects, speech, hearing, eyesight, memory, or ability to concentrate, learn or understand, and the perception of the risk of physical danger.

The Act places obligations on employers and service providers to make '*reasonable adjustments*' to the work environment or when providing access to goods, facilities, services, and premises. The Act is lengthy but easily accessible. Readers who require detailed information should pursue further reading.

The role of the nurse—in relation to the DDA, the nurse should be aware of the major areas covered by the Act so that they can contribute to supporting people with ID who may be discriminated against, so that they could advocate on their behalf. Nurses who have some responsibility for service provision should ensure that any necessary *reasonable adjustments* are made as outlined in the Act.

Further reading

HM Government (1995). *Disability Discrimination Act 2005*. HMSO: London.

Human Rights Act

The Human Rights Act 1998 is an Act of Parliament that came into force on 2 October 2000. The Act makes the ECHR (see 📖 European Convention of Human Rights, p.478) enforceable in UK courts. In effect the Act does not create any new rights but provides ways for cases to be heard in UK courts, rather than the European Court of Human Rights. The human rights covered under the Act are:

- The right to life
- Prohibition of torture
- Prohibition of slavery
- The right to liberty and security
- The right to a fair trial
- The right not to be held guilty of a criminal offence that did not exist in law at the time at which it was committed
- The right to privacy, family life, home and correspondence
- The right to freedom of thought, conscience and religion
- The right to freedom of expression
- The right to freedom of assembly and association
- The right to marry
- The right to the protection of property
- The right to education
- The right to free elections
- The right to the rights and freedoms set out above without discrimination on any grounds.

Not all of these rights are absolute, as some may be conditional and could be denied in certain circumstances. This is partly because a key purpose of the Act is to balance the rights of the individual against the rights of another individual and the greater public good. The Act is not designed to bring actions against private individuals. The purpose of the Act is to affect the way public authorities behave, and to ensure that they attend to the human rights listed above.

It is recognized that adults with ID constitute a client group that is vulnerable to having their human rights compromised or denied. The government's JCHR has acknowledged this, and in March 2007 called for evidence to support this assertion. The JCHR commented that:

'The extent to which the rights of adults with learning disabilities are currently being respected raises fundamental issues of humanity, dignity, equality, autonomy and respect. It also raises important issues of substantive human rights law such as the right to life, the prohibitions on inhuman/degrading treatment and unjustified discrimination, and the right to respect for family life.'[1]

The views of the JCHR reflect that there is an increasing awareness that the human rights of people with ID can be denied. There is an expectation that the Human Rights Act will contribute to a growing 'rights culture' within public services in relation to how people with ID are treated. The DDA (see 📖 Disability Discrimination Act 2005, p.474), and *Valuing People*[2] (see 📖 Principles and values of social policy and their effects on intellectual disability, p.22) both supplement the Human Rights Act in supporting a rights culture.

The nurse's role

Working within a person-centred multidisciplinary and multiagency context in relation to the Human Rights Act the nurse should:
- where necessary question care practices within organizations if it is felt that they violate human rights
- understand 'whistle blowing' policies and procedures—the NMC Code of Professional Conduct[3] and the right to freedom of expression covered by the Human Rights Act both support the right to 'whistle blow'
- ensure that you receive appropriate training and support.

Nurses who are concerned that the human rights of an individual with ID are being breached can:
- take the individuals concerns seriously
- seek advice from the CAB or an advocacy group
- seek advice from a social services care manager or CLDT
- contact the Social Services Inspection Team or Community Health Council.

1 Joint Committee on Human Rights (2007). *Press Notice—The Human Rights of Adults with Learning Disabilities: Call for Evidence*. HMSO: London.
http://www.parliament.uk/parliamentary_committees/joint_committee_on_human_rights.cfm.

2 Department of Health (2001). *Valuing People: a New Strategy for Learning Disability in the 21st Century*. Cmnd 5086. HMSO: London.

3 Nursing and Midwifery Council (2008). *Nursing and Midwifery Council Code of Professional Conduct, Performance and Ethics*. Nursing and Midwifery Council: London.

European Convention of Human Rights

The ECHR was developed by the Council of Europe in 1950 with the intention of protecting human rights and fundamental freedoms. The Convention established The European Court of Human Rights, which can examine the case of any person who feels that their rights have been violated under the Convention. The ECHR forms the basis of the Human Rights Act 1998 (see 📖 Human Rights Act, p.476) which made the ECHR enforceable in UK courts. Along with the DDA and other legislation such as *Valuing People*,[1] the ECHR contributes to the developing 'rights culture' within the field of ID. The convention covers the following rights/articles:

Articles

- The obligation to respect human rights
- The right to life
- The prohibition of torture
- The prohibition of slavery
- The right to liberty and security
- The right to a fair trial
- No punishment without the law
- The right to respect for private life
- The right to freedom of thought, conscience, and religion
- The right to freedom of expression
- The right to freedom of assembly and association
- The right to marry
- The right to effective remedy
- The prohibition of discrimination.
- The right to property, education and free elections.

Protocol 1

The government has concerns that the rights listed above may be denied to some people with ID. The JCHR has concerns in the following areas:

Article 1—because of fundamental issues associated with humanity, dignity, equality, respect and autonomy

Article 2—because of the very poor standard of medical care, which poses a risk to life

Article 3—because of the way some people with ID are treated, particularly in health care settings

Article 8—due to a variety of factors, including barriers to participating in community activities, which is covered under this article of the convention.

Nurses should examine their personal practice and the operation of the services they provide by using the human rights outlined above as a checklist.

Further reading

Joint Committee on Human Rights (2007–08). *A Life Like Any Other? Human Rights of Adults with Learning Disabilities*. Joint Committee on Human Rights: London. 🖳 http://www.publications.parliament.uk/pa/jt200708/jtselect/jtrights/40/40i.pdf

1 Department of Health (2001). *Valuing People: a New Strategy for Learning Disability in the 21st Century*. Cmnd 5086. HMSO: London.

Race relations

Baxter *et al.* 1990 recognized that people from ethnic minority groups and who have ID may experience double discrimination.[1] Chapter 6.10 of *Valuing People* also stated that this client group is at a particular risk of discrimination in gaining access to healthcare, due to language and cultural issues, and the use of English-based assessment tools.[2] The Race Relations (Amendment) Act 2000 is aimed at eliminating racial discrimination. The Act makes it unlawful to discriminate against anyone on the grounds of:

- Race
- Colour
- Nationality (including citizenship)
- Ethnic origin
- National origin.

The Act applies to:

- Jobs
- Training
- Housing
- Education
- The provision of goods, facilities, and services.

Importantly it is unlawful for public bodies to discriminate in the provision of their services, and in carrying out any of their functions. The amended Act also imposes a general duty on all public bodies to promote equality of opportunity and good race relations.

The role of the nurse

Nurses can:

- work in person-centred ways with clients from ethnic minorities to help them meet their individual needs
- evaluate whether the public bodies they have contact with operate in a non-discriminatory way, and seek to promote good race relations
- work with advocacy groups to produce guidance on matters pertaining to healthcare and ethnic minority groups.

1 Baxter C, Poonia K, Nadirshaw Z (1990). *Double Discrimination*. King's Fund: London.

2 Department of Health (2001). Valuing People: *A New Strategy For Learning Disability For The 21st Century. HMSO*: London. Y http://www.dh.gov.uk/en/Publicationsandstatistics/Publications/PublicationsPolicyAndGuidance/DH_4082493

Diversion from custody schemes

Diversion from custody is a method of redirecting people with ID and mental disorder from the criminal justice system to hospital or suitable community settings, where they can receive treatment appropriate to their needs. There are 3 principal reasons why this is necessary:

- Those with ID and/or mental disorder can fall through the net of support services and gravitate into the criminal justice system. The standard of care for this client group in prison is recognized as being poor. Prisons are not classified as hospitals for detention under the MHA 1983, and therefore people cannot be detained under the Act for appropriate treatment in prison.
- There have been a number of policy initiatives within the past 4 decades as follows:
  - The Butler report 1975 was influential in the development of medium secure units[1]
  - Home Office circular 66/90 of 1990 recommended diversion from custody wherever possible[2]
  - The Reed Report 1992 recommended nationwide provision of appropriately resourced court assessment and diversion schemes as well as other measures that support diversion[3]
- The Reed report has been influential, and it has resulted in an increase in the number of people being diverted from the criminal justice system. Nacro report that in 2004 approximately 136 court diversion schemes were operating nationally.[4] There is quite a degree of flexibility in how schemes operate, and a number of models of delivery have developed as follows:
  - Community mental nurses (or input from ID nurses) based in court
  - Psychiatric assessment teams based in police stations, and/or the court, and/or with input in A&E departments
  - Community teams with direct links to the court
  - Standalone consultant-led teams.

Within these models of delivery Birmingham identified elements of best practice likely to result in successful diversion schemes, as follows:[5]

- Being nurse-led and closely linked to appropriate local services
- The existence of good working relationships with magistrates and the prosecution
- Access to suitable interview facilities
- The use of appropriate screening/assessment tools
- Direct access to available hospital beds/specialized community facilities
- Involvement of senior psychiatrists
- Being integrated with police and other liaison teams.

How people can be diverted

The MHA 1983 allows for a number of mechanisms to be used to divert people from custody. Readers should consult the MHA 1983 and associated literature in order to understand in detail how each one of the following apply in practice:

Section 2—admission for assessment

Section 3—admission for treatment

Section 4—emergency admission for treatment

Section 35—remand to hospital for report on mental condition

Section 37—hospital and guardianship order

Section 37/41—restricted hospital order

Section 38—interim hospital order

Section 45A—hospital direction order

Section 47—removal to hospital of sentenced prisoners for treatment

Section 48—removal to hospital of other (remand) prisoners (for urgent treatment)

Section 136—removal of mentally disordered persons found in public places. This is used by the police to take people to a place of safety i.e. a mental health unit rather than into custody.

It is important to understand that diversion from custody does not, in most instances, equate to the discontinuation of criminal proceedings. Clearly diversion from custody schemes present the opportunity for nurses to work in a specialized role as designated diversion 'officers' or through involvement with the process as part of a broader remit. Nurses working in this specialized role will need to be able to carry out thorough assessments of individual need, including that of risk and its management, and this can be done by accessing:

• educational history—including evidence of special educational need
• level of literacy/numeracy
• access to official documents from health, social services, and criminal record information
• interviews with the individual and carers
• the use of appropriate assessment tools such as the HASI.[6]

From this, the nurse can draw up or contribute to pre-sentencing reports that offer options for diversion from custody. In order for this to work successfully the nurse or team will need access to beds in specialist facilities.

1 Home Office and Department of Health and Social Security (1975). *Committee on Mentally Disordered Offenders.* HMSO: London.

2 Home Office (1990). *Provision of Mentally Disordered Offenders* (circular 66/90). HMSO: London.

3 Department of Health (1992). *Reed Report: Review of Mental Health and Social Services for Mentally Disordered Offenders and Others Requiring Similar Services: Vol. 1 : Final Summary Report.* (Cm 2088). HMSO: London.

4 Nacro (2004). *Findings of the 2004 Survey of Court Diversion/Criminal Justice Mental Health Liaison Schemes for Mentally Disordered Offenders in England and Wales.* Nacro: London.

5 Birmingham L (2001). Diversion from custody. *Advances in psychiatric treatment* **7**, 198–207.

6 Hayes S (2000). *Hayes Ability Screening Index.* University of Sydney: Sydney.

Appropriate adult

The PACE 1984[1] stipulates that all people <17yrs and those >17yrs with mental health problems and ID must have an appropriate adult (AA) present when they are being questioned by the police, or asked to provide or sign a written statement while in police custody. The purposes of this are to assist and protect the welfare of vulnerable people who have difficulty in understanding their legal rights, and may be at risk of providing unreliable and misleading information. It is the responsibility of the custody officer to identify those who require an AA and to arrange it so that procedures relating to the detained person are conducted in the proper manner. The custody officer must inform the detained person of their rights, and this includes the circumstances in which it is deemed appropriate for an AA to be present.

An appropriate adult can be:
- A parent
- A guardian
- Any responsible person who is at least 18yrs and is neither a police officer nor employed by the police
- Those with experience of helping people with ID
- A social worker or RNLD who is not involved with the offence as a witness, victim, or suspect, and who has not received either admissions or denials from the detained person before attendance at the police station.

The role and function of the appropriate adult
- To assist with communication between the police and the detained person
- To advise, support, and generally assist the detained person, particularly when they are being questioned
- To ensure that the police are acting properly and fairly
- To observe that the police are respecting the rights of the detained person and to tell them if it is believed they are not doing so.

What the appropriate adult should avoid doing
- Acting as a passive observer
- Discussing the alleged offence with the detained person
- Answering questions on behalf of the detained person
- Giving legal advice—this the responsibility of a solicitor.

The rights of the appropriate adult
- To intervene during an interview if it is felt necessary and in the best interest of the person, in order to help them communicate with the police
- To speak privately to the detained person at any time
- To be informed why the detained person is being held
- To inspect the written records (the custody record) of the person at any time
- To see copies of the Codes of Practice that outline the powers and responsibilities of the police

- To request a break in any interview if the person is distressed or ill, to seek legal advice, or consult with the detained person
- To be present during any procedure that requires the detained person to be given information or have it sought from them.

Further reading

Leggett J, Goodman W, Diani S (2007). People with learning disabilities experiences of being interviewed by the police. *British Journal of Learning Disabilities* **35**(3), 168–173.

1 Home Office (1984). *Police and Criminal Evidence Act,* London: HMSO.

The Representation of the People Act 2000

The RPA 2000 amended the RPA 1983; its principal aim is to increase voter participation in elections. Historically people with ID and/or a mental disorder were excluded from voting. It is a widely held assumption that these client groups were and still are not eligible to vote. This was not the case for many people detained in hospital; however, the RPA 1983 made voting extremely difficult for those detained under the MHA 1983, because in order to vote a person must have been resident at a voting address for 6mths. For those detained for lengthy periods under the MHA 1983 this effectively prevented them from voting as psychiatric hospitals were not recognized as voting addresses. In 1999 Mind submitted a case to the ECHR claiming that this situation violated Protocol 1 of the Convention. Subsequently Clause 4 of the RPA 2000 amended this issue, and now states that patients (both voluntary and detained) who live in a mental hospital and have mental capacity can register to vote at the hospital address or another address with which they have a local connection.

Exceptions

Please note that these arrangements only apply to patients in mental hospital who are not detained offenders, and that therefore those detained on remand or the following sections (MHA 1983) are ineligible to vote:
- Section 37
- Section 38
- Section 44
- Section 45A
- Sections 46, 47 or 51(5).

RPA 2000 criteria for entitlement to register as a voter:
- Citizenship—British, other Commonwealth, or a citizen of the Republic of Ireland
- Age—18yrs, although if not 18yrs you may be able to register to vote in elections following the 18th birthday
- Residency—you must be resident in the constituency where you will vote
- You must be on the electoral register.

You must not be subject to any legal incapacity to vote

The RPA 2000 does not make specific reference to ID. This client group is covered under the generic term 'mental disorder'. Whereas the Act does not categorically state that people with mental impairment, significant mental impairment and/or a mental disorder are ineligible to vote, they can be prevented from doing so if they are deemed to lack mental capacity (see ⬚ Mental Capacity Act 2005, p.490).

Arrangements for voting
The RPA 2000 stated that patients detained under the MHA 1983 can only vote via **proxy** or by **post**.[1]

The role of the nurse
Nurses may be in a position to:
- inform individuals of their right to vote
- explain the process
- be involved in assessment of mental capacity
- liaise with advocacy/legal and other services
- escort voluntary patients who can vote to the polling station.

1 HM Government (2000). *Representation of the People Act.* HMSO: London.

Employment law

Most issues that apply to employment law and ID relate to the DDA 2005 (see 📖 Disability Discrimination Act 2005, p.474)

The employment of people with ID is complicated by the benefits system, as the way that it is organized indicates an assumption that most people with ID will never work. The main welfare benefits for people with ID are:

- Income support (IS)
- Disabled living allowance (DLA)
- Incapacity benefit (IB)
- Severe disability allowance (SDA) (no longer available to new claimants)
- Job seekers allowance (rarely as most people with ID are likely to need support to find work).

Complications can arise when people receiving benefits seek to work. Some people with ID undertake 'permitted work'. Under 'permitted work' anyone claiming benefit based on incapacity can do some paid work for less than 16hrs/wk without approval from a doctor for a 12mth period. Those receiving IB or SDA can earn significantly more per week than those claiming IS. When a person is in receipt of benefits and moves into paid work, usually their means-tested benefits are reduced or withdrawn. This includes housing benefit and council tax benefit. They may also become responsible for their own care charges. Inevitably this can cause people to be significantly worse off than they would be on benefits. They can claim working tax credits, but only if they work more than 16hrs/week. This divide at 16hrs limits choice, and the potential contribution of people for whom part-time work is the most appropriate option.

Consent to examination, treatment, and care

Consent in relation to people with ID is a potentially contentious issue due to a variety of interrelated factors. People with ID are often perceived to lack the capacity to give valid consent; they are often in unequal power relationships in which others consent on their behalf. Due to the complexities relating to consent, readers should consult the recommended reading. For the purposes of this section, consent will be divided into:

• Seeking consent—people with capacity
• Consent when adults lack capacity
• Compulsory treatment under the MHA 1983.

Seeking consent—people with capacity

For consent to be valid a person must be:

• capable of taking that particular decision (in other words 'competent)
• acting voluntary and not under coercion, duress, or pressure from others
• provided with enough information to enable them to make a decision.

People who have given their consent to a procedure/intervention can withdraw their consent at any time. If they appear to withdraw consent during treatment, then it is good practice to stop it unless it puts the person's life at risk. Those with capacity can refuse treatment, even if to do so is detrimental to their health and well-being. Legally it is irrelevant whether a person signs a form to give consent, or does so orally or non-verbally. The key factor in valid consent is whether the person has capacity (see 📖 Mental Capacity Act 2005, p.490). Succinctly, for people to give valid consent for treatment they must be able to:

Comprehend and retain information relevant to the decision, particularly in relation to the consequences of having or not having the treatment, and use and consider this information in the decision making process.

Nurses and others should see seeking consent and ascertaining capacity as a process that involves individual person-centred ways of explaining treatments. This can be done via augmented communication methods, using easy to understand language, pictorial guides, or conveying information through a close carer or family member.

Consent when adults lack capacity

Some people with ID lack the capacity to give valid consent; however, it is possible for treatment to be lawfully provided if the treatment is deemed to be in the person's best interests. No one can give consent on behalf of an adult who lacks the capacity to give consent, and this includes their parents. Legally it is the health professional responsible for the treatment who decides whether the treatment is in the person's best interests. In practice most decisions taken by the responsible professional will be after discussion with and agreement from a multidisciplinary team, carers, and family. A decision on what is in a person's best interest should not be based on medical treatment/intervention alone. Matters such as general well-being, relationships, social issues, and spiritual/religious beliefs should also be considered. When a proposed treatment is controversial e.g. sterilization, and interested parties strongly oppose it, then the doctor responsible for the treatment can and should seek a court decision on best interest.

Compulsory treatment under the Mental Health Act 1983

The consent to treatment provisions are covered under Sections 56–64. Some key areas are outlined below in relation to those who have capacity but refuse to consent to treatment.

Section 58 specifically applies to medication and ECT. It requires consent or a second opinion, and applies to detained patients. It allows for medication to be given without a second opinion for a period of 3mths after it was first given. It is mandatory that the RMO discusses the treatment plan with the person in order to gain consent before this period elapses. If consent is not gained then a second opinion must be sought. If there is agreement from a second doctor then treatment can continue after the initial 3mths.

Section 62 allows for treatment that is immediately necessary as long as it is not irreversible or hazardous. The treatment should be carried out under the direction of the RMO, but in practice this is not always possible. There are no limitations to the treatments that may be given.

Section 63 allows for any treatment to be given without consent that is not covered by Sections 57 (the implantation of hormones) and 58. Treatment under this section can cover many things, including care, rehabilitation, and psychotherapy. Once again this should be done under the direction of the RMO; however, nurses may be involved in the delivery of these treatments.

Further reading

Department of Health (2001). *Seeking Consent: Working with People with Learning Disabilities.* HMSO: London.

Wheeler P (2003). Patients' rights: consent to treatment for men and women with learning disability or who are otherwise mentally incapacitated. *Learning Disability Practice* **6**(5), 29–37.

Mental Capacity Act 2005

The MCA 2005 is a hugely influential policy initiative that has the potential to affect many aspects of the lives of people with ID. One such aspect is that of consent, and you are strongly advised to read 📖 Consent to examination, treatment, and care (p.488), in conjunction with this section. The MCA 2005 received Royal Assent in April 2005, some parts of the Act became active in April 2007, but most of the Act came into force in October 2007. The main aim of the Act is to provide a statutory frame-work to empower and protect people (>16yrs) who may lack capacity to make some decisions for them—including those with ID. Section 1 of the Act sets out 5 underpinning principles as follows:

A presumption of capacity—every adult has the right to make their own decisions, and they must be assumed to have capacity to do so unless it is proved otherwise.

Individuals being supported to make their own decisions—an individual must be given all practicable help before anyone treats them as not being able to make their own decisions.

Unwise decisions—just because an individual makes what could be considered to be an unwise decision, they should not be treated as lacking capacity to make that decision.

Best interests—an act done or decision taken under the Act for or on be-half of a person who lacks capacity must be done in their best interests.

Least restrictive option—anything done for or on behalf of a person who lacks capacity should be the least restrictive of their basic human rights and freedoms.

What the Act does

Assessing lack of capacity—it sets out a single clear test for assessing whether a person lacks capacity at a particular time. The Act states that no one can be judged to lack capacity as a result of a medical diagnosis, condition, age, appearance, or behaviour.

Best interests—the Act provides a checklist of factors that decision makers must work through in order to decide what is in a person's best interests. Under the Act those involved in caring for the person lacking capability have the right to be consulted in relation to best interest.

Acts in connection with treatment—Section 5 of the Act gives statutory protection from liability where a person is performing an act connected to caring for the person who lacks capacity.

Restraint—the Act defines restraint in relation to those who lack capac-ity as any restriction of liberty or movement whether or not the person resists. Restraint is permissible if those using it reasonably believe it is necessary to the individual and that it is a proportionate response. (see 📖 Use of restraint, p.426).

Lasting powers of attorney—the Act allows for a person to appoint an at-torney to act on their behalf should they lose capacity in the future.

Court appointed deputies—deputies are able to take decisions on welfare, healthcare, and financial matters as authorized by the new Court of Protection.

New Court of Protection—this new Court has jurisdiction over the whole Act. The court can make declarations, decisions, and orders affecting those who lack capacity. It is particularly important in resolving complex and disputed dilemmas relating to consent and best interests.

A new Public Guardian will be responsible for the supervision attorneys and deputies, and liaise with other agencies such as the police and social services to respond to any concern relating to attorneys and deputies.

Independent Mental Capacity Advocate—an IMCA is someone appointed by a person who lacks capacity to act and speak for them if they do not have anyone, such as family or friends, who can do this for them. IMCAs are involved only where decisions need to be made about serious medical matters or a change in the person's accommodation.

Advance decisions to refuse treatment—the Act has created statutory rules so that people can make a decision in advance to refuse treatment should they lack capacity in the future.

A criminal offence—the Act has created a new criminal offence, which is that of ill treatment or neglect of a person who lacks capacity.

Research—the Act introduces rules about research and allows for it to be carried out and involve people who lack capacity, so long as it is approved by an ethics committee.

Exclusions—the Act acknowledges that some decisions cannot be made by someone on behalf of a person who lacks consent, because they are governed by other laws or are of a very personal nature. These include marriage, sexual relationships, and voting. People can also still be treated compulsorily under the MHA (see 📖 Consent to examination, treatment, and care, p.488).

Code of Practice—a statutory COP that accompanies the Act provides comprehensive guidance for all those who work with or care for those who lack capacity. It clearly sets out in 16 chapters the responsibilities of all relevant parties, with specific reference to nurses. Readers are strongly advised to review the COP.

Further reading

The Mental Capacity Act, The Code of Practice, and other related documents can be found at
🖥 http://www.dca.gov.uk/menincap/legis.htm

Healthcare Commission

The role of the HC is to promote improvements in the quality of healthcare and public health in England and Wales, although its role varies between the 2 countries. The aims of the HC are to:

- safeguard patients and promote continuous improvement in healthcare services for patients, carers, and the public
- promote the rights of everyone to have access to healthcare services and the opportunity to improve their health
- be independent, fair, and open in decision making, and consultative about processes.

Statutory roles are to:

- Assess healthcare provision in the NHS and independent sector
- Produce an annual rating for each NHS trust in England
- Regulate the independent sector through registration and inspection
- Examine and carry out independent reviews of complaints
- Investigate serious service failings
- Coordinate the healthcare inspections of others.

The aims and roles listed above indicate that the HC is an important body with considerable influence. It has produced reports and audits relating to ID practice, and these can be seen at the HC website:

🖳 http://www.healthcarecommission.org.uk

Some reports are specific to one particular service, but the findings are often indicative of a broader picture, such as the Commission's report (3 December 2007) on progress following lapses in care within the Bromley ID service. A combination of reports that identified significantly poor practice (Cornwall Partnership NHS Trust in July 2006, and Sutton and Merton PCT in January 2007) led to an extensive, major and far-reaching inquiry into healthcare services for people with ID. The report is called *The Healthcare Commission's Audit of Specialist Inpatient Healthcare Services*. This and subsequent recommendations can be accessed via the website above. In summary the audit was for the most part highly critical of services, and below is listed the audit's main findings:

- Insufficient attention is paid to safeguarding vulnerable people across all aspects of their care.
- Services are not monitored by the organization that commission them.
- There is lack of stimulating activities and opportunities.
- There is a lack of leadership.
- Care is poorly planned and does not involve people with ID.
- Residential care is provided in institutionalized settings.
- Physical restraint procedures were appropriate.

The HC commented that major changes are required to meet the standards of care expected in the 21st century, and that even in the best services the safety and quality of care were not adequate. The HC also commented on the institutionalized nature of services that denied people with ID of their human rights and dignity in many instances. Poor physical environments were found to contribute to this negative picture. Services were found to be of low priority within the healthcare system, and characterized by poor leadership, poor training, and no framework with which to measure performance. After auditing 154 services the HC has recommended the closure of all 'NHS campus' accommodation by 2010, and it made no fewer than 2548 recommendations to improve care, grouped under the following headings:

- Choice
- Environment
- Relationships
- Money
- Monitoring
- Person-centred care
- Physical interventions
- Safeguarding
- Staffing.

The HC has offered an extensive list of detailed recommendations under each of the above headings, and these can be accessed through the website above under 'table of recommendations'.

Common law and duty of care

Common law is based on decisions made by judges that are derived from previous cases that have set precedents/legal principles that other judges follow. It is an ancient form of law that is grounded in jurisprudence. It is different from statute law, which is law made by Parliament. The notion of duty of care stems from common law and some of the cases that set legal principles are important in influencing nursing practice, and are outlined in this section. Duty of care can be considered to be a formalization of the implicit responsibilities held by an individual towards another individual in society. It is not a requirement that duty of care is defined by law, but it often develops through the jurisprudence of common law. In summary there is a strong connection between common law, duty of care, and negligence.

Duty of care is a key element of the NMC code of professional conduct, which in Paragraph 1.4 states that:[1]

'You have duty of care to your patients and clients, who are entitled to receive safe and competent care.'

This would seem self-evident, and requires further explanation. The common law that underpins duty of care comes from the 1932 case of *Donoghue v Stevenson*, from which the judge stated that:

You must take reasonable care to avoid acts or omissions which you can reasonably foresee would be likely to injure your neighbour.' (Cited in Dimond 2005, p38).[2]

In other words there is a duty of care if a person can see that their actions are reasonably likely to cause harm to another. In the field of nursing this underpins the duty of care that a nurse has to the patient. The code of conduct also states in Part 1.3 that:

'You are personally accountable for your practice. This means that you are answerable for your actions and omissions, regardless of advice or directions from another professional.'

The issue of accountability is extremely important in nursing, as nurses can be called to account for their actions in a court of law. If this occurs, then the proceedings are very likely to be based on the nurse giving an account of their actions relating to a breach of their duty of care, which is often construed as negligence. Common law via the law of tort (this includes negligence) provides a framework for how care should be delivered and whether it falls short of the required standard. The common law principle that underpins decisions on the standard of practice is the Bolam Test (Bolam *vs* Friern Hospital Management Committee 1957). The key principle of the Bolam Test is:

'The test is the standard of the ordinary skilled man exercising and professing to have that special skill. A man need not possess the highest expert skill at the risk of being found negligent, it is sufficient if he exercises the skill of an ordinary competent man exercising that particular art.' Cited in NMC *Advice Sheet: Duty of Care* 2006, p2[3]

In other words, the standard against which a nurse is judged is that of a reasonably competent practitioner working within accepted parameters. In some instances an expert witness may be called on to give their opinion as to whether a nurse was performing their duties to the standard of a reasonably competent practitioner. Duty of care may be owed by a number of different professionals and organizations to the same individual. The nurse who actually delivers care or performs the task in question has a primary duty of care to the individual. Where a task has been delegated by a more experienced nurse, it may be this person who has the primary duty of care (guidance on this can be found in the Code of Conduct in Paragraph 4.6).

Vicarious liability

An organization providing care and employing nurses may owe a duty of care to the individual being cared for, as will the nurses themselves, and the organisation may be liable for systemic errors. An example of this would be harm caused to a person who had been physically restrained because an organization had not ensured that staff were adequately trained in control and restraint techniques.

Withdrawing care

It is acknowledged that in some circumstances nurses may withdraw their duty of care. Such circumstances should be agreed and set out within local policies, such as:
- where a nurse fears physical violence
- where there are environmental health and safety issues involved in providing care
- where a nurse is being racially or sexually harassed.

Situations off duty

In the UK if a nurse encounters an emergency while not on duty they do not have a legal duty to intervene. If the nurse does decide to intervene then they take on a legal duty to act reasonably and within the parameters of their best skills and knowledge. Although the nurse does not have a legal duty to intervene, the code of conduct (Paragraph 8.5) places a professional duty on nurses at all times. In the event of an emergency outside of work it is reasonable for a nurse to act in a proper manner e.g. giving support and comfort without direct intervention.

1 Nursing and Midwifery Council (2008). *The Code: Standards for Conduct, Performance and Ethics For Nurses and Midwives.* Nursing and Midwifery Council: London.

2 Dimond D (2005). *Legal Aspects of Nursing.* 4th edn. Pearson Longman: Harlow.

3 Nursing and Midwifery Council (2006). *Advice Sheet: Duty of Care.* Nursing and Midwifery Council: London.

Safeguarding adults

Up to 2000, there had been no coordinated guidance on the protection of vulnerable adults from abuse. The UK government document *No Secrets: Guidance on developing and implementing multiagency policies and procedures to protect vulnerable adults from abuse* set out to address this issue.[1] The main intention of this document was to offer guidance on how the protection of vulnerable adults should be organized. *No Secrets* is applicable to any vulnerable client group or adult, and for the purposes of the guidance a vulnerable person is someone 18yrs or over and:

'who is in need of community care services by reason of mental or other disability, age or illness, and who is or may be unable to take care of him or herself, or unable to protect him or herself against significant harm or exploitation.' No Secrets, p.8[1]

Clearly most people with ID will fall within this definition.

Abuse

Abuse is a generic term that is open to wide interpretation. It can be a single act or it can be systematic repeated acts. It can occur within institutions and as a result of institutionalization. It can occur within families and in public places. It is a violation of one person's human and civil rights by another. It is customary to categorize forms of abuse under the following headings:

- Physical abuse
- Sexual abuse
- Psychological abuse
- Financial or material abuse
- Neglect and acts of omission
- Discrimination.

Abusers can be anybody and from any walk of life, and they can be family members, nurses, doctors, paid carers, transport escorts, volunteers, strangers, and those who deliberately target vulnerable people. Often perpetrators use positions of power to abuse or work in close proximity to, and provide intimate care for, vulnerable people.

  No Secrets suggested that there are different levels of abuse, and that not all abuse justifies intervention.[1] It goes on to suggest that the following factors should be considered when assessing the seriousness of abuse:

- The vulnerability of the person
- The nature and extent of the abuse
- The length of time it has been happening
- The impact on the vulnerable person
- The risk of repeated or increasingly serious acts.

Dealing with abuse is dealt with in ▢ Dealing with abuse, p.544. This section is focused on a more general overview of abuse, and the interagency framework for managing it. Section 3 of *No Secrets* outlines guidance for setting up an interagency framework, and identifies the relevant agencies who should be involved:[1]

- Health and social care providers
- Providers of sheltered and supported housing

- Service regulators
- Commissioners of health and social care services
- The police and other relevant law enforcement agencies
- The voluntary and private sector
- Housing and education departments
- Benefit agencies
- Carer support groups
- User groups
- Advocacy groups.

In essence, as broad a representation as possible should be achieved. *No Secrets* also recommends that the interagency committee should then:[1]

- identify roles, responsibilities, authority, and accountability
- establish mechanisms and *modus operandi*
- draw up procedures
- develop guidance, implement equal opportunity, and antidiscriminatory training
- balance the sometimes conflicting requirements of confidentiality
- identify mechanisms for monitoring and review.

Readers should consult *No Secrets*[1] for extensive guidance in relation to the above and what can be done when individual abuse has been identified (some of this is alluded to in 📖 Dealing with abuse, p.544).

POVA register—this is a recent safeguard measure. In 2004 the Department of Health launched The Protection of Vulnerable Adults (POVA) scheme—a key aspect of which is the POVA list of care workers who have harmed vulnerable people in their care. From 26th July 2004 it became a requirement for all registered care providers to request a check against the POVA list when considering a person for a care position.

Nurse's role—interagency committees designate different people to have roles to protect vulnerable adults. One such role is that of the 'alerter'. Alerters are responsible for reporting suspected incidents of abuse to the appropriate person; they are unlikely to be investigators.

1 Department of Health and the Home Office (2000). *No Secrets—guidance on developing and implementing multiagency policies and procedures to protect vulnerable adults from abuse.* HMSO: London.

Medicines—the role of the nurse

In the UK the control and administration of medicines in the UK is governed by the Medicines Act 1968. Under the original Act nurses could not prescribe medicines. This situation was altered by the Medicinal Products: Prescription by Nurses etc Act 1992[1] that amended section 58 of the 1968 Medicines Act to allow some limited nurse prescribing. This Act came into force in 1994, and stipulated that nurse prescribing would be limited to RGNs, midwives, and health visitors. In 1999 the Department of Health extended the range of potential prescribers,[2] and this has enabled RNLDs to become nurse prescribers. Nurses can become either supplementary prescribers or independent nurse prescribers.

Supplementary prescribers

These nurses can prescribe any medication listed in the BNF,[3] identified on a clinical management plan, and within their scope of practice. Supplementary prescribing legally allows nurses to prescribe from a wider range of medication applicable to the field of ID than that available within the formulary of independent nurse prescribing. Supplementary prescribing is based on clear limitations set out in the clinical management plan, which must be agreed with the individual patient, and in consultation with an independent prescriber, who must be a doctor or dentist.

These plans must be signed by both the nurse and doctor.

Independent nurse prescribers

These prescribers can prescribe any licensed medicine for any medical condition within their competence, including some controlled drugs.

The Department of Health has laid down criteria regarding the eligibility of those wishing to become nurse prescribers.[4] In summary, they should be able to study at degree level, have 3yrs post-registration experience (the preceding one in the clinical area they wish to prescribe in), and have the ability to assess client need.

The development of nurse prescribing in the field of ID is in its infancy, with the first RNLD becoming an independent and supplementary prescriber in 2003.

The benefits of nurse prescribing include:
- Professional flexibility
- Recognition of the nurse's increased skills and responsibilities
- Improved multidisciplinary working
- Removing some barriers to patients accessing medication
- More effective/efficient/timely healthcare
- Improved ability to help patients and carers manage medication
- Early intervention.

1 *Medicinal Products: Prescription by Nurses etc Act 1992 (commencement No 1 order 1994) Statutory Instrument 1994 No.2408 (C.48).* HMSO: London.

2 Department of Health (1999). *Review of Prescribing, Supply and Administration of Medicines.* Crown Report II. HMSO: London.

3 British Medical Association and the Royal Pharmaceutical Society of Great Britain. *British National Formulary.* British Medical Association and the Royal Pharmaceutical Society of Great Britain: London.

4 Department of Health (2006). *Patients' Access to Medicines: A Guide to Implementing Nurse and Pharmacist Independent Prescribing within the NHS in England.* HMSO: London.

Research

Introduction

This chapter examines research and ID nursing. Nursing is relatively new to the world of research. Although nurses have used research findings for many years, it is only in recent decades that they have been required to undertake research, or to study it systematically during pre and post registration nurse education. In the 1990s British nursing education moved from hospital based schools of nursing to universities, and this brought with it a requirement that all nurses engage with research. This primarily has taken the form of nurses ensuring that their practice is evidence based, but for a smaller group it has led to the direction of and participation as researchers in research projects.

This chapter is an introduction to some of the key concepts in nursing research that are most relevant to ID nursing. The major methodologies of quantitative and qualitative research are discussed, to help in identifying and evaluating their use in practice. Some of the stages of the research process are outlined so that you will know what to look for when reading research, or what to start with if you want to pursue your own research ideas. Finally, the chapter examines some of the issues that are important to ID nursing research. These include ethical issues that are fundamental to all research as well as working with people with ID, carers, and children.

Definitions of terms

Readers who are not familiar with research may find some of the terms difficult. Most are like a lot of nursing terms that are simply shorthand to mean things that would take a great deal of time to explain every time that they are used. Some of the terms used in this chapter will be explained in the context that they are used, but this section defines some of the main ones that are used.

Research is the systematic approach to discovering or developing knowledge.

Participatory research is research that involves its participants as an integral part of its method.

Methodology is the intellectual framework that is used in a research project.

Research methods are the techniques that are used within the methodological framework.

The two primary methodologies are quantitative and qualitative research.

Quantitative research uses experimental methods. Research is particularly concerned with reliability, generalization, control of variables, testing hypotheses, and statistical association between variables, and is often large scale in nature.

Qualitative research uses naturalistic methods and examines the social world or 'lived experience' of people. Research is less concerned with reliability and generalization, and is descriptive in style, small scale in nature, and engages directly with participants.

Defining areas for research

An area for research must be clear, achievable, and manageable within the available resources. This section will concentrate on how to bring clarity to areas of research.

Most researchers start with a broad question or vague area of enquiry. Readers can probably think of their own examples, and they may be similar to the following:
- Why do people with ID have poorer health than the rest of the population?
- How can people be encouraged to adopt healthy lifestyles?
- How can a nurse be sure that they are adopting the correct interventions for someone whose behaviour disturbs others?

The first step in defining an area for research is to think carefully about your idea(s), and to discuss this with colleagues. A literature review is then required to find out what has already been written (see 📖 Undertaking a literature review, p.504). The literature review will unearth research that has already been carried out, and may provide answers to your question. It is more likely going to lead to a refinement of the area of research.

However, sometimes it is found that the literature related to your question is sparse. This may require you to re-examine the original broad area for your research; it will possibly need to be broken down to more discrete questions to ensure that it is clear, and that you are clear about the parameters.

As an illustration the first question, from the examples above, is now going to be broken down.
- Why do people with ID have poorer health than the rest of the population?

There are several elements to this broad question that have to be broken down. For the sake of simplicity this will be done through a series of questions.

What is meant by 'people with ID' in this context?
The researcher needs to be very clear about the remit of their enquiry. Is the definition going to include all people with ID? Is there a difference between the health of people with profound and complex disabilities and those with less complex needs? It may be that this is what the research is really trying to tease out. Perhaps the comparison will be with people with ID and the general population, in which case both will still need to be defined. This is often referred to as inclusion and exclusion criteria.

What is the evidence for the underlying assumption that people with ID have poorer health?
There is a clear assumption behind the broad research question, and the researcher needs to be quite clear that there is a body of evidence to demonstrate that this assumption is correct. It may be demonstrated adequately within the literature, but even so the researcher needs to be sure that it is right for the question being asked. If it is not in the

literature then can it be demonstrated through statistics, observation, or is it simply a 'gut' feeling? If the evidence is not clear then the area for research will have to be significantly refined to:

• Do people with ID have poorer health than the rest of the population?

What is meant by health?

Health is a very difficult concept to define, although there are some generally accepted measures that help to clarify the health status of groups. Morbidity and mortality figures tend to be used to draw broad lessons. Morbidity refers to the incidence of a particular disease; mortality refers to a measure of the number of deaths due to a particular disease/cause. You may be more interested in positive states of health, in which case evidence based on a method such as quality of life surveys may be more useful. Other issues to consider are whether your interest is in the health status from the individual point of view, or whether there needs to be an attempt to introduce objective measures.

What is the general population?

There are figures published for illness rates in the general population, and these are nationally defined. Reference to these will help in making broad comparisons, but the research will still need to be very clear about the nature of the comparisons to be made and between which groups.

In this example a broad research question has been turned into several smaller questions that need to be addressed in order to define the area for research. It may be that one of the narrower questions becomes one that develops into the final research question for a specific research project.

Whatever is decided, the research area needs to be achievable. This will require you to consider:

• Can the question be answered?
• Is enough known about the background to the topic?
• Is enough known about all the elements of the research question?

The research area to be studied then needs to be manageable within the available resources of the research team. It is of little use having an achievable project that can be managed only by a much larger research team, unless you can successfully bid for the resources.

Undertaking a literature review

At its simplest, a literature review is a systematic summary of what is already known about a subject.

A literature review involves two main stages:

- A literature search
- Making sense of the findings of the research.

Literature search

First of all you need to know what you are looking for. There is an enormous amount of literature published about some subjects and very little about others, and it is important to start with a clear idea of what you want to find out. Most literature searches are now conducted with computerized databases, and while this has made searching the literature much more accessible, the amount of material retrieved can be overwhelming. If you are lucky you may have a library in the organization where you work, and if so you are well advised to use the services of the librarian or information specialist to help you. If not, you can undertake a simple search for material using an internet-based search engine such as Google Scholar. However, please be aware that searches using popular search engines throw up a large number of references, and it is not always easy to discriminate between different forms of material. It is important to use your critical skills in assessing the important from the unimportant material.

Some simple tests to use:

- Has the article been subject to peer review?
- Does the article say how it came to the findings?
- Is the article a piece of journalism or opinion based?
- Is the article written by a professional?
- Has the author written anything else?
- Is the author's work referenced by others?

These questions can help you to assess whether an article is useful for your literature review and whether the information is reliable. Of course you may find that your search reveals that there have already been reviews written about the subject you are interested in; such reviews will be your first port of call, although there may be more recent material in print and you will have to find this.

You will need to establish criteria for inclusion in your literature search. Most search engines will help you with this. Typically you may wish to restrict your search to a particular time period and to a particular language. The search engine will do this for you if you set the parameters to the search that you think is necessary. You may also wish to restrict your search to particular types of research, such as large-scale studies, or smaller in-depth research using only a few subjects. It is usual to refine search criteria as you find out the amount of material that you are dealing with.

Making sense of the findings of the research

Once you have completed your initial search you will need to make sense of the material. In an ideal world you will have unearthed enough material to tell you what you need to know without being overwhelmed. However, you may find that you need to further refine your criteria in order to be able to make use of the material. You can do this by narrowing the dates, by restricting your criteria to primary research papers, or possibly to a narrower subject. Whatever you decide will involve a critical analysis of the material that you have found.

When you have done this, and have satisfied yourself about the quality of the research that you have found, you will need to arrange it in a way that makes sense to you and to others. This will become the literature review itself. It is usually helpful to develop a table or some other means of grouping the research by categories such as:
- Method used
- Number of subjects
- Key findings
- Limitations.

Once you have done this it is time to write up your review. Your table or list of themes may be sufficient for what you need. If you wish to publish your literature review, however, or put it into a report, you will need to include an account of how you conducted your review as well as the main findings. Key questions to ask about the papers that you have considered are:
- Are there any trends?
- Are there any gaps in the literature?
- Does the literature lead to new research questions?

Further reading

Parahoo K (2006). *Nursing Research: Principles, Process and Issues*. 2nd edn. Palgrave Macmillan: London.

Qualitative approaches

Qualitative research encompasses research designs and methods such as:
- Grounded theory
- Descriptive and interpretative phenomenology
- Interpretative phenomenological analysis
- Narrative analysis-based approaches.

Qualitative approaches are guided by an inductive approach in which the research seeks to discover, identify, describe, and usually interpret, information provided by participants. These approaches are underpinned by a view that individuals and social processes contrast and reconstruct the 'worlds' that people and groups inhabit, and it does not accept that there is a single objective world.

Within these designs the aim is to explore the 'world' as perceived by individuals and groups.[1] In doing so it seeks to provide insights into the complex individual and social experiences and phenomena. The overall aim of qualitative approaches is the desire to seek to understand perceptions, experiences, emotions, and social processes. Given the diversity of designs and methods that may be used within qualitative approaches, together with approaches to analysis and interpretation, it will be necessary to refer to authoritative text books such as those in the 📖 Further reading.

Ethical approval

All research projects, including small local projects, have ethical aspects that need careful consideration in relation to aspects such as voluntary participation, confidentiality, anonymity, security of data, and the use of findings. Given the personal and often sensitive nature of the information collected in qualitative projects, care must be taken in developing and undertaking projects in an ethically defensible manner. Researchers should clarify local research governance requirements, and must ensure that all necessary approval from local or regional ethical committees has been obtained before any recruitment to or data collection within a project commences.

Sampling

All sampling within qualitative projects is non-random. In seeking to generate a sample, the focus is on identifying people who have undergone the experience which is being researched, e.g. parents of children with ID, or people living in independent accommodation. Therefore approaches such as purposive, snowballing, or theoretical sampling may be used. The numbers of participants within a qualitative study will be smaller than quantitative projects, with an emphasis on the depth and richness of data obtained rather than the quantity or ability to represent an overall population. Many qualitative studies have samples of less than 20 participants, and some have used single case study designs.

Data collection

Qualitative data may include words, songs, poetry, still or moving images, and will depend on the research aim of the specific project. Often a combination of approaches is used to collect data, including:

- Semi-structured interviews
- Unstructured interviews
- Diary entries
- Focus groups
- Observations (participant, non-participation, video recorded)
- Questionnaires (largely for biographical information).

Data may be collected on one occasion, but in many projects participants are interviewed on more than one occasion to provide opportunities to explore their experiences in depth, or changes over a period of time.

Data analysis

The framework for data analysis will largely be determined by the specific research design used within the project. A number of analysis frameworks exist with differing approaches, a different number of steps, and different titles of steps, but which are similar overall in so far as moving from initial thoughts about key points, to identifying themes and sub-themes. Data analysis in qualitative projects is not reliant on figures and statistics for meaning. The detail of individual analysis frameworks, and the need for robustness and clear audit trails in data analysis is discussed fully in research texts in the 🕮 Further reading.

Further reading

Denscombe M (2003). *The Good Research Guide for Small-scale Social Research Projects*. 2nd edn. Open University Press: Maidenhead.

Patton M (2002). *Qualitative Research and Evaluation Methods*. 3rd edn. Sage: Thousand Oaks, California.

Vitae 🖳 http://www.vitae.ac.uk/

Intute 🖳 http://www.intute.ac.uk/

The British Library 🖳 http://www.bl.uk/

University of Bristol Norah Fry Research Centre 🖳 http://www.bristol.ac.uk/norahfry/

1 Fox M, Martin P, Green G (2007). *Doing Practitioner Research*. Sage Publications: London.

Quantitative approaches

Quantitative approaches to research can be located in the positivistic paradigm of understanding the world, and use experimental methods to study (research) it. Quantitative research incorporates a range of approaches that adopt a deductive approach to generating knowledge, that includes (an) observable relationship(s) between independent and dependent variable(s).

An independent variable is something that can be manipulated to bring about some kind of predicted effect (hypothesis), and this can be accounted for by some change to an independent variable—this is often referred to as a cause and effect relationship.

In quantitative research further work conducted under the same experimental conditions should result in this cause and effect relationship being replicated. This is important because this implies an ability to generalize findings; research in this genre attempts to emulate the natural sciences, and is concerned with the generation and testing of knowledge, and thereby the construction of theory. Within ID research, quantitative approaches may be used to undertake studies in aspects of teaching, behavioural interventions, factors affecting attitudes towards people with ID, skills development (if measured on scales), and effectiveness of medications. It should be remembered, however, what quantitative research does not purport to do, and that is it does not study research questions in natural settings, it does not try and interpret 'real and lived' experiences, it is not exploratory in nature, and it does not seek to engage with participants involved in the research.

Understanding quantitative research requires time, patience, and a detailed knowledge of design, sampling, methods of analysis and statistics, the power of the experiment, and the attendant levels of significance of any finding, and for this reason the reader is strongly advised to refer to authoritative text books, such as that shown in the 📖 Further reading.

Quantitative research designs
- The experiment or randomized controlled trial (RCT)
- Quasi-experimental design
- Surveys
- Cohort studies
- Factorial
- Systematic reviews and meta-analyses.

Sampling
Probability
Probability refers to a range of sampling approaches used by the researcher to select a random sample of respondents or subjects from the population being studied e.g. simple random sampling, systematic random sampling, and stratified random sampling.

Non-probability
Non-probability refers to a range of sampling approaches used by the researcher to select a non-random sample of respondents or subjects

from the population being studied e.g. convenience sampling, purposive, and snowball sampling.

Data collection
- Questionnaires
- Structured interviews
- Systematic observation schedules—these have usually been validated and held reliable.

Data analysis
The extent and type of analysis is dependent on sample, level of measurement—nominal, ordinal, interval or ratio, research design and variables. The data can be analysed either through descriptive or inferential statistics.

Descriptive statistics
Measure of central tendency—mean, median and mode; also used are distribution of data, standard deviations, and ranges.

Inferential statistics
Statistical analysis of data could include bivariate or multivariate analysis; however, this is determined by whether parametric or non-parametric tests are used, and this is equally determined by factors in measurement decisions and type of research design.

Further reading
Gates B, Wray J (2000). The problematic nature of evidence. In: Gates B, Gear J and Wray J. *Behavioural Distress: Concepts and Strategies.* Baillière Tindall: London, 283–300.

Parahoo K (2006). *Nursing Research: Principles, Process and Issues.* 2nd edn. Palgrave Macmillan: London.

Vitae ▣ http://www.vitae.ac.uk/

Intute ▣ http://www.intute.ac.uk/

The British Library ▣ http://www.bl.uk/

Unversity of Bristol Norah Fry Research Centre ▣ http://www.bristol.ac.uk/norahfry/

Ethical issues in research

Arguably all research with human subjects should comprise a range of ethical issues, and typically includes:

- *Beneficence* (to do good)
- *Non-maleficence* (not to cause harm)
- *Autonomy* (to treat people with respect and provide them with the kinds of information they need to make informed decisions)
- *Justice* (to try and ensure that through the research some justice is served).

Due regard must be given to and acted upon to obtain consent from people with ID before they become involved in research.[1] Even if the proposed methods are not invasive, the research must still be conducted within the general ethical conventions of social research at all times.[2] Research must always be conducted in a manner that respects the people who participate in the process, and will demonstrate concern for their dignity and welfare.

Seeking permission

In order to involve people with ID in research it is good practice to ensure that ethical approval is obtained from an established ethical committee e.g. in a university, local authority, or health authority. Within the NHS, for example, as a general rule all research projects require Local Research Ethics Committee (LREC) approval. If the research is to be undertaken as a national study, then review is undertaken by a Multi-centre Research Ethics Committee (MREC); these exist across England, Scotland, Wales, and Northern Ireland.

In nearly all cases that involve people with ID, this will require the researcher to demonstrate how they will ensure that they have obtained informed consent, as well as giving due consideration to capacity to consent; this is usually achieved through the development of 'accessible' information sheets about the research, along with 'accessible' consent forms (Fig. 14.1). These are usually in the form of straightforward information sheets that use simple language and are frequently supported with pictures from picture databases such as Change.[3]

Bracknell Forest PCT

**MENTAL HEALTH RESEARCH
PROJECT
CONSENT FORM**

If I decide that I do not want
to continue being part of the
project, I can stop at any time

NAME:

I agree to take part
in the mental health
research project.

I understand that
anything I say will
be recorded.

This form has been
explained to me by
Mary or Bob.

I understand that
anything I say will
not be told to
anyone else with my
name attached to it.

SIGNED
DATE

Fig. 14.1 An example of an accessible consent form. Images from www.
changepeople.co.uk, with permission.

Further reading

Parahoo K (2006). *Nursing Research: Principles, Process and Issues.* 2nd edn. Palgrave Macmillan:
London.

Department of Health (2004). *Research Governance in Health and Social Care: NHS permission for
R&D involving NHS patients.* Department of Health: London. ⌨ http://www.dh.gov.uk/en/Publicati
onsandstatistics/Publications/PublicationsPolicyAndGuidance/DH_4122563

1 Department of Health (2001). *Seeking Consent: Working with People with Learning Disabilities.*
Department of Health: London.

2 Haber J (1998). Legal and ethical issues. In: LoBiondo-Wood G and Haber J (Eds.) *Nursing
Research: Methods, Critical Appraisal and Utilisation.* 4th edn. Chapter 11. Mosby-Year Books:
Missouri.

3 Change ⌨ http://www.changepeople.co.uk/

Involving people with intellectual disabilities in the research process

The role of people with ID within research has changed over the past 20yrs. Historically people with ID have had research done to them—they have been the subjects of the researcher, the studied, the analysed, but never the participant.[1,2,3] Today contemporary researchers are charged with the responsibility of making their research accessible and inclusive to people with ID.

Kinds of involvement

Since the development of the concepts of participatory research[4] that led to emancipatory research[5] within the general disability field, a natural progression has been to incorporate these principles into research with people with ID.[6] The following are some examples of methodological approaches to research that embrace the principles of involving people with ID:

- Personal narratives
- One-to-one interviews
- Focus groups
- Consumer researchers
- Research groups.

The first of these approaches was initially demonstrated by the use of personal narratives to illustrate life experience.[7,8,9,10] This approach has provided us with authentic accounts of people's lives, as well as placing them at the centre of the research. Extensive one-to-one interviews were used to study parenting by people with ID.[11,12] In the case of the Booths' approach this provided new insights into the lives of parents with ID as well as their children.[11] Additionally, focus groups are now increasingly popular for research.[13] Here a group of people with a shared interest e.g. gender, age, ethnicity, religion, life experience, expertise, are brought together to discuss a particular issue. Yet another approach to involving people with ID is that of engaging them as active consumer researchers.[14] Increasingly, academic researchers are pairing up with people with ID and forming research groups able to unite their various strengths and respond to calls for research proposal from a range of bodies commissioning such work.

Researchers are responsible for making their research accessible and inclusive to people with ID. It should be noted, however, that it is not always possible to involve all people with ID.

1 Kiernan C (1999). Participation in research by people with learning disability: origins and issues. *British Journal of Learning Disabilities* **27**(2), 43–51.

2 Walmsley J (2001). Normalisation, emancipatory research and inclusive research in learning disability. *Disability and Society* **16**(2), 187–205.

3 Dye L, Hendy S, Hare DJ, Burton M (2004). Capacity to consent to participate in research – a recontextualisation. *British Journal of Learning Disabilities* **32**(3), 144–150.

4 Northway R (2000). The relevance of participatory research in developing nursing's research and practice. *Nurse Researcher* **7**(4), 40–52.

5 Hanley B (2005). *Research as Empowerment.* Toronto Group Joseph Rowntree Foundation: York.

6 Walmsley J (2004). Inclusive learning disability research: the (non disabled) researcher's role. *British Journal of Learning Disabilities* **32**(2), 65–71.

7 Goodley D (1996). Tales of hidden lives: a critical examination of life history research with people who have learning difficulties. *Disability and Society* **11**(3), 333–49.

8 Atkinson D, Walmsley J (1999). Using autobiographical approaches with people with learning difficulties. *Disability and Society* **14**(2), 203–216.

9 Gray B, Ridden G (1999). *Lifemaps of People with Learning Disabilities.* Jessica Kingsley Publishers: London.

10 Atkinson D (2005). Narratives and people with learning disabilities. In: Grant G, Goward P, Richardson M, Ramcharan P, Eds. *Learning Disability: A Life Cycle Approach to Valuing People.* Open University Press: Milton Keynes.

11 Booth T, Booth W (1996). Sounds of silence: narrative research with inarticulate subjects. *Disability and Society* **11**(1), 55–69.

12 Knox M, Mok M, Parmenter TR (2000). Working with the experts: collaborative research with people with an intellectual disability. *Disability and Society* **15**(1), 49–61.

13 Gates B, Waight M (2007). Reflections on conducting focus groups with people with learning disabilities: theory and practice. *Journal of Research in Nursing* **12**(2), 111–126.

14 Feldner C, Gregory C, Vakaria A et al. (2007). People with learning disabilities as consumer researchers: a case study. *Learning Disability Today* **7**(2), 9–14.

Working with people with intellectual disabilities in the research process

Why involve people with intellectual disabilities?

In the era of policy objectives such as inclusion, it may seem inappropriate to ask why people with ID should be involved in research into their lives and services. However, in every research project it is important to consider who should be involved in order that the research aims and objectives can be achieved. When it is clear that in order to answer the research questions being asked that people with ID need be involved, then concerted efforts should be made to actively involve them in the research process.

How may people with intellectual disabilities contribute?

With opportunities and support, people can contribute to all stages of the research process, including being involved as co-researchers in the development of the research question, the data collection, analysis and dissemination phases. It is necessary, therefore, to consult with people with ID at the start of the research process when research questions are being developed.[1] In doing so the opportunity exists to identify questions that are of relevance to the lives of people and their families, and guard against projects that are focused on the personal interest of the person undertaking the research. Such collaborative working with voluntary and not for profit organizations may also provide access to funding opportunities that are not available to statutory or private sector services alone.

Conducting ethical research

All research must be undertaken in an ethically defensible manner, and when working with people with ID, specific consideration needs to be given to additional challenges and vulnerabilities that may be present. It is also important that all research proposals, including those for local small-scale projects, have been reviewed in line with local research governance requirements, and received the necessary ethical approval in writing before any recruitment or data collection commences.

In undertaking research with people with ID, the ethical principles listed below should be followed, and a clear audit trail of how this was achieved should be maintained.[2]

The professional integrity of the researcher

People undertaking research must at all times behave in a professional manner and objectively seek to answer the research question and report all findings, including those that may not support their personal views. They should be open about the limitations of the research and their own competence in undertaking the research, seeking independent support when necessary.

Respect for the rights and dignity of participants

All people participating in the research should have the necessary information in a format accessible to them (using pictorial cues, signs and symbols—see ⌨ Inclusive communication, p.294) and the time necessary to make a decision about participation. They must know that they have the option not to participate in the project, to decide how much information they wish to share, and that they may withdraw at any time. When involving children, consent must be obtained from parents.

Throughout the project participants should be kept up to date with the process of the project, and be involved in consultation at key points in the research process if appropriate. They should also have contact information if they wish to receive an update during or following completion of the project. There should be an agreement as to how the time, effort, and costs of contributing to the project will be appropriately acknowledged, and if payment will be made how this will be organized.

The well-being of all those involved

Participants should be aware of the limits of confidentiality when participating in a project,[3] while every effort should be made to maintain confidentiality and anonymity when storing and reporting findings.

Participants and researchers should not suffer any adverse effects from their involvement in the research. All people involved should be aware of the focus of the project, and any potential difficulties should be considered in advance and agreed plans should be in place as to how these will be addressed.

Participants and researchers should remain safe throughout the project, and a risk assessment should be undertaken when appropriate, with an agreed risk management plan in place before a project commences. Researchers should also have ongoing access to appropriate supervision and support during the project.

1 Emerson E, Hatton C, Thompson T, Parmenter TR (2004). *The International Handbook of Applied Research in Intellectual Disabilities.* John Wiley and Sons: Chichester.

2 Connolly P (2003). *Ethical Principles for Researching Vulnerable Groups.* Office of First and Deputy First Minister: Belfast.

3 Nursing and Midwifery Council (2008). *The Code: Standards of Conduct, Performance and Ethics for Nurses and Midwives.* Nursing and Midwisery Council: London.

Mixed methods

Traditionally research has been viewed as fitting into either a quantitative 'positivistic' or a qualitative 'interpretative' paradigm. At times these two paradigms have been portrayed as completely separate and not compatible to being used together. However, in the past decade that view has been regularly challenged. While both approaches have important contributions to research projects and have been used in most previous studies within ID, they are only able to provide a partial view of what may be complex situations. There is now a growing awareness of the potential contribution of a mixed methods design, sometimes also referred to as an integrated design.[1]

Rationale for using mixed methods design

When planning research, nurses need to consider in detail the research question(s) being asked, and in light of that, the various approaches that may be used to 'answer' the research question(s). A mixed methods design recognizes that in real-life experiences there is no 'single real world', but rather a number of perceived 'real worlds', and the challenge is to gain an understanding of these worlds and their interconnectedness.

With the increased recognition of the complexity of most human experiences and the limitations of other more traditional research designs, the use of a mixed method design provides an opportunity to gain broader insights into the wider experience and identify the potential connections and influences that may exist, which will not be illuminated by using purely quantitative and qualitative approaches.

The use of a mixed methods approach provides the opportunity to:
- enhance validity of research findings through providing corroboration of these across different research methods (triangulation)
- illustrate, clarify, and amplify the meaning of constructs or relationships
- gain a further understanding of the complexity of issues which can be taken forward through exploring the inconsistencies across differing research perspectives (development)
- enhance theoretical insights, hypothesis generation, and instrument development through providing alternative views and perspectives of the area under investigation.

Sampling, data collection, and data analysis

When using a mixed method design, the procedures for sampling, data collection, and data analysis will be guided by whether that aspect of the study is qualitative or quantitative in nature. However, 4 key decisions are:
- Which approach (quantitative or qualitative) has priority in the overall mixed methods design?
- How will the quantitative and qualitative aspects of the overall study be sequenced?
- How will the qualitative and quantitative aspects of the study fit together, will the overall design keep these as separate components of the study, or will each preceding phase directly influence what comes after it within a more integrated approach?

- How will data analysis be undertaken? As with sequencing of data collection, will data analysis be dealt with in separate components (combined only in final discussion) or presented as an integrated process?

Some notes of caution

As with all research designs, the selection of the design and methods must be linked to research questions and not selected on the basis of which approach the researcher prefers, or whether it is a 'new fad'. Likewise the use of a mixed method design must be justified in light of the research question being asked. Care must be taken to select approaches that are consistent with the aspect of the project to be addressed, and not to breach the logic of each individual component of the research design, in order that they could be defensibly applied, or else the resultant research design will be best described as 'mixed up methods'.

Mixed methods designs are also more complex than single quantitative or qualitative designs. Nurses considering using them should remember that although the outcome may be more comprehensive, mixed methods studies can take longer to complete, may have additional costs involved for time and equipment, and require an understanding (in researcher or supervisor) of both quantitative and qualitative paradigms, and how these may be blended together.

Given the diversity of designs and methods that may be used within mixed methods approaches, together with approaches to analysis and interpretation, to build on the overview provided in this section it will be necessary to refer to authoritative text books, such as those shown in 📖 Further reading.

Further reading

Fox M, Martin P, Green G (2007). *Doing Practitioner Research*. Sage Publications: London.

Tashakkori A, Teddlie C (2003). *Handbook of Mixed Methods*. Sage: Thousand Oaks.

---

1 Creswell JW (2003). *Research Design: Quantitative, Qualitative and Mixed Methods Approaches.* 2nd edn. Sage: Thousand Oaks.

Audit

Audit has similarities to research. Both need to be carried out in systematic ways, and aim to find things out. They also have to have regard for ethical principles. The fundamental difference is that research is defined by the aim of creating new knowledge. Audit can be defined by the aim of measuring existing service provision. Informal audit, like research, should be part of the work of every nurse because it helps answer the question about how the individual's and the organization's practice is affecting care.

NICE have defined audit as follows:[1]

A quality improvement process that seeks to improve patient care and outcomes through systematic review of care against explicit criteria, and the implementation of change.

Audit uses research methods and research findings to investigate existing practice, and usually makes comparisons with practice elsewhere or with specific benchmarks. In other words, is the organization doing what it should be doing, says it's doing, or aspires to do?

Clinical audit is closely associated with improving patient care. NICE makes this clear in their guidelines, in which they include the following questions as part of a clinical audit cycle:[1]

1 What are we trying to achieve?
2 Are we achieving it?
3 Why are we not achieving it?
4 Doing something to make things better?
5 Have we made things better?
6 Back to 1. What are we trying to achieve?

Audits do not normally need formal ethical approval but should still follow ethical guidelines e.g. data should be confidential, and users of services should not be coerced in any way into taking part in an audit. It has been suggested that some research studies may have been changed into audits in order to avoid complex ethical scrutiny.[2]

Many organizations have audit teams, and it is important to consult them prior to undertaking audits within your organization. They will likely have clear guidelines to be followed. NICE suggests that audit needs to be properly supported both financially and with appropriate time. It should be part of the organization's work, and it should involve people who use the service, who may have different priorities than the professionals.[1]

In the absence of organizational guidelines, the following need to be taken into account:
• What is the aim of the audit (what are you trying to find out)?
• Is the issue important enough for an audit?
• Is the issue an organizational priority?
• Are there any benchmarks to be measured against?
• How can the information that you need be obtained?
• Is it going to be possible to change things following the audit?
• How is the audit to be carried out?
• Are there sufficient resources for the audit?

Methods that can be used for an audit are very similar to those used in research projects. Some typical methods are:

- Reviewing case notes
- Analysis of complaints
- Analysis of critical incident reports
- Direct observations of care settings or waiting areas
- Satisfaction surveys
- Review of admission and discharge statistics
- Workload analysis.

Quite apart from research and audit there is the process of 'service development'. This approach does not fit neatly into either 'research' or 'audit', but generally service development does adopt systematic approaches. These might include collection and analysis of previous literature, taking baseline measurements, and comparing these with post-service changes. Therefore, such approaches often attempt to describe/measure the impact of a particular service development e.g. changes to the well-being of a person with ID, or improvements in organizational effectiveness.

1 NICE (2002). *Principles for Best Practice in Clinical Audit*. Radcliffe Medical Press: Oxford.

2 Paxton R, Whitty P, Zaatar A, Fairbairn A, Lothian J (2006). Research, audit and quality improvement. *International Journal of Health Care Quality Assurance* **19**(1), 105–111.

Evidence-based care

All health and social care should be based on the best available evidence. Arguably, most recipients of care, given the chance to express an opinion, would expect, or at least hope that this was so. However, nurses will sometimes struggle to cite the evidence behind some of their practice. This problem is not specific to nurses: many professionals when put 'on the spot' will find it difficult to cite the evidence behind some of their decisions. It will be reassuring to know that to be an evidence-based practitioner does not require us to be able to make reference to a peer-reviewed article every time we make a decision about our practice. However, nor does it mean justifying decisions for practice by arguing that 'we've always done it this way' or 'this is the way I was taught' or 'it's common sense'.

There is not a consensus about the definition of evidence-based practice in nursing. French has highlighted this in a paper that reviews the development of evidence-based nursing.[1] He suggested that there is 'insufficient evidence to demonstrate that evidence-based nursing is a single construct or process that can be distinguished from its other concomitants'. This supports anecdotal evidence that evidence-based practice in nursing is frequently seen as the use of a range of evidence to support clinical decision making, and that such evidence is not restricted to published research findings.

All nurses need to be able to use research. Thompson et al. have suggested that nurses should be able to:[2]
- accept research as a normal and integral aspect of nursing practice
- read and understand research reports
- apply research findings to clinical practice
- influence colleagues on the use of research data
- accept responsibility for their own professional development.

There are a variety of ways in which evidence-based care can be fostered. Some of them are dependent on the organization who employs the nurses, but there is also a responsibility for individual nurses to ensure that they are up to date with practice. There is now a wealth of information available, and it is probably more of a task to sift through the material than to find it in the first place. The following are ways in which nurses can keep up to date, and help ensure that they are adopting evidence-based practice:
- Regularly reading journals relevant to the specific area of practice
- Maintaining links with electronic discussion networks
- Searching library databases (the NHS library is ideal for this—
  ⌨ http://www.library.nhs.uk/evidence/
- Discussing research with colleagues
- Participating in a journal club.

Whereas nurses should be able to evaluate research critically for themselves, it is important to remember that papers published in peer-reviewed journals have already been through critical review and are likely to be more reliable than other publications or internet resources. Many researchers would go much further than this and suggest that there is a clear hierarchy of evidence. French cited a Canadian report that considered the following types of evidence acceptable:[1]

- Experimental (randomized clinical trials, meta-analyses, and analytic studies)
- Non-experimental (quasi-experimental, observational)
- Expert opinion (consensus, based on published literature and consensus process, commissioned reports)
- Historical or experiential.[3]

1 French P (2002). What is the evidence on evidence-based nursing? An epistemological concern. *Journal of Advanced Nursing* **37**(3), 250–257.

2 Thompson *et al.* (2002). Research in nursing. In: Daly J, Speedy S, Jackson D and Darbyshire P. *Contexts in Nursing: An Introduction*. Blackwell Publishing: Oxford.

3 Tranmer JE, Squires S, Brazil K *et al* (1998). Factors that influence evidence-based decision making. National Forum on Health. Canadian Health Action: Building on the legacy. Volume 5. *Making Decisions: Evidence and Information*. Multimondes: Quebec.

National occupational standards and professional requirements

QA statement of intellectual disability nursing

Intellectual disability nursing for England, Scotland, Wales, and Northern Ireland

'Programmes in the learning disabilities branch of nursing prepare nurses to work with people with a range of learning disabilities and with their families and significant others. Learning disability nurses' work is under-pinned by the concepts of partnership, inclusion and advocacy. The role of the learning disability nurse, specifically, is to assist and support people to become and remain healthy, to improve their competence and quality of life, and to fulfill their potential. Learning disability nurses work with people with a spectrum of needs and abilities in a wide variety of settings, often working collaboratively with professionals from a range of health and social care agencies. This support may take place in the National Health Service (NHS), voluntary or independent sector, or in the patient/client's own home'.[1]

1 Quality Assurance Agency for Higher Education (2001). *Benchmark Statement Health Care Programmes Phase 1 Nursing*. Quality Assurance Agency for Higher Education: Gloucester.
⌨ http://www.qaa.ac.uk/academicinfrastructure/benchmark/health/nursing-final.asp
[accessed April 2009]

Nursing and Midwifery Council (UK)

Origins of the NMC

The NMC was set up by Parliament in 2002 as a result of the Nursing and Midwifery Order 2001. The powers of the NMC are detailed in the The Nursing and Midwifery Order 2001. The work of the NMC is governed by this and other associated legislation. The NMC replaced the previous professional body, which was called the United Kingdom Central Council for Nursing, Midwifery and Health Visiting (UKCC).

Remit of the NMC

The key areas of responsibility of the remit of the NMC is set out in the Nursing and Midwifery Order (2001), the primary responsibility of which is to protect the public. The NMC seeks to achieve this broad aim by undertaking a number of key tasks as outlined below.

Key tasks undertaken by the NMC

The NMC has the responsibility to:
- maintain a register of nurses and midwives eligible to practice in the UK (nurses must register on an annual basis)
- set criteria for entry to the register for all nurses who have been educated in the UK, or wishing to register in the UK. The specific requirements for overseas nurses wishing to enter the register can be found on the NMC website (www.nmc-org.uk)
- set standards and information for nursing and midwifery conduct, performance, and ethics
- quality assure nursing and midwifery education
- consider allegations of misconduct, lack of competence, or unfitness to practise due to ill health
- set standards and provide guidance for local supervising authorities for midwives.

Two key areas that have a direct bearing on the education and practice of nurses and midwives are considered below. More detail on all the key tasks of the NMC can be accessed on their website at www.nmc-uk.org.

Fitness for practice

The primary responsibility of the NMC is to protect the health and wellbeing of the public. The NMC publish and periodically update standards, which all nurses and midwives registered with NMC are required to adhere to. These are contained within a publication entitled *The Code: Standards of Conduct, Performance and Ethics for Nurses and Midwives* and their related documents. All registered nurses and midwives are personally accountable for their practice.

It is the responsibility of the NMC Fitness to Practise procedures to investigate all allegations of impairment of fitness to practise made against nurses and midwives on grounds including misconduct, lack of competence, and ill health. If misconduct has occurred, the NMC has the authority to issue a number of sanctions, including removal of the nurse or midwife from the NMC Register, preventing them from practising as a nurse or midwife in the UK. The NMC may also put in place suspensions of registration, cautions, and conditions of practice orders.

Education and quality assurance

The NMC sets and monitors the standards for all nursing courses that lead to a registered or recorded qualification within the UK. In doing so they put in place and periodically review standards of education for practice, including outcomes to be achieved by students by the end of the Common Foundation programme, and competencies for entry to the register. They also have arrangements for the quality assurance of education, they approve courses, programmes and educational institutions, and provide guidance for educational institutions on the good health and good character of nurses undertaking their education. In additon, they also produce periodic guidance and set standards related to the provision of education in university and clinical practice settings.

Support available from the NMC

The NMC provide an online registration confirmation service for employers, a free and confidential advice service for nurses and midwives, free publications to keep practitioners, students and the general public informed about the Council's work, a range of events including exhibitions, seminars and conferences, a quarterly news magazine called NMC News is mailed to all registrants in the UK and overseas (to the address held by NMC for the registrant), provide online advice sheets and a wide range of guidance in relation to the practice of nurses and midwives, all of which are downloadable from their website. All nurses and midwives should regularly visit the NMC website for the latest news and publications.

NMC address   Nursing and Midwifery Council
23 Portland Place
London
W1B 1PZ

NMC website   ▢ www.nmc-uk.org

An Bord Altranais—requirements

Requirements and standards for registration

An Bord Altranais (ABA) is the statutory body responsible for the regulation of nursing practice, including ID nursing in the Republic of Ireland. It operates under the provisions of the Nurses Act (1985). The general concern of ABA is the promotion of high standards of education, training, and professional conduct among nurses. Registration with ABA is mandatory in order to practice as a registered ID nurse. This assures the public, the employer, and colleagues that you are accountable to the Board for meeting and maintaining the competencies and standards of the nursing profession.

The primary function of the registration section of ABA is to maintain the register of nurses in accordance with both Part IV of the Nurses Act (1985), and in accordance with appropriate Nurses Rules. It also issues standards for professional behaviour (see 📖 Codes of practice, p.530).

Regulations can change over time; it is important, therefore, to refer to the ABA documentation current at the time of your application. At the time of writing this section the regulations below were in place.

In order to obtain registration with ABA you must submit:
* A completed application form detailing your nursing experience from graduation to date
* Details of the educational institute where you undertook nurse training
* Details of the registration you hold with the relevant nursing registration authorities,
* Birth certificate, photograph and appropriate application fee.

You must arrange to have the Verification of Registration and Good Standing Document (Form C in application form) sent directly from the relevant registration authorities to ABA.

Information for nurses qualified outside the Republic of Ireland

ID nurses who have completed their training and gained registration in countries outside the Republic of Ireland must apply for admission to the register maintained by ABA prior to practising in Ireland.

All overseas application requests must be made in writing, and each application will be considered on an individual basis against the regulations and criteria in place at the time of application. An Bord Altranais cannot state in advance if an application will be accepted.

In order to be granted direct registration, your training programme must meet with the educational requirements and standards of Irish trained nurses. Information regarding the rules, syllabi and criteria under which Irish nurses are trained can be accessed at 🖥 www.nursingboard.ie.

Translations—if original documents are not in the English language they must be submitted to ABA together with an original translation bearing the stamp/seal of the official translator. If other documents received directly as part of your application (Verification of Registration and Good Standing, References, Transcripts of Training) are not submitted in English or together with an English translation, you will be responsible for the translation costs.

English language competency (non-EU applicants)—non-EU applicants for registration are required to demonstrate proof of English language competence, if English is not their first language or primary language of expression, at a level that supports communication and enables the applicant to practice nursing safely and effectively in Ireland. Applicants need to demonstrate that they have reached specified standards in the International English Language Testing System (IELTS), Academic Test or Test of English as a Foreign Language (TOEFL)/Test of Written English (TWE)/Test of Spoken English (TSE).

Further reading

An Bord Altranais (The Nursing Board) ▣ www.nursingboard.ie

Nurses Act (1985). Stationary Office: Dublin.

ABA address and contact details

An Bord Altranais (The Nursing Board)
18/20 Carysfort Avenue
Blackrock, Co. Dublin. Ireland.
Tel: 00353-1-639 8500
Fax: 00353-1-639 8595

Codes of practice

What is a nursing code of professional conduct?

A code of conduct or ethics is usually issued by the statutory body that governs registered nurses in all countries, and provides guidance on the expected standards of behaviour of those nurses. Nursing codes of conduct develop over time, and may vary between countries; therefore nurses should always be familiar with the latest edition of the code of conduct or ethics issued by the body with which they are registered, and also the code of conduct for nurses in the country in which they are working.

The function of the code is viewed as:

- A guideline for practice, establishing boundaries and rules, and providing professional standards
- Upholding/preserving/safeguarding public protection
- A representation of the profession and the professional
- Promoting professional status
- A benchmark against which a disciplinary committee can judge professional practice in deciding if professional misconduct has occurred.

The Code: Standards of Conduct, Performance, and Ethics for Nurses and Midwives

The code of conduct for nurses and midwives in the UK issued by the NMC in April 2008 provides standards that are expected from all nurses and midwives on the NMC Register.[1] It states that: *'the people in your care must be able to trust you with their health and well-being. To justify that trust, you must:*

- *make the care of people your first concern, treating them as individuals and respecting their dignity*
- *work with others to protect and promote the health and well-being of those in your care, their families and carers, and the wider community*
- *provide a high standard of practice and care at all times*
- *be open and honest, act with integrity, and uphold the reputation of your profession'.*

Within the code of conduct, additional guidance as to how nurses should implement the above standards are provided. The code of conduct also highlights that each nurse or midwife as a professional is: *'personally accountable for actions and omissions in your practice and must always be able to justify your decisions'* and *'must always act lawfully, whether those laws relate to your professional practice or personal life'.*

The code of professional conduct for nurses in Republic of Ireland

The Code of Professional Conduct for each Nurse and Midwife[2] defines 'patient' and 'nurse' as follows: a 'patient' is broadly interpreted as individuals or groups who have contact with the nurse in his/her professional capacity. It does not necessarily denote or imply ill health. A 'nurse' is a person registered in the Live Register of Nurses as provided for in Section 27 of the Nurses Act (1985),[3] and includes a midwife, and nursing includes midwifery.

The code formulates the following duties and responsibilities on nurses:
- Fitness to practice
- Accountable for practice
- Provide safe standards of care
- Maintain confidentiality
- Foster/endorse informed judgement
- Maintain competency
- Practice within scope of practice
- Acknowledge one's own limitations
- Responsibilities to junior staff
- Overall responsibility of care in relation to student nurses
- Collaboration with other healthcare professions
- Preserving human life, both born and unborn
- Regulations relating to statements, promotion of commercial products, and accepting gifts
- Professional misconduct
- Safeguarding research activities.

At times specific issues are considered by An Bord Altranais when they arise, and may be the subject of further interpretative statements issued.

1 Nursing and Midwifery Council (2008). *The Code: Standards of Conduct, Performance and Ethics for Nurses and Midwives.* Nursing and Midwifery Council: London. ▣ www.nmc-uk.org

2 An Bord Altranais (The Nursing Board) (ABA) (2000). *The Code of Professional Conduct for each Nurse and Midwife.* ABA: Dublin. ▣ www.nursingboard.ie

3 Nurses Act (1985). Stationary Office: Dublin.

Unsafe standards of care

There is continual emphasis in healthcare to improve the quality of care provided and thus to eliminate poor practice, particularly unsafe standards of care. This is achieved through standard settings at different levels, which should be continually monitored. A number of initiatives and strategies have been put in place to do this e.g. clinical governance, benchmarking, integrated care pathways, care standards, and national service frameworks. These approaches set safe standards of care, which staff should follow; this is particularly important in the field of ID, where clients may have little concept of what safety means.

Unfortunately due to a variety of reasons e.g. poor management, lack of competence and training, poorly developed and implemented care plans, and lack of resources, standards may fall short of what is considered safe practice. Areas in ID nursing that have been known to have had concerns raised regarding unsafe standards of care include:

- Use of restraint
- Administration of medication
- Manual handling of clients with profound and multiple learning disabilities
- Feeding
- Poor communication
- Bathing and personal care
- Developing independent living skills (road safety, cooking, gardening activities etc.)

(Many of these reasons highlighted above have been identified in both the recent inquiries undertaken in Cornwall, and Sutton & Merton Trusts.)[1,2]

As a registered nurse your first consideration in all activities must be the people in your care, who you should treat as individuals and respect their dignity. The NMC (2008) code of conduct further states that: '*You must work with colleagues to monitor the quality of your work and maintain the safety of those in your care*'.[3] Safety must never be compromised, and there is no middle ground with safety. A practice standard is either safe or unsafe, it cannot be just a little bit or moderately safe. Therefore you should never knowingly engage in practice once it has been deemed to be unsafe. Practice should also always be based on the best available evidence.

As a registered nurse you are personally accountable for your actions and omissions in practice and you must keep your skills and knowledge up to date. You should know the limits of your competence and you should strive to take part in appropriate training that develops your competence and performance in practice. Safety is everyone's concern, and should be promoted as a positive and essential activity. In caring for people with ID, some activities carry inherent risks, which properly managed can help enormously in the development of the client. However, every risk has to be properly assessed, using a risk assessment approach.

A risk assessment should:
- identify what is unsafe
- identify who is likely to be harmed and how
- evaluate the risks and put an action plan together
- record the steps taken
- review the actions taken and revise if necessary.

If you cannot remedy the unsafe standard of care then you must:
- act quickly to protect all those likely to be harmed (client, carers, colleagues and visitors)
- in an emergency, provide care in or outside the work setting as long as you do not put yourself or others at further risk
- follow set procedures for reporting risks and harm (policies, guidelines, health and safety procedures)
- report concerns regarding the environment of care to an appropriate person and put it in writing
- offer reassurance to those in the immediate environment.

Further reading

Nursing and Midwifery Council (NMC) 🖳 www.nmc-uk.org

Health and Safety Executive (HSE) 🖳 www.hse.gov.uk

National Patient Safety Agency (NPSA) 🖳 www.npsa.nhs.uk

1 Commission for Healthcare Audit and Inspection (2006). *Joint Investigation into the Provision of Services for People with Learning Disabilities at Cornwall Partnership NHS Trust.* Commission for Healthcare Audit and Inspection: London.

2 Commission for Healthcare Audit and Inspection (2007). *Investigation into the Service for People with Learning Disabilities Provided by Sutton and Merton Primary Care Trust.* Commission for Healthcare Audit and Inspection: London.

3 Nursing and Midwifery Council (2008). *The Code: Standards of Conduct, Performance and Ethics for Nurses and Midwives.* Nursing and Midwifery Council: London.

Recording and reporting

Good record keeping is an essential component of effective and safe nursing practice. It helps to protect the welfare of clients, identifies risks, promotes high standards, and aids communication. It should also provide a pen picture of the assessment, planning and delivery of individualized care. Increasingly, records are now being shared with other members of the healthcare team to produce one single comprehensive record of the client's healthcare journey.

There is no single form for recording every incident, although most organizations have standardized forms for various events.

Key features to observe when completing a record

You must:

- do it as soon as possible after the incident has occurred
- accurately date and legibly sign the record
- be clear, accurate and concise
- follow a methodical and logical sequence
- sign, date and time all entries
- ensure it is readable when copied
- record in terms that the client can understand
- identify risks/problems and actions taken to rectify such areas
- provide evidence of assessment, care planning, decision making, care delivery, effectiveness of treatment, and sharing of information
- ensure that if you make an entry in an electronic record, that it is clearly identifiable.

You must not:

- make alterations without a record of change
- use abbreviations, jargon or meaningless phrases
- make offensive or subjective statements.

If it is appropriate, every effort should be made to involve the client with ID, and/or carer, in the completion of the record; it therefore should be written in an understandable format. Increasingly, clients are also being encouraged to look after their own records.

Important points to remember

- Records should be held securely and confidentially
- When delegating responsibility for completing records you should ensure that the person is competent to do so (registered nurses remain accountable for doing this)
- In law the view tends to be that *'if it is not recorded, it has not been done'*
- Record events on appropriate forms or documents and avoid making notes on scraps of paper
- In community settings you need to be particularly careful when sharing and transporting records. They should be kept securely, and you should ensure that only authorized personnel have access to them
- The loss or damage of records should be reported immediately to the appropriate person.

Access to records

The 1998 Data Protection Act gives clients the right to access their own health records (paper or computer based records). In some exceptional circumstances it may not be in the client's best interests for them to view the record made about them. If you make such a decision to withhold information then a record needs to be made of the reasons for doing so.

Further reading

Important and up-to-date information for registered nurses on record keeping can be obtained from the Nursing and Midwifery Council (NMC) website at ▣ www.nmc-uk.org

Complaints

A complaint can be made by anyone e.g. a service user, advocate, carer, or person affected or likely to be affected in some way by the actions/decisions of an individual or organizsation. The complainant is usually unhappy about the level of service provided and they want an answer to their concerns. All organizations should have a complaints procedure for you to follow, and many have complaints personnel who deal with such matters.

There are generally two types of complaints—informal and formal.

Informal complaints

Most complaints are informal and made verbally in person or over the telephone, and can be dealt with on the spot without the need to formalize proceedings. Often an explanation of why things may have gone wrong, and an apology if they did, is all that is needed to satisfy the complainant. Every effort should be made to resolve the complaint at this stage; help may be required from your line manager. If the complaint cannot be resolved at this stage, then you should ask the complainant to put it in writing as soon as possible.

Formal complaints

Formal complaints are made in writing or by electronic means such as email or by text. The complainant needs to write down the exact nature of what they are complaining about. They should be advised that they also need to put down how they would like their complaint to be satisfactorily resolved.

General principles when dealing with complaints

You must:
- maintain confidentiality
- be polite and courteous
- LISTEN carefully to what is being said
- act promptly
- remain neutral
- be fair and open minded
- give a constructive and honest response
- cooperate with internal and external investigations.

You must not:
- be angry or annoyed
- ignore the complaint in the hope it will go away
- make personal judgements about the complainant
- make promises that you or the organization cannot keep
- treat people detrimentally because they have complained.

Remember that dealing with complaints effectively often leads to improvements in practice. Many of the past and recent inquiries into abuses of people with ID highlighted that complaints were made but were not acted upon or dismissed.[1,2,3] It was also highlighted that very little information was made available on how to complain, or produced in an easy to read and accessible format for people using services, and their carers and relatives.

People with ID must be supported to make complaints. For example, they may need the support of family and friends, or may require the services of an independent advocate. It is important that their complaint should be treated sensitively and without prejudice. It can be very stressful to speak out about aspects of care, particularly against the people providing such care. It should be viewed as good practice to develop client assertive skills in this area within a culture that promotes client empowerment. A major barrier faced by people with ID is the dismissive attitude of others towards them. All complaints need to be acted on, and the actions taken need to be reported back to the complainant within a specified time scale.

If an individual wishes to complain about an aspect of the NHS, then they can access information from the Department of Health website or the following complaints policy document from:

📖 www.dh.gov.uk/en/Policyandguidance/Organisationpolicy/Complaintspolicy/NHScomplaintsprocedure/DH_4080900

Members of the public have the right to complain about the fitness to practise of any registered nurse, and can do so by contacting the Nursing and Midwifery council (NMC). For advice on how to complain, the following document can be obtained from:

📖 www.nmc-uk.org/aFrameDisplay.aspx?DocumentID=204

1 Committee of Inquiry (1969). *Report of the Committee of Inquiry into Allegations of Ill-treatment of Patients and Other Irregularities at the Ely Hospital, Cardiff, Cmd 3975*. HMSO: London.

2 Commission for Healthcare Audit and Inspection (2006). *Joint Investigation into the Provision of Services for People with Learning Disabilities at Cornwall Partnership NHS Trust*. Commission for Healthcare Audit and Inspection: London.

3 Commission for Healthcare Audit and Inspection (2007). *Investigation into the Service for People with Learning Disabilities Provided by Sutton and Merton Primary Care Trust*. Commission for Healthcare Audit and Inspection: London.

Right to independent advocacy

Independent advocacy is associated with the role of citizen or peer advocates. It has been a legal right in particular circumstances. For example, there exists the right of access to an 'appropriate adult', who could be a professional, friend, or family member, to assist a person with ID in understanding aspects of legal proceedings including police interviews. A mentally vulnerable detainee is defined for the purposes of the Codes of Practice under the Police and Criminal Evidence Act (PACE) 1984 as 'any detainee who, because of their mental state or capacity may not understand the significance of what is said, of questions or of their replies'. (Code C, Guidance Note 1G). The PACE Codes make specific provision for detainees who are mentally disordered or mentally vulnerable to receive the support of an appropriate adult during their time in police custody (Code C 1.7).

Appropriate adults have an important role to play in the custody environment by ensuring that the detained person whom they are assisting understands what is happening to them and why. An appropriate adult might be:

- a parent or guardian or, if the person is in the care of a local authority or voluntary organization, somebody representing that authority or organization
- a social worker of a local authority social services department
- if no person falling within the first 2 categories is available, any responsible person 18yrs or over who is not a police officer or a person employed by the police.

The Mental Capacity Act 2005, which applies to anyone 16yrs or over in England and Wales, provides for the appointment of 'independent mental capacity advocates' by an 'appropriate authority'. The equivalent law in Scotland is the Adults with Incapacity Act 2000, and there is currently no equivalent law in Northern Ireland pending the outcome of the Bamford Review of Mental Health and Learning Disability. The Mental Health Act 2007 places a duty on the appropriate national authority to make arrangements for help to be provided by independent mental health advocates.

Citizen advocates in England have no legal recognition currently. Citizen advocates may be affiliated to a recognized advocacy group that provides training and support. An individual who is not a member of a group may still be recognized but should be aware of code of practice, and consent and complaint issues. Citizen advocacy works most effectively for vulnerable people when its role is understood and recognized by their carers and families.

The role of the citizen advocate or peer advocate

Citizen or peer advocates enable advocacy partners to express their views, wishes, and choices, and through this support them in pursuing their rights, safeguarding their interests, and achieving their goals.[1]

- Citizen or peer advocates should always respond to the opinions of their advocacy partner as far as these can be ascertained and not their own opinions.
- Where an advocacy partner's views, wishes or choices cannot be ascertained, the citizen advocate uses insight gained from the advocacy relationship to speak up for what the advocacy partner would be likely to decide if able to do so.
- In speaking up for advocacy partners, citizen advocates should state whether they are conveying what the partner has actually said or indicated, or whether they are using their own insight.
- The citizen advocate's first loyalty is to the advocacy partner, advocates should always approach situations from the partner's perspective.
- Citizen advocates should not be in or enter into such a position that a conflict of interest arises between the citizen advocate role and any other activities they pursue or intend to pursue.
- The citizen advocate must at all times respect the right to confidentiality of the advocacy partner as expressed in the confidentiality policy of the supporting advocacy group.
- The citizen advocate should be vigilant on behalf of the advocacy partner, and where there is any suspicion that the partner is at risk must alert the supporting advocacy group and the appropriate staff.
- Citizen advocates support their advocacy partner in obtaining advice and information, but are not responsible for providing them.
- Citizen advocates must be independent from those who provide services to their advocacy partners, and also from the families of partners.
- Citizen advocacy is not befriending, although friendship may well arise naturally out of the advocacy relationship.
- Service staff, families and others may at times be unclear about the role of the citizen advocate. It is the responsibility of the citizen advocate to explain their role, where necessary with support from the local advocacy group.

Further reading

BILD (2001). *The Advocacy Workbook.* BILD: Kidderminster.

1 Oxfordshire Learning Disability NHS Trust/Oxfordshire Advocacy Development Group 2004. *Guidelines for the Recognition of Citizen Advocates.* Oxfordshire Learning Disability NHS Trust: Oxford.

Emergencies

Emergency management of a person in a seizure

Most epileptic seizures self-terminate, lasting <2mins (see 📖 Epilepsy, p.156). When supporting a person who has epilepsy it is advisable to have an individual epilepsy management plan that informs staff when to either contact emergency services or administer emergency medication if pre-scribed (see 📖 Epilepsy, p.156). It is advised that emergency medication or emergency services should be contacted if seizures last >5mins.

Status epilepticus

Emergency management of seizures outside of the acute hospital is to prevent status epilepticus. Tonic–clonic status epilepticus is defined as a condition in which prolonged or recurrent tonic–clonic seizures persist for 30mins or more. It may result in permanent neurological damage, cognitive decline, and further brain damage. Death may occur. The risk of morbidity is increased the longer the duration of the seizure, therefore the earlier treated the better. Non-convulsive status epilep-ticus is less common, and can be difficult to diagnose, with the person often presenting with abnormal mental state—changes in behaviour or cognition with diminished responsiveness. Diagnosis requires evidence of continuous or near continuous discharges on EEG.

Emergency management plan

Any person prescribed emergency medication should have in place an EMP designed to provide clear instruction for carers. The EMP should be agreed by the prescriber, the individual where they have capacity to consent, parent/guardian, employer, and carers. Registered nurses who delegate the administration of emergency medication should follow local policy ensuring care staff receive appropriate training, and consult the guid-ance of their registration body (NMC/ABA). A detailed recording system is necessary to review use of the emergency medication. This should include time of administration of the emergency medication to seizure stopping, together with a description of the actual seizure activity.

EMP should detail:
- Description and duration of seizure type for which medication is prescribed
- Indications for the use of emergency medication e.g. after certain time and/or number of seizures
- The initial dose of emergency medication
- If and when a second dose can be given
- Who should administer the medication
- Usual response to treatment if known
- When emergency assistance should be sought
- Consent
- Other relevant information e.g. when medication was last administered.

Individuals in any seizure are vulnerable, more so in the emergency situation. When it has been possible gain the individual's prior consent to treatment, it is essential to recognize individual needs while managing the emergency. Ensure dignity and privacy as far as possible and explain all actions to the individual, who may at any time regain consciousness. When the person regains consciousness, which will depend on the individual's response to treatment, reassure and explain what has occurred and action taken. In some circumstances e.g. in public, it may not be appropriate to administer emergency medication if privacy and dignity cannot be provided; in such situations emergency services must be sought in the first instance.

Emergency medication

Benzodiazepines in the form of rectal diazepam or midazolam (midazolam in the form of Epistatus®) are unlicensed for use in epilepsy at time of writing; however, some doctors may prescribe it for particular individuals, for use by family and care staff. Rectal diazepam administered into the rectum or midazolam administered into the buccal cavity of the mouth, passes across the thin mucosal lining, is absorbed directly into the bloodstream and travels directly to the brain. It reduces the brain excitability by strengthening the brain inhibitory systems. Most seizures are stopped within minutes. Side effects of benzodiazepines include sedation, hypotension, cardiorespiratory depression, and respiratory arrest. It is advised to contact emergency services on first use of these drugs if not under medical supervision. A second dose may be prescribed depending on the age, weight, and other relevant factors of the individual. A third dose is not advised given the long half-life in particular of rectal diazepam. Oral benzodiazepines may be prescribed for cluster seizures when the individual regains consciousness between seizures, and seizure history identifies a pattern.

Emergency services—acute hospital

Emergency services should be contacted if full prescribed emergency medication fails to stop the seizure, or a person not prescribed emergency medication has recurrent seizures or does not appear to be making an expected recovery within a few minutes. Information should be provided on the medication already administered, prescribed AEDs, and seizure history. Management of early status in the acute clinical setting involves—securing airway, oxygen, assessing cardiorespiratory function, establishing intravenous access and AED treatment in accordance with local protocols. See also NICE Guidelines Appendix C for guidelines on treatment of tonic–clonic status epilepticus.[1]

Further reading

Nashef L (1997). Sudden unexpected death in epilepsy: terminology and definitions. *Epilepsia* **38**(Suppl.11), 56–58.

1 Stokes T, Shaw EJ, Juarez-Garcia A, Camosso-Stefinovic J, Baker R (2004). *Clinical Guidelines and Evidence Review for the Epilepsies: Diagnosis and Management in Adults and Children in Primary and Secondary Care.* Royal College of General Practitioners: London.

Dealing with abuse

Abuse of people with ID is widespread, and the likelihood is that ID nurses will come across it at some point in their career and will need to deal with it. Abuse can be categorized into 'types', and these are listed in 📖 Safeguarding adults, p.496. *No Secrets*[1] gives comprehensive guidance on how services should respond to the abuse of vulnerable people from an organizational and collaborative perspective, but does not advise on how individuals should react if they come across abuse. It is likely that locally agreed interagency procedures for dealing with abuse divide the roles and responsibilities of professionals into the following categories:

- People raising the alert (alerters)
- Investigators
- Managers.

It is most probable that nurses will be alerters, it is the responsibility of the police to investigate allegations of abuse, and *No Secrets* identifies the local social services as the lead agency for co-coordinating protection frameworks. Nurses should therefore consider how they should respond in individual cases of abuse and 'alert' the appropriate people through the recognized channels, who will then investigate the issue and take necessary action. Although there are different types of abuse, there are some universal principles that can be applied in all instances. Therefore, if a nurse comes across a disclosure of abuse they should:

- be empathic
- stay calm
- be aware that medical evidence may be required and act accordingly to secure this following advice and in collaboration with police services
- let the person know that they have done the right thing, it is not their fault, you are taking it seriously, and that other people may need to know
- inform them that in some circumstances the police and social services may be informed without their consent
- record as soon as possible what has been said/occurred
- consider who to report the information to
- make sure the person is and remains safe.

Nurses should not:

- breach confidentiality by passing on information to anyone other than on 'a need to know basis'
- press the person for more detail by asking overly leading questions
- be judgemental or blaming.

There have been occasions when people who have raised an alert have felt that the abuse has not been dealt with adequately by line managers or that their line managers/supervisors are involved in that abuse. If this is the case then nurses are required to report to a more senior person within the organization.[2] Nurses can also report directly to the CSCI, social services, regional body responsible for inspection of services, or the police.

If nurses have the responsibilities of a line manager and they receive information from an alerter of abuse they should consider the following actions:

- Discuss with the person raising the alert what has happened, what action to take, and whether the matter will be referred to the police and/or social services for investigation
- Decide how best to support the victim of abuse
- Maintain contact with the person raising the alert, and the victim where appropriate
- Report the matter to CSCI if you are a registered manager
- Maintain a confidential record of all events and actions
- If the alleged abuser is a staff member, take any necessary action as stipulated in organizational policies e.g. suspension from duty
- Organize, monitor, and evaluate regular staff training on abuse
- Contribute to and implement policy guidelines
- Clearly understand their role within the interagency framework for managing abuse
- Ensure that all job applicants are checked against the POVA / POCVA register.

Readers are strongly advised to make themselves aware of local interagency frameworks that have been developed to protect vulnerable adults.

1 Department of Health (2000). *No Secrets: Guidance on Developing and Implementing Multi–agency Policies and Procedures to Protect Vulnerable Adults from Abuse.* HMSO: London.

2 Nursing and Midwifery Council (2008). *The Code: Standards of Conduct, Performance and Ethics for Nurses and Midwives.* Nursing and Midwifery Council: London. ▣ www.nmc-uk.org

Self-harm

Self-harm is a term defined as 'self-poisoning or injury, irrespective of the apparent purpose of the act'.[1] People with ID also engage in this type of behaviour, although the term self-injury is usually used (see 📖 Self-injury, p.550).[2]

There is a danger that people who engage in self-harming behaviour may incur censure and rejection from those around them when it is deemed a deliberate act. In supporting people who have self-harmed, the focus should also be placed on the care, support, and development of the individual. The nursing process (assessment, planning, implementation, and evaluation) can be used to organize care for individuals who engage in self-harm. Understanding the motivation for the self-harm is crucial to helping a person, although it can be very difficult to determine whether the act was intentional or not in people with ID. Nursing assessment and care should be structured and holistic. While it is important to gain insights into the possible motivations for self-harm, this should not be the sole focus, and care should be taken to avoid negative assumptions being made about motivations, as it is not helpful.

Some reasons why people may self-harm

- Low self-esteem
- Feelings of isolation
- Feeling stressed
- Past or current abuse
- Being bullied
- Suffered a bereavement
- Problems with sexuality
- Experiencing social rejection
- A desire to end one's life
- Severe mental illness i.e. command hallucinations during a psychotic episode.

It can be very difficult to understand why people should want to self-harm. For some it may provide a sense of release from emotional pain or may act as a type of coping mechanism. It may be a way of communicating to others the distress that the individual is feeling. Self-harm is often carried out in private and on parts of the body that are usually covered with clothing. As such it can be difficult to tell if someone is self-harming, but other signs might be that the person becomes withdrawn, irritable, lacking energy, covering up, and not taking part in certain activities e.g. swimming. People with ID may not conform to the usual pattern of self-harming and will often self-harm quite openly and injure parts of their body that are not usually covered up by clothing, such as the face.

Some specific expressions of self-harming behaviour

- Swallowing poisonous substances or objects
- Burning or scalding
- Cutting.

Practitioners need to LISTEN to the messages that clients try to communicate when they self-harm—you can listen with all your senses, particularly your eyes and ears. Remember it can be very distressing for other clients and you should offer reassurance to those in the immediate environment.

Important considerations when nursing an individual who engages in self-harming behaviour

The individual should be:
- treated with respect and dignity
- treated for their injuries
- consulted and included in all decisions
- given privacy during consultation and treatment
- shown understanding with their coping mechanism
- assessed for further risk
- assumed to have mental capacity unless there is evidence of doubt.

They should not be:
- discriminated against
- forced to disclose why they self-harmed
- automatically considered a dangerous person
- punished for self-harming.

Interventions

Interventions would be similar to self-injury (see 📖 Self-injury, p.550).

Further reading

Mental Health Foundation 🖥 www.mentalhealth.org.uk

Mind 🖥 www.mind.org.uk

1 National Institute for Clinical Excellence (2004). *Self-harm. The Short-term Physical and Psychological Management and Secondary Prevention of Self-harm in Primary and Secondary Care.* Clinical Guideline 16. National Institute for Clinical Excellence: London.

2 Jones V, Davies R, Jenkins R (2004). Self-harm by people with learning difficulties: something to be expected or investigated. *Disability & Society* **19**(5), 487–500.

Risk of suicide

Suicide is one of the most common causes of premature death in all age groups. About 5000 deaths/yr are caused by suicide in England. In the 20yr period 1980–2000, suicide rates fell in women and older men but rose in young men.[1] There have been very few studies to investigate suicide in people with ID.

Prevalence

A study in Finland followed up a nationwide sample of 2677 people with ID over a 35yr period.[2] During this period only 10 suicides occurred. This is much lower than the national suicide rates in England and lower still in relation to the rates in Finland where the study was undertaken.

Risk

There are no indications in the literature to suggest any significant differences between the factors that are indicative of risk of suicide in the general population from risk in the ID population. The clearest single indicator for risk of suicide is the wish to die. In clinical practice this is often referred to as suicidal intent or suicidal ideation.

Risk factors

Factors that are statistically linked with an increased risk of suicide are:
- Being male and <35yrs
- Being in a lower socioeconomic group
- Presence of mental illness and particularly depression
- Unemployment
- Alcohol and drug misuse
- Deliberate self-harm in the previous year
- Serving a prison sentence for the first time, particularly in the early stage.

Risk assessment tools

There are currently no known grounds to adapt assessment tools that are used generally to assess for risk of suicide:
- In clinical practice the CPA, which incorporates a general assessment of risk to self and others, is the most common framework for assessing risk.
- Where the CPA is not used, a policy regarding general risk assessment should be in place.
- The Pierce Suicide Intent Scale or Beck's Suicidal Intention Scale can be used following an attempted suicide to focus specifically on future suicide risk.[3,4]

Risk management

- All people who engage in deliberate self-harm should be asked, as far as possible, to explain in their own words why they have harmed themselves in order to assess for risk of suicide.
- A thorough assessment should be undertaken to identify underlying causes for suicidal thoughts and behaviour.
- Underlying causes should be treated where possible e.g. depressive illness.

- Appropriate support should be provided to assist the person to address circumstances and situational factors that contribute to suicidal thoughts and behaviour. This may include signposting and support to access other health and welfare services.
- Plans may include access to listening or support services on a 24hr basis. This may include mainstream psychiatric services, emergency services and helplines (e.g. the Samaritans, Saneline).
- External management of risk may be required to prevent serious harm or death including:
  - Admission to hospital for a period of assessment and/or treatment
  - Close observations or supervision during periods of increased risk
  - Preventative environmental adaptations i.e. removal of ligature points
  - Limited access to means of attempting suicide.

Deliberate self-harm

Deliberate self-harm, sometimes called parasuicide, is differentiated from attempted suicide on the basis that it is inflicted with no intent to die. This can be difficult to ascertain in people with ID who may have problems describing their own thoughts, motivations and intentions.

Further reading

Riding T, Swann C, Swann B (2005). *The Handbook of Forensic Learning Disabilities*. Chapter 6. Radcliffe Publishing: Oxford.

Department of Health (2008). *Care Programme Approach* Department of Health: London. www.dh.gov.uk/en/Publicationsandstatistics/Publications/DH_083650

National Institute for Clinical Excellence (2004). Self-harm. *The Short-term Physical and Psychological Management and Secondary Prevention of Self-harm in Primary and Secondary Care*. Clinical Guideline 16. National Institute for Clinical Excellence: London.

Jones V, Davies R, Jenkins R (2004). Self-harm by people with learning difficulties: something to be expected or investigated. *Disability & Society* **19**(5), 487–500.

Mental Health Foundation www.mentalhealth.org.uk

Mind www.mind.org.uk

1 Department of Health (2004). *National Suicide Prevention Strategy for England*. Department of Health: London.

2 Patja K (2004). Suicide cases in a population based cohort of persons with intellectual disability in a 35 year follow-up. *Mental Health Aspects of Developmental Disabilities* **7**(4), 117–123.

3 Pierce DW (1997). Suicidal intent in self-injury. *British Journal of Psychiatry* **130**, 377–85.

4 Beck A, Schuyler D, Herman J (1974). Development of suicidal intent scales. In *The Prediction of Suicide* (eds Beck A, Resnik H, Lettieri DJ), pp.45–56. Charles: Bourie, MD.

Self-injury

The term self-injurious behaviour is commonly used in services for people with ID to describe self-harming behaviour particularly motivated by biological factors. It may also be a learnt behaviour reinforced by responses of others, or biological responses to pain in the body. It may also be worth considering the idea that people deliberately injure themselves. For instance if the risks of pica (eating inedible material) or poison are not known then it would not be self-injury. However, in mental health care the preferred term is self-harm, although both terms mean that the individual has injured or harmed themselves in some way (see 📖 Self-harm, p.546). Individuals who self-injure should be treated with the same respect, dignity, and privacy as other clients, regardless of whether the act of self-injury was intentional or not.

Biological causes of self-injury in people with intellectual disabilities

- Genetic syndromes such as Cornelia de Lange, Lesch–Nyhan, Fragile X, and Prader–Willi
- Neurochemistry defects such as a low level of dopamine.

Remember that just because an individual has a particular syndrome does not mean that they will automatically engage in self-injurious behaviour. There is evidence that interventions such as those that relieve pain or treat gastric reflux may reduce the incidence of self-injurious behaviour. Individuals are also susceptible to the same external triggers as the general population such as:

- Impoverished environments
- Abuse
- Lack of activities
- Frustration.

People with ASD may also engage in self-injurious behaviours due to:

- Having a low pain threshold
- Obsessive and compulsive behaviours
- Self-stimulatory behaviours
- Inquisitiveness—experimenting to see what will happen.

Again they are also susceptible to the same external triggers as the general population.

Some common types of self-injurious behaviours displayed by some individuals with ID:

- Head banging and face slapping
- Biting, pinching and scratching
- Eye poking and hair pulling
- Repeated vomiting
- Consuming inedible foods (pica) e.g. cigarettes, faeces, paper etc.

Interventions

Short-term interventions

In an emergency, assess the severity of self-injury and respond accordingly. (When dealing with a serious incident of self-injury e.g. poisoning, breathing difficulties, head injury or loss of blood, you need to act quickly to prevent loss of life). Full emergency procedures should be initiated if appropriate—medical help, phone ambulance, A&E unit, and providing emergency services with full information of the incident and client history (e.g. exact injuries, method used, timescales, complicating factors such as alcohol, methods used to respond, and their effectiveness). It is also important to remember to provide psychological support throughout the event.

Longer term interventions

- Chemotherapeutic e.g. medication such as naltrexone and/or fluoxetine
- Behavioural e.g. PBS
- Humanistic e.g. gentle teaching
- Cognitive e.g. CBT, counselling.

The same principles apply as with self-harm (see 📖 Self-harm, p.546) in that the individual who self-injures has the right to be treated with the same respect and care as other clients.

Further reading

Gates B (2007). Theory and practice of managing self-injurious behaviour in people with learning disabilities. In: Gates B (Ed). *Learning Disabilities Toward Inclusion* (5th edn). Churchill Livingstone: Edinburgh, 445–457.

Hare D, Leadbeater C (1998). Specific factors in assessing and intervening in cases of self-injury by people with autistic conditions. *Journal of Learning Disabilities for Nursing, Health and Social Care* **2**(2), 60–65.

Physical assault

A 'zero tolerance' campaign towards assault of staff has been introduced in many health services with the intention of minimizing the risk to staff.[1] The initiatives advocated by the government covered all NHS staff and environments. The campaign documentation describes violence as: 'any incident where staff are abused, threatened or assaulted in circumstances related to their work, involving an explicit or implicit challenge to their safety'.[1]

A note of caution is necessary in relation to zero tolerance, in so far as nurses and other professionals must remain alert to the possibility that behaviour which involves the threatening, abuse or assault of staff may have another cause, e.g. a head injury, confusional state, or metabolic disorder. It is essential that staff clearly assess possible reasons for such behaviour, and are not blinkered by a blind adherence to 'zero tolerance'.

Working with people with ID can present challenges that are in some cases different from other areas of nursing practice. Some people with ID:
- have learned to respond in inappropriate ways to their environment, and the consequences of this behaviour have been reinforcing for individuals
- display behaviour that may be viewed by some people as threatening or abusive to communicate their needs that would otherwise remain unmet
- show threatening or abusive behaviour that may be associated with a condition (e.g. mental illness, epilepsy)
- show behaviour that is a response to abuse
- may use behaviour to draw attention to something e.g. pain.

The above is not an exhaustive list but indicates the complexity of distressed behaviours that some people with ID use in order to communicate their distress. Physical assault in the field of ID might include:
- Biting
- Scratching
- Nipping
- Grabbing
- Slapping
- Punching
- Poking
- Hair pulling
- Head butting
- Throwing objects
- Using weapons
- Choking
- Inappropriate touching.

The management of physical assault in ID can be outlined from the perspectives of clinical aspects and organizational responses. Nurses involved with working in direct contact with people who may physically assault need to consider clinical and management aspects.

From a clinical perspective the management of and limitation of physical assault can be aided by:
- training—staff working in environments where physical assault may occur should receive mandatory training in restraint, break away techniques and de-escalation (see 📖 De-escalation, p.554)
- adequate staffing levels so that clients and staff are safe from harm
- the ability to be able to closely observe people to identify and respond promptly to triggers that may lead assault
- functional analysis—the process of gaining an understanding as to why people may become physically aggressive (record antecedents, behaviours and consequences for individual)
- access to and the ability to provide clinical supervision
- the use of self as a therapeutic tool in order to build relationships with clients
- good communication techniques including augmented communication
- the ability to work within an interdisciplinary framework
- knowledge of the appropriate use of medications prescribed for the person
- structured interventions to help clients manage their anger
- recording and reporting of incidents using appropriate incident reports
- individual client risk management.

From an organizational perspective the management of and limitation of physical assault can be aided by:
- producing and disseminating robust policies
- involving criminal justice/forensic services (see 📖 Chapter 13, pp.459–498)
- adopting strategies for risk management
- managing resources so that staff engaged in individual client work can operate safely given the considerations outlined above
- structured post-incident support/staff counselling
- providing systematic collation and interpretation of trends emanating from incident reports
- managing the environment to ensure it is as therapeutic as possible/commissioning of services based on best practice
- ensuring staff have the necessary knowledge, skills and confidence to competently undertaken their role, including staff with a specific role in responding to threatening, abusive or assaultive behaviour.

Further reading

Gates B, Gear J, Wray J, (eds.) (2000). *Behavioural Distress: Concepts and Strategies*. Baillière Tindall/RCN: London.

De-escalation

Challenging behaviour, physical assault and some self-injurious behaviours can sometimes be avoided through the use of de-escalation. For the vast majority of people aggression and physical assault is an uncommon occurrence that usually arises due to an environmental trigger, and results in some physiological changes that can make an aggressive outburst almost inevitable. This phenomenon is part of the 'assault cycle',[1] which has the following phases:

- Baseline behaviour—this is a person's usual pattern of behaviour, which for most people does not include violence
- Trigger phase—something in the person's environment causes them to become increasingly agitated
- Escalation phase—the person deviates more and more from their baseline behaviour and they become increasingly less likely to respond to any form of rational behaviour
- Crisis phase—physical assault is likely to occur and the least effective response is to attempt to reason with the person
- Plateau/recovery phase—a gradual reduction in agitation
- Post-crisis or depression phase—this is when the person dips below their usual baseline behaviour and they may feel exhausted and depressed.

The assault cycle is linked to physiological changes, particularly in the trigger, escalation and crisis phases when adrenaline is being quickly released into the body for 'flight or fight'.

De-escalation is based on intervention before a person reaches the crisis phase so that a violent incident can be avoided. Nurses need to be vigilant for any changes from baseline behaviour in the trigger and escalation stages and for any known triggers that cause a person to become violent. Experienced nurses with extensive knowledge of the people in their care will usually be able to recognize the triggers that affect individuals and behavioural changes that signify entry into the trigger phase. Such behavioural changes might include:

- Pacing
- Hand wringing
- Fist clenching
- Muttering
- Being red faced or pale
- Standing tall
- Making gestures
- Rapid breathing
- Direct and prolonged eye contact
- Any major change in behaviour
- Tensing of muscles.

To avoid a violent incident the nurse can use the following techniques.

Non-verbal
- Create a distance between self and client
- Move towards a safer place and avoid corners
- Consider access to exits
- Mood matching
- Mirroring
- Intermittent eye contact
- Open posture/avoid squaring up
- Keep both hands visible
- Display calmness
- Avoid sudden movements.

Verbal
- Speak slowly, gently and clearly; if more than one member of staff is involved only one should speak and give instructions
- Lower your voice
- Do not argue, confront, make threats or give ultimatums
- Listen
- Give clear, brief and assertive instructions
- Use open questions
- Show concern/empathy
- Do not patronize
- Acknowledge grievances and frustrations
- Depersonalize issues.

The above are all well recognized de-escalation techniques, and can be used with people with ID, particularly those with verbal speech. For some people with more profound and complex needs de-escalation may involve identifying and altering environmental triggers, such as:
- Temperature—too hot or cold
- Noise levels
- Over stimulation/under stimulation
- Inability to communicate a need e.g. hunger, thirst, need to go to the toilet
- Lights—too bright/or too dim
- Too many people
- Too many demands being placed on the person
- Illness/pre-existing condition
- Change in routine (often in autism).

1 Doy R (2006). The ABC of community emergency care: 16 Mental Health. *Emergency Medicine Journal* **23**, 304–312.

Use of restraint

It is widely acknowledged that the use of physical restraint is an undesirable but sometimes inescapable practice, but that it can be used as long as it is the last resort, a proportionate response, and the method is the least restrictive form of restraint. It is imperative, therefore, that nurses make sure that both staff and those who may be subject to being restrained know how and why someone may be restrained. Readers are advised to consult Chapter 19 of the Mental Health Act Code of Practice[1] because it provides comprehensive guidance on the legality of restraint and how it should be used, and the wide array of resources available via the BILD website.[2] It is also probable that local policies on restraint that nurses must work to have been developed from this code of practice and the BILD guidelines on restraint.

Restraint can take many forms:
- Physical restraint—by members of staff
- Use of mechanical devices/equipment
- Seclusion/time out
- Manipulation of the environment e.g. baffle locks
- Medication.

In summary, restraint can be a spectrum of interventions ranging from the insidious to physical restraint. The code of practice states that restraint is most likely to be used for behavioural management issues that include:[1]
- Physical attacks on others
- Self-injurious behaviour
- Destructive behaviour
- Refusal to participate in treatment programmes
- Prolonged verbal abuse and threatening behaviour
- Going missing
- Risk of physical injury by accident
- Prevention of harm to others
- Severe and prolonged over-activity likely to lead to exhaustion.

Restraint can be justified if it is likely to prevent significant harm to others, and it should also be noted that it can often be in the client's best interest to use restraint. Restrictive interventions can either be:
- Planned—as part of an agreed multidisciplinary treatment/care plan, which will include explicit detail on the process of restraint, risk assessment(s), the condition/vulnerability of the individual, and roles and responsibilities of staff
- Emergency and unplanned interventions that must still be guided by best practice principles.

The purposes of restraint are to:
- take immediate control of a dangerous situation
- contain/limit the patient's freedom for no longer than is necessary
- end or reduce significantly the danger to the patient or others
- administer an appropriately prescribed treatment, where necessary.

Physical restraint is distressing for both staff and clients, and its use can lead to physical harm and psychological damage; it can be counter productive in a therapeutic sense. Therefore, if restraint is carried out it must be done within the parameters of defined policies as suggested above, and it must wherever possible be explained to those who may be restrained how and why restraint could be used. Readers should therefore access the restraint policies that govern their work in their own locality, and those nurses who work in areas where restraint is commonly used must receive mandatory training on control and restraint, and break away techniques. It is also the case that all preventative measures should be taken to minimize the need for restraint, and that de-escalation should be attempted (see 📖 De-escalation, p.554). Local policies will advise on how physical restraint should be carried and by whom. Most policies will include the following:

- Make a visual check for weapons
- Arms and legs should be restrained from behind if possible
- Attempt to immobilize quickly and safely
- Continually explain the reason for the restraint
- Offer reassurance throughout
- Attempt to get the individual to regain voluntary control as quickly as possible
- Avoid neck holds
- Avoid placing excess weight on any area, particularly the stomach and neck
- Methods such as using a blanket or tying to furniture must not be used
- Monitor the client for signs of injury during and after the restraint
- The necessity for debriefing after the event
- Rigorous record keeping/reporting procedures.

Situations when control and restraint should not be used:
- When behaviours can be averted by verbal request
- Where a modification in the environment or a relocation to a low stimulus environment could prevent escalation
- In most circumstances when property is being damaged and unless there is an intention to use it as a weapon or for self-injury
- For verbal abuse.

1 Department of Health (1999). *Code of Practice: Mental Health Act 1983*. London. HMSO.

2 British Institute of Learning Disabilities (2002). *Easy Guide to Physical Interventions: for people with learning disabilities, their carers and supporters*. British Institute of Learning Disabilities: Kidderminster. 🖳 www.bild.org.uk

Missing person

People with ID go missing for a wide variety of different reasons. This can result in serious anxieties, particularly if the person is considered vulnerable or there are concerns that they may harm other people. In some situations those responsible for the care of the person will have specific authority to take action to locate and return them. In other circumstances i.e. supported living situations, the response will be the same as would be available for any other missing person.

Emergency situations can often be predicted from previous behaviour. A detailed understanding of individual needs and past behaviour will assist greatly in the development of plans that reduce the necessity to respond to emergencies, and inform the most effective responses when/if an urgent situation arises.

Terms and definitions

Care should be taken to include a description of the circumstances when recording and reporting incidents that involve people going missing. Incident reports are an important source of information for risk assessment, and inform decisions about people's care and management. Inappropriate use of language may affect important decisions and could result in overly restrictive management or plans that do not adequately reflect the nature and degree of risk.

Absconding—use only to describe incidents that involve people absenting themselves without the necessary consent i.e. where others have authority over their movements and have not given consent to a period of leave or unescorted activity. This can include detention under the MHA, bail conditions, license conditions following a prison sentence, conditions subject to the sex offenders register, or conditions of residence subject to community supervision by the probation service and deprivation of liberty under the MCA 2005 (revised 2007).

Absent without leave (AWOL)—people who are subject to the provisions of the MHA are considered absent without leave if:
- They have left the hospital or failed to return without their absence being agreed by their responsible clinician (under section 17 MHA)
- They are absent without permission from a place they are required to reside as a condition of guardianship under the provisions of section 7 or 37 MHA 1983
- They have failed to return to the hospital if their leave under section 17 has been revoked or
- The Secretary of State (Ministry of Justice) has recalled them from conditional discharge (section 41 MHA)
- A patient who is subject to Supervised Community Treatment (section 17A) fails to return to hospital upon being recalled or absconds from the hospital following recall.

Missing—used when people absent themselves and their whereabouts is unknown.

Risk assessment

For some people with ID 'going missing' or 'absconding' will be an identified area of risk. Where this is the case a thorough assessment specific to this area of risk should be undertaken using as many sources of information as possible. All information should be checked for factual accuracy.

The best indicators for future risk will come from information about previous incidents. Areas for particular attention include:

- Circumstances when risk has occurred in the past, including setting conditions, antecedents and specific triggers
- Likely destinations and likely contacts from previous incidents
- Evidence regarding planning/preparation
- Person's vulnerability/ability to manage independently
- Evidence regarding potential risks to others
- Evidence regarding the likelihood of safe return without intervention.

(see 📖 Risk assessment and management, p.400)

Risk management

Individual assessment information should be used to inform plans to address risk. Ensure that plans:

- are developed and agreed jointly between those who are responsible for the person's care
- reflect the assessed level of risk and the personal circumstances of the person i.e. living situation, legal framework, abilities and personal rights
- recognize that the likelihood, immediacy, frequency and consequences of the risk may be subject to change
- are regularly reviewed and amended as required to address changes in identified risk and personal circumstances, including vulnerabilities
- provide a balanced approach, including preventative strategies, plans for managed risk taking, and emergency management strategies.

Local policies

All care settings, including hospitals, should have a policy regarding actions to be taken when a vulnerable person goes missing. Actions will differ depending on whether the person concerned is detained under the Mental Health Act,[1] whether they are detained under a criminal section,[2] and other circumstances, including:

- Immediate actions to be taken by staff who become aware that a patient is missing, including responsibilities for reporting this to superiors/responsible clinician
- Circumstances/timescales in which a local search should be undertaken
- Circumstances in which the police and others should be informed, and the information that should be made available, including vulnerability and risk of harm to others.

1 Department of Health (2008). *Revised Mental Health Act Code of Practice*. Department of Health: London.
2 Stone N (2003). *A Companion Guide to Mentally Disordered Offenders*. Shaw & Sons: Kent.

Allergies

A true allergy is a sensitization of the human immune system to a specific allergen, mediated by immunoglobulin E. The body produces antibodies against these allergens, with subsequent exposure leading to severe reactions. There is overreaction of the body's defense mechanism to something that is usually harmless; the most common reactions include sneezing, watery eyes, coughing, itchy rashes, and swelling of the lips and tongue. More severe reactions result in lowering of blood pressure, difficulty in breathing, and anaphylactic shock.

Many 'allergic' reactions are not true allergies. Some food 'allergies' are due to direct effects of substances within the food on the body in predisposed individuals. Heat, sun, and cold allergies are similar, in that the body has not produced antibodies against heat/cold, but instead, the individual is predisposed to respond by releasing histamine from cells in the skin, producing urticaria.

An allergen is any substance that the body mistakenly perceives as a threat that triggers an allergic reaction.

Some of the most common allergies are to:

- Pollen and moulds (often found indoors where humidity is high and can easily become airborne), dust mites, insect stings or bites, peanuts and tree nuts, penicillin, latex, cosmetics e.g. make-up, creams, lotions, sprays, perfumes, powders, deodorants, bath oils, and bubble baths.

Some precautions in trying to prevent an allergic reaction

- Keep a record of known allergens for an individual and try to avoid where possible
- Check food labels for allergy causing ingredients
- If the person is affected by hayfever then monitor the pollen report
- Consider immunotherapy for desensitization to a known allergy—under medical supervision.

Signs and symptoms of an allergic reaction:

- Shortness of breath, tightness of the chest or chest pain, wheezing and/or coughing, a runny nose, sneezing, itchiness, hives, redness of the skin, a rash, nausea, diarrhoea, stomach cramps, itchy eyes, swelling, puffiness or red eyes, swelling of the face, lips, tongue or throat.

Action in the event of an allergic reaction

- Assess the severity of the allergic reaction and ask the person and/or carers whether the person is known to suffer from an allergy
- Identify if the person has been prescribed medication for allergic reactions and encourage them to take it if available
- Seek medical advice should any signs or symptoms be detected or persist after taking prescribed medication for allergic reaction
- Ensure arrangements are made for person to visit GP for advice and treatment as necessary
- Contact GP out-of-hours service if outside of normal working hours

- Provide reassurance, support, and information to person with ID
- Depending on the severity of the symptoms i.e. difficulty in breathing, severe rash, altered consciousness, or history of severe reaction symptoms, contact emergency services or attend the local A&E department, providing all relevant information.

Types of medications that can be used in the management of allergies

- Antihistamines
- Decongestants
- Corticosteroids and non-steroidal anti-inflammatory drugs
- Bronchodilators.

Anaphylactic shock

This is a severe allergic reaction that affects the whole body. It may develop within minutes of contact with a trigger factor, and is potentially fatal. Triggers may be:

- Airborne or contact with particular materials
- A specific drug
- Insect sting
- Ingestion of a particular food substance, e.g. peanut.

Signs and symptoms of anaphylactic shock

- Anxiety, widespread red/blotchy skin, swelling of the tongue and throat, puffiness around eyes, impairment in breathing that may result in gasping for air, signs of shock.

Action in the event of an anaphylactic shock

- Dial 999/emergency number and describe the person's symptoms
- Aid breathing and minimize shock
- Provide reassurance and support
- Help person to take any necessary medication they may be carrying
- If person is conscious, help to sit up to help with breathing
- If person becomes unconscious, check breathing and seek to maintain open airway
- If necessary give rescue breaths and chest compressions as per local policy
- Treat any symptoms of shock until help arrives.

Further reading

Resuscitation Council (UK) 🖳 http://www.resus.org.uk

McArthur J (2006). Allergen avoidance. *Practice Nurse* **31**(5), 14, 17–19.

Adverse reactions to medications

Definition

An ADR is an untoward, unintended, and unwanted or harmful reaction that is experienced by an individual, which is suspected as being related to the medication being taken. This reaction may be physical and/or psychological in nature. It is estimated that 10,000 serious drug reactions and 1,200 deaths are caused by prescribed medicines each year.

The simplest classification of ADRs is type A and type B.

Type A (most common)

- Predictable from the pharmacology of the drug
- Are dose related (occurring at a dose that is too high for an individual), and reactions are usually slow in onset
- Increased risk in the elderly and neonates
- Usually a reduction in dose will suffice; however, a severe reaction requires the drug to be stopped.

Type B

- Reactions are not predictable from the drug pharmacology
- Susceptibility to this type of reaction is individualistic
- Usually rapid in onset and are often allergic
- Reactions can involve anaphylaxis (see 📖 Allergies, p.560) and usually requires causative drug to be stopped.

Reducing the risk

- Is there clear indication for the need of the medication, if so, identify recommended dose range
- Review information available on possible ADRs of the drug, and identify if there are any risks of drug interactions i.e. polypharmacy
- Establish patient susceptibility e.g. pharmacokinetic issues, and any pre-disposing factors
- Patient medical history of allergies and any previous ADRs
- Try and establish dose range that allows effective control of the disease/illness.

Monitoring ADRs

- Introduce a systematic approach to patient surveillance and maintain ongoing monitoring
- Identify and use an appropriate scale for identifying adverse reactions, e.g. DAI-10, LUNSERS, UKU Side-effects Scale, Quality of Life Scale
- Education and training for person with ID and/or their carers to recognize ADRs.

Considerations
- ADRs have the potential to impact on the person's physical, psychological and social well-being, resulting in impaired quality of life
- Be aware that a black triangle next to a drug in the BNF indicates that it is either new, under intensive surveillance, or an old drug marketed in a new combination or formulation
- Act in accordance with the NMC's standards for medicines management.

Reporting ADRs
- If a serious ADR is suspected, then report via the Yellow Card (available from the back of the BNF) voluntary scheme supervised by the MHRA.

Response to an ADR
- Respond rapidly to any suspected ADR by providing first aid treatment as required, e.g. anaphylactic shock (see 📖 Allergies, p.560)
- Immediate contact to be made with GP, prescribing professional or emergency services, as assessed necessary given the gravity of the situation or type of reaction, i.e. type A or B
- Keep the person with ID informed and reassured, and involve them in making decisions about their treatment; consider relevant legislation, i.e. The MCA 2005
- Keep others involved in the person's care informed
- Give appropriate advice in respect of response to ADR and treatment to the person with ID and/or carers
- Be vigilant in monitoring and early detection of unwanted effects
- Maintain effective interventions that address empowerment, understanding of their illness/condition, quality of life, physical and psychological well-being
- Maintain an up-to-date knowledge of adverse reactions in order to exercise duty of care, and ensure evidence-based practice in respect of treatment and management
- Document incident in person's case notes, and complete all other relevant paperwork as required by local policies and procedures
- Make sure a clear note is made on the person's prescription chart in respect of the medication causing an ADR.

Further reading
The Yellow Card Information Service—The MHRA provides free advice and information on suspected ADRs. Tel. 0800 731 6789

🖥 www.mhra.gov.uk provides detailed information on reporting, and a list of products currently under intensive monitoring.

Medication error

Definition

'Any preventable event that may cause or lead to inappropriate medication use or patient harm while the medication is in the control of health professional, patient or consumer'.[1]

The NMC require competency in drug administration to be an integral criterion for entry to the professional register. Nurses should also apply the principles of the standards for medicine management in their own areas of practice.[2] Therefore, good practice by nurses in drug administration would incorporate recognizing why potential near misses and actual medication errors occur. Reasons why near misses and actual errors occur are multifaceted, and ways to reduce these must be considered. The impact of a medication error could be significant for the nurse and for the patient. It is important, therefore, that an open culture exists encouraging the immediate reporting of errors or incidents in the administration of medicines. However, it may be that an error is not identified immediately but is highlighted some time after the incident. This should again result in immediate reporting. The aim of the nurse should be to promote the safety of the person with ID at all times (see 🕮 Medicines management, p.208).

Some factors that cause near misses and drug administration errors

- Poor mathematical skills that result in overdosing or underdosing
- Poor knowledge of the drug being administered and its actions and side effects
- Illegibly written records
- Dispensing errors
- Inappropriate drug choice by prescribing person
- Lack of knowledge in respect of the uptake and therapeutic efficacy of the drug
- Environmental issues, such as being distracted, noise, unpredictability, and stressful conditions
- Medication records not kept up to date, resulting in overdosing i.e. no signature on medication records to signify administration
- Complacency in practice of medication prescribing and administration
- Tiredness and lack of attention to detail.

Minimizing the risk of a medication error

- Complex calculations should be second checked by another practitioner
- Attend training provision and structured revision sessions to develop and maintain mathematical competence for drug calculations
- Recognize the limitations of your own knowledge and professional competence
- Seek out information when in doubt
- Administer medication in the form in which it is packaged and be aware of the risks and professional implications of tampering with drugs, such as covertly administering in food and drink.

- Maintain good communication mechanisms with doctors, other nurses, pharmacists, and patients
- Immediately report near misses and errors
- Seek clarification of any uncertainties regarding prescription or dose regimen
- Take the necessary time and avoid rushing the process of calculating and administering medication
- Document administration on completion
- Act in accordance with the NMC standards for medicine management.

Responding to a medication error

- Respond rapidly to any actual or suspected medication error
- Provide first aid treatment as required
- Immediate contact to be made with GP/A&E/hospital medical staff for advice as to recommended actions
- Keep the person with ID informed and reassured
- Keep others involved in the person's care informed
- Document incident in the person's nursing notes, and complete all other relevant paperwork as required by local policies and procedures.

Professional and legal requirements

This requires that medicine is given to the right person, at the right time, in the correct form, using the correct dose, via the correct route.[2] Nurses are accountable for their actions/omissions and therefore need to be aware of their professional responsibility with regard to drug administration. Nurses need to be aware, therefore, of the Medicines Act (1968) and the Misuse of Drugs Act (1971), as failure to abide by these could lead to criminal prosecution and professional conduct hearings by the NMC, as well as disciplinary action by the employer.

Final thought

Any nurse is potentially at risk of making a medication error. It is important that, whether you are the contributor or an observer, you report the incident as soon as possible to minimize patient harm, and to ensure appropriate advice and response.

Further reading

Audit Commission (2002). *A Spoonful of Sugar: Medicines Management in NHS Hospitals.* Audit Commission for Local Government and NHS in England and Wales, London.

---

1 National Coordinating Council for Medication Error Reporting and Prevention (2005). *NCC MERP: The First Ten Years –Defining the Problem and Developing Solutions.* NCCMERP: Maryland USA. 🖳 http://www.nccmerp.org/pdf/reportFinal2005-11-29.pdf [accessed December 2007].

2 Nursing and Midwifery Council (2007). *Standards for Medicine Management*
🖳 http://www.nmc-uk.org/

Needle stick/sharps injuries

A needle stick/sharps injury is a puncture to the skin or a percutaneous injury. Nurses are at risk of exposure to infections such as HIV, hepatitis B and C within their practice due to blood-borne pathogens. Approximately 16% of accidents to NHS staff are caused by needle stick/sharps injuries, and there are ~35,000 reported incidents a year.

Causes of needle stick/sharps injuries

- Incorrect use of equipment
- Failure to dispose of used needles properly in puncture-resistant sharps containers
- Recapping of needles
- Accidental—resulting from an unexpected movement by the patient.

Reducing the risk of needle stick/sharps injury in practice

- Be aware and familiar with the local needle stick/sharps injury policy which should cover:
  - Education and training
  - Safe working practices
  - Safe disposal of devices
  - Procedures in the event of a needle stick injury
  - Monitoring and evaluation
  - Procedures for reporting needle stick injuries
- Undertake any necessary risk assessments
- Access training to refresh knowledge and skills in the correct use and disposal of sharps and in respect of infection control
- Where available use sharps with built-in safety features rather than conventional needles
- Eliminate needle re-capping
- Promptly dispose of contaminated sharps immediately in sharps collection boxes, and ensure these are not full prior to undertaking procedure
- Use appropriate personal protective equipment i.e. gloves
- Remain up to date with hepatitis B immunization status
- Avoid distractions while undertaking the intervention
- Inform your employer of any needle stick/sharps hazards you observe.

Actions in the event of a personal needle stick/sharps injury

- Immediate first aid and decontamination of the wound by washing with soap and large amounts of warm water, without scrubbing.
- **Do not suck**
- Free bleeding should be encouraged
- Appropriate dressing should then be applied
- Inform your line manager
- Immediately contact the relevant occupational health department for advice and support regarding appropriate medical investigations/actions
- Outside of usual office hours, immediate attendance at the nearest minor injury unit or A&E department.

- If known that there is a significant risk of transmission of an infectious disease then immediate attendance at the nearest A&E department
- Complete the relevant accident and/or incident form as per local policy and procedure.

Actions in the event of witnessing a needle stick/sharps injury

- Provide immediate assistance and support in respect of first aid.
- **Do not suck**
- Ensure person contacts occupational health department, attends minor injury unit or A&E department as appropriate
- Ensure that an accident form and/or incident form is completed
- Provide support for any distress.

Further reading

Health and Safety Executive website 🖳 http://www.hse.gov.uk/healthservices/needlesticks/

Needle Stick Injuries: A guide for Local Government safety representatives. Available from: 🖳 http://www.unison.org.uk/acrobat/10840.pdf

Trim JC, Elliott TSJ (2003). A review of sharps injuries and preventative strategies. *Journal of Hospital Infection* **53**(4), 237–242.

Resources

UK-wide intellectual disability and health networks

There are a number of UK-wide ID networks that offer a valuable and free resource to ID nurses.

Networking in ID circles is a well established and useful way of sharing and disseminating information rapidly, in a cost effective way. The idea of the development of UK wide electronic networks that deliver collaborative advantage is an essential tool to improve services and outcomes, and is underpinned by the hypothesis that by working together we can be more effective than by working alone.

The UK health and learning disability network hosted by The Foundation for People with a Learning Disability

A national network concerned with health issues and people with ID. This is an open forum with a wide range of membership, predominantly from health services.

To join log on to 🖥 www.learningdisabilities.org.uk/ldhn

Access to Acute (A2A) network

Acute hospitals and people with ID.

To join log on to 🖥 www.nnldn.org.uk/a2a/

The Mental Health in Learning Disability Forum at the Estia Centre

The aim is to develop a support network that helps meet the mental health needs of people with ID.

To join log on to 🖥 www.estiacentre.org/mhildnetwork.html

The National Health Facilitation network

The purpose of the network is to freely share our knowledge, experiences, and skills relating to health facilitation, as described in *Valuing People*.[1]

To join log on to 🖥 www.networks.nhs.uk/nhfnetwork

The National Network for the Palliative Care of People with Learning Disabilities

To join log on to 🖥 www.helpthehospices.org.uk

The National Learning Disability Nurses Network (NNLDN)

A 'network' of networks which aims to support networks and nurses within the field of ID.

To join log on to 🖥 www.nnldn.org.uk

The Profound and Multiple Learning Disability Network

This forum discusses the support of people with profound and multiple ID.

To join log on to 🖥 www.learningdisabilities.org.uk/information/have-your-say/pmld-network/

NHS networks

A means of promoting and connecting the many networks that exist throughout the NHS.

To join log on to 🖥 www.networks.nhs.uk

These next networks all operate from 🖬 www.jan-net.co.uk

- UK disabled children's network, a network to support children with complex and continuing health needs
- UK CAMHS
- Learning Disability Network
- UK Lecturers Network—a network for university lecturers in ID
- UK Forensic and Learning Disability Network—a network for people with ID in criminal justice systems or forensic services
- UK Continuing Care network—a network for people meeting NHS continuing care criteria.

To join these networks log on to 🖬 www.jan-net.co.uk and complete electronic joining forms relating to network of interest.

1 Department of Health (2001). *Valuing People: a New Strategy for Learning Disability in the 21st Century.* Cmnd 5086. HMSO: London.

British Institute of Learning Disabilities

Work of the BILD

BILD is a UK-wide charity working to improve the quality of life of people with ID. Its vision is a world where people with ID are accepted as equal citizens with the potential to make a positive contribution to our communities.

It believes that services offered to people with ID should be person centred. This means seeing the person and not just the disability. It also means finding out what each person wants and how their individual needs can be met, and helping people to make choices that are important to them. Finally it means ensuring that the views of people with ID influence those around them—including carers, service providers, and government.

To try and achieve this, BILD works with government and other organizations, and tries to include people with ID in everything it does.

Some of BILD's services
- An extensive programme of conferences and training events
- A catalogue of over 50 publications and training resources, including material supporting Learning Disability Qualifications
- Providing bespoke training for organizations in both the public and private sector
- Supporting The Quality Network—a framework for service user led quality review of services
- Publishing a range of journals and information resources
- Providing a membership scheme for access to information, networking opportunities, and other benefits e.g. free journals
- Work in behaviour support, including the publication of a code of practice for the use of physical interventions, and the accreditation of training organizations
- Working with advocacy groups, and have administered funding schemes on behalf of Department of Health and Welsh Assembly Government.

How to find out more

The website ▣ www.bild.org.uk contains much more information about BILD and other news and information, with a section devoted to stories about people's lives. It also includes many links to other useful sources of information.

Many BILD products and services may be purchased online, including membership, journal subscriptions, and BILD publications.

Fact sheets

Fact sheets are available for download from the website or available by post. Topics include:
- Intellectual disabilities
- Advocacy
- Chemical restraint
- Seclusion
- Self-injurious behaviour.

Partners
- BILD works in partnership with many other organizations in the ID field
- BILD is a member of the **Learning Disability Coalition**—10 ID organizations who have come together to form one group with one voice
- BILD is a member of the **PMLD Network**—working together to improve the lives of people with profound and multiple ID
- BILD is a partner of **Scottish Consortium for Learning Disability**, building respect in the Scottish community.

How to contact them
BILD,
Campion House
Green Street
Kidderminster,
Worcestershire DY10 1JL
UK

Tel: 01562 723010
Email: enquiries@bild.org.uk
Website: www.bild.org.uk

BILD is a registered charity (number 1019663) and the company is registered in England and Wales (company number 2804429). BILD is a member of the Fundraising Standards Board. They promise to treat the public with respect, fairness, honesty, and clarity in fundraising activities.

Learning Disability Specialist Library

⌨ http://www.library.nhs.uk/learningdisabilities/

What is it?

The LDSL is one of a number of specialist sites that are part of the NLH, which provide access to current knowledge for a range of health topics.

LDSL aims to meet the information needs of healthcare professionals, including carers, nurses, librarians, students, and anyone else who has an interest in key documents and evidence on ID.

Whereas the NLH is committed to the highest standards of evidence throughout the site, there is recognition that there may be few meta-analyses or systematic reviews of trials currently available within the field of ID. LDSL features those reviews that are available, as well as single studies, and qualitative evaluations.

What can I find on it?

The LDSL site contains the best available evidence for decision makers supporting people with ID including:

- Guidance from NICE, Department of Health and Valuing People Support Team
- Systematic reviews from the Cochrane Centre
- Key publications from Research Institutes.

In addition the library team produces a monthly evidence bulletin, which presents findings from published articles in peer-reviewed journals. From the electronic version of the bulletin, users of the site can link to extended summaries of those articles.

Each of the specialist libraries also manages a 'National Knowledge Week', part of the NLH programme. Each specialist library focuses on a small set of topics, systematically searches for the evidence in relation to that topic, and presents the findings on the library site.

For 2007 the focus was on the health needs of people with ID, looking at:

- Cancer
- Coronary heart disease
- Epilepsy and challenging behaviour
- Respiratory illness.

The knowledge week summaries will be updated annually.

How do I use it?

The homepage of the LDSL has a menu, loosely based on the key issues covered in *Valuing People*.[1] The menu has 16 options, including:

- What is learning disability?
- Challenging behaviour
- Health
- Person-centred services.

This menu links to all the documents in the library. Each section is also by document type, e.g. 'Guidelines', 'Evidence', 'Reference' and 'Patient information'. If you prefer, you can use the search bar. The search is 'free text' and will deliver results by publication type.

As well as the subsections, the homepage can also link you to monthly evidence bulletins, an email group for library users, and latest additions (available as an RSS feed) to Social Care Online.

How do I get involved?

Contact the LDSL team using the form on the website:
🖳 http://www.library.nhs.uk/learningdisabilities/ContactUs.aspx

Join the email group:
🖳 http://groups.google.com/group/nlh-learning-disabilities-specialist-library?lnk=li

1 Department of Health (2001). *Valuing People: a New Strategy for Learning Disability in the 21st Century*. Cmnd 5086. HMSO: London.

Mencap and Enable

Their work

On their website Mencap state that they are the voice of ID. They state that their work is exclusively about valuing and supporting people with ID, and their families and carers. They work in partnership with people with ID, and their services support people to live life as they wish to. Their work includes:

- providing high-quality, flexible services that allow people to live as independently as possible in a place they choose
- providing advice through helplines and websites
- campaigning for the changes that people with ID want.

They are an individual membership organization, with a local network of more than 500 affiliated groups. Their work is developed from what the membership inform the organization as to their needs and wishes.

Some of their services

Mencap work with people with ID to bring about changes to existing legislation and services, they publicly challenge prejudice, and provide direct support to many people to live their lives as they choose. Some of their existing services are:

- Providing support for people with ID to get a job or take a college course, or they can help them find a place of their own to live in
- Offering advice about things like respite care, individual budgets or transport services
- Running residential/day-care services and leisure groups that are important to so many people with ID, and their families and supporters
- Supporting people with ID to be part of their local communities
- Lobbying the government to change laws so that more and more people with ID can have control over their own lives.

Enable in Scotland helps people by campaigning, providing services, supporting people to do things in new and innovative ways, and by helping children, young people, and adults to have a say in the decisions which affect them. Like Mencap they ensure that people with ID are at the centre of their work.

Enable is committed to improving life opportunities for people with ID by providing services that support people to live, work, and enjoy a meaningful role in everyday life. They operate across Scotland, and in most areas they have local managers who work alongside people with ID and their families to design and develop the kinds of services that they want.

Enable supports people with ID to:

- live in their own house, either on their own or with a friend
- find the job they want
- develop an active social life
- get away for a holiday or short break
- use inclusive day services in local areas.

How to find out more

Mencap and Enable have websites that contain much more information about the organizations, and other news and information, with sections devoted to stories about people's lives. They also include many links to other useful sources of information.

Many products and services are available online, including membership, journal subscriptions, and publications.

Fact sheets and resources

Mencap offer an extensive range of resources that includes: audio material, fact sheets, links, national organisations, publications, videos, and other general documents.

How to contact them

- England 🖳 http://www.mencap.org.uk/
- Scotland 🖳 http://www.enable.org.uk/
- Wales 🖳 http://www.mencap.org.uk/page.asp?id=2146
- Northern Ireland 🖳 http://www.mencap.org.uk/page.asp?id=1928

The vision of all of these organizations is a world where people with ID are valued equally, listened to, and included. They aspire to everyone having the opportunity to achieve the things they want out of life.

Foundation for People with Learning Disabilities

Who they are
The aims of the FPLD are to:
- stick up for the rights of people with ID, and their families
- help get good chances in life for people with ID, and their families.

What they do
FPLD work with people with ID, their families, and those who support them to:
- do research and projects that help people be included
- support local people and services to include people with ID
- improve services for people with ID
- spread knowledge and information.

Within all their work they seek to address diversity and to challenge discrimination. They continue to seek ways of increasing the numbers of people with ID, and family carers, who work with them as colleagues.

You can find lots of information about the work of the FPLD on the website: ⌨ www.learningdisabilities.org.uk. The site offers information and good practice publications, and DVDs to download or order online. It provides a range of information on ID, a daily news service, and directories of organizations, websites, and events. Website visitors can ask questions and share ideas through the electronic forums, join the mailing list, and find out how to support the organization.

Examples of their work
The FPLD sustains a strong programme of projects and contracts.

Promoting the rights of people with ID to play a full part in society
- Working with faith communities to improve their responsiveness to people with ID
- Research on implementation of the MCA
- Research on antenatal screening to improve the information available to pregnant women and their partners.

Helping ordinary services and communities to include people with ID more
- Supporting people with ID to start small businesses
- Creative approaches to securing better opportunities for people with high support needs
- Supporting creative approaches to community capacity building
- Facilitating the National Advisory Group on Learning Disability and Ethnicity.

Empowering people with ID and their families to take control of the planning and delivery of their support
- Leadership programmes for people with ID, and family carers.

Promoting person-centred practice, services, and systems
- Project work on people with ID becoming carers for their ageing parents
- Research on direct payments
- Longer-term contracts to support the development of person-centred approaches
- Extending person-centred planning to people with ASD
- Improving the range of short-term breaks
- Research on improving day opportunities
- Supporting local authorities to transfer work into the third sector, and to develop new models of working (e.g. brokerage)
- Supporting older families, including person-centred approaches to planning ahead.

Helping to get improvements in people's physical and mental health, so they can lead fuller lives
- Work on access to health services (primary care, acute hospitals and mental health services)
- Action learning sets (e.g. on improving access for young people and adults to mental health services).

How to contact them
The Foundation for People with Learning Disabilities
Sea Containers House
20 Upper Ground
London SE1 9QB
UK

Tel: 020 7803 1100
Email: fpld@fpld.org.uk

Scotland:
Merchants House
30 George Square
Glasgow G2 1EG

The Foundation for People with Learning Disabilities is part of the Mental Health Foundation, registered charity no. 801130

Down's Syndrome Association

Their work

The DSA is the main campaigning and information-providing organization in the UK focusing solely on all aspects of living with Down syndrome. The DSA is a membership-led organization, with over 20,000 members, which provides information and support for people with Down syndrome, their families, and carers, as well as professionals who work with them. The DSA strives to improve knowledge of the condition and champions the rights of people with Down syndrome at a national level.

Some of their services

- A regular journal with useful advice on all stages of life, together with a colour supplement written for and by people with Down syndrome
- Helpful booklets and fact sheets, which look at all aspects of living with Down's syndrome, plus information on new developments in policy and services
- Inexpensive conferences and training days, which cover a comprehensive range of topics e.g. health, education and social care
- A telephone helpline and advocacy service with access to specialist advisers in benefits, education, health, speech, and language
- Information on pioneering research to benefit people with Down syndrome
- Provides contact details for DSA's affiliated groups throughout the UK.

How to find out more

Their website contains much more information about the DSA and other news and information. It also includes many links to other useful sources of information. Every month a group of young adults with Down syndrome gather at the DSA Head Office to meet; they are known as the Down 2 Earth group, and they act as a very important focus group—by letting the DSA know about their experiences, so they can make sure they are addressing the right issues for them. The vision of the DSA is to assist people with Down syndrome to live full and rewarding lives.

Down's Syndrome Association
Langdon Down Centre
2A Langdon Park
Teddington
Middlesex TW11 9PS
UK

Tel: 0845 230 0372
Fax: 0845 230 0373
Email: info@downs-syndrome.org.uk
Website: www.downs-syndrome.org.uk

Training, conferences and consultancy services
- Organize training courses and conferences, and act as consultants to organizations who wish to develop and expand their services for people with ASD.

How to find out more
- The NAS website Autism Data is a vital research tool for any researcher looking at ASDs
- The Autism Services Directory is a UK-wide database of autism-specific services across the UK
- Signpost provides information tailored to an individual's needs
- The online shop sells carefully selected books, leaflets, videos, DVDs and CD-ROMs
- Current awareness subscription services keep you up-to-date with the latest updates on research
- Helpline email service is an online advice and information service.

The National Autistic Society
393 City Road,
London, EC1V 1NG
UK

Tel: +44(0)20 7833 2299
Fax: +44 (0)20 7833 9666
Email: nas@nas.org.uk
Website: http://www.nas.org.uk/

Index

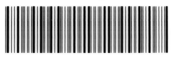
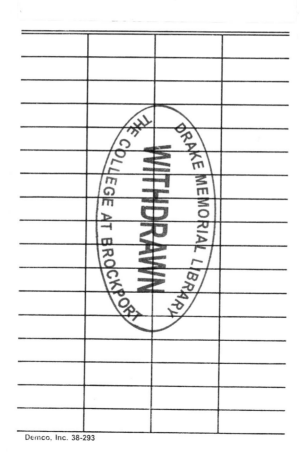

THE COLLEGE AT BROCKPORT

DRAKE MEMORIAL LIBRARY

WITHDRAWN